The Sociology of the Caring Professions

The Sociology of the Caring Professions

2nd edition

edited by

Pamela Abbott
and
Liz Meerabeau

Routledge
Taylor & Francis Group
LONDON AND NEW YORK

First published in 1998 by Routledge
2 Park Square, Milton Park, Abingdon, Oxfordshire OX14 4RN
711 Third Avenue, New York, NY 10017

First issued in hardback 2016

Routledge is an imprint of the Taylor and Francis Group, an informa business

British Library Cataloguing-in-Publication Data
A CIP catalogue record for this book is available from the British Library.

Library of Congress Cataloging-in-Publication Data are available

ISBN 13: 978-1-138-14969-4 (hbk)
ISBN 13: 978-1-85728-903-9 (pbk)

Typeset in 10/12pt Baskerville
by Graphicraft Limited, Hong Kong

Contents

Acknowledgements

The first edition of *The Sociology of the Caring Professions* was jointly edited by Pamela Abbott and Claire Wallace. We would like to acknowledge Claire's contribution to the original idea for the volume.

Chapter 2 in this edition contains material that was originally in Chapter 9 of the first edition. Pamela and Claire would like to thank Roger Sapsford for agreeing to its inclusion here.

'Conflict over the grey areas: district nurses and home helps providing community care', by Pamela Abbott, is a slightly modified version of an article that originally appeared in *Journal of Gender Studies*. We should like to thank the editors of the *Journal* and Carfax Publishers for permission to reproduce it in this collection.

The chapter by Mavis Kirkham, 'Professionalization: dilemmas for midwifery', is developed from a chapter which appeared as 'Professionalization past and present: With women or with the powers that be?' in *Midwifery Care for the Future* (London: Baillière Tindall), edited by Debra Kroll, and appears by permission of the publishers, W. B. Saunders Co. Ltd, London.

List of Contributors

Pamela Abbott is Professor and Director of Social Sciences at the University of Teesside.

Davina Allen is a Research Fellow in the Nursing Research Unit, School of Nursing Studies, University of Wales College of Medicine, Cardiff. She is a nurse and holds degrees in sociology from the University of Nottingham.

Jill Annison obtained her CQSW in 1978 and has worked as a probation officer and specialist social worker. She is currently undertaking a PhD at the University of Plymouth.

John Clarke is Professor of Social Policy at the Open University.

Richard Hugman is Professor of Social Work and Head of School at Curtin University, Perth, Western Australia.

Mavis Kirkham is Professor of Midwifery in the Sheffield Centre for Health-Related Research at the University of Sheffield.

Lesley Mackay is a Lecturer in the School of Health Care Studies at the University of Leeds.

David McCallum teaches sociology and social policy at the Victoria University of Technology in Melbourne.

Tim May is a Lecturer in Sociology and Social Policy at the University of Durham.

Liz Meerabeau is Professor of Health Care and Head of the School of Health at the University of Greenwich.

Kate Robinson is Pro Vice-Chancellor at the University of Luton and Dean of the Faculty of Health and Social Studies.

Claire Wallace is a Fellow at the Institute for Advanced Studies in Vienna and a Professor of Social Research at the University of Derby.

Introduction

This book is concerned with developing a sociological perspective on the caring professions. While a number of occupations may claim to be members of this group, the articles in this collection focus on nurses, midwives, health visitors, social workers and probation officers. This is because, arguably, these occupational groups present paradigm cases of caring professions which in their work have a primary commitment to care for their clients; personalized care is central to their practice as professionals. The needs of clients are said to take precedence in their work. There is still a feeling, especially with respect to nursing, that the work is vocational, suggesting a selfless dedication to duty and putting the needs of others first – that is, they are professions imbued with a service ideology (see Lesley Mackay, Chapter 3 of this volume). The professional ethos of social work is profoundly 'client-centred', with a strong commitment to respect the individual, to be 'non-judgemental', to 'start where the individual is at' and to allow 'client determination'.

A key question is, of course, the extent to which these two occupational groups are in fact able to deliver personalized care to clients. Both are generally employed within bureaucratic organizations and have to adhere to regulations of the agency which might conflict with what are seen as the needs of the client. Social workers have statutory duties which may require them to take actions which may be opposed to the wishes of the client. Nurses, health visitors, midwives, probation officers and social workers all tend to work with individualistic theories about the causes of social problems (see David McCallum, Chapter 4 in this volume) and intervene at the level of the individual. This often means that the root causes of the client's problems – such as poverty, unemployment, bad housing, and so on – are beyond the scope of their professional practice. Nursing and social work share certain characteristics and problems: they had their origins in nineteenth-century philanthropy and expanded with the advent of the welfare state into what have been termed 'professional' occupations (see Abbott and Wallace, Chapter 2 of this volume); they are concerned with the 'human qualities' of clients to a greater or lesser extent; they are created and sustained through the identification of a particular social problem and the treatment developed for it – in other words the regulation and control of problematic areas of social life. Related to this last point, they share particular kinds of knowledge base, aspects of which are derived from sociology as well as from other social sciences such as psychology (see David McCallum). They are often termed 'the semi-professions', being situated within state bureaucracies rather than being represented by independent 'collegiate' organizations in the same way as law or medicine, and this is indicative of the rather fragile status which they hold, their status as 'professions' being often disputed (see Abbott and Meerabeau, Chapter 1 of this volume). Related to this, perhaps, is the fact that these are very often seen as careers for women, and therefore intersect with gender ideologies in particular ways. Indeed, they still survive with a penumbra of unqualified and volunteer helpers surrounding the career professionals.

The articles in this collection are all concerned with issues relating to the professional status of social work, probation, nursing, midwifery, social work and health visiting. Each contributes to the contemporary debates about the status of these occupations and the strategies used to enhance the standing of their members. In Chapter 1 Pamela Abbott and Liz Meerabeau briefly review the issues surrounding professionals and professionalization, highlighting both the difficulty of definition and the uncertain status of the occupational groups under consideration.

The chapters that follow develop specific issues and debates. In Chapter 2 Pamela Abbott and Claire Wallace trace the historical development of nursing, midwifery, health visiting and social work, demonstrating how they grew from the philanthropic endeavours of nineteenth-century reformers concerned with morality and hygiene into state occupations, underpinned by scientific discoveries in the twentieth century. In Chapter 3 Lesley Mackay examines issues relating to nursing recruitment and nursing as a vocation. David McCallum, in Chapter 4, looks specifically at the ways in which psychology came in the twentieth century to define 'the case' for social work. The theme of the importance of a knowledge base for professional practice is taken up and developed in the chapters by Liz Meerabeau and Kate Robinson: Liz Meerabeau (Chapter 5) considers how recent reforms in nurse education relate to professionalizing strategies, while Kate Robinson discusses the issue of evidence-based practice in Chapter 6. In Chapter 7 Mavis Kirkham considers the professional dilemmas for midwifery, while Chapter 8 (Tim May and Jill Annison) and Chapter 9 (Richard Hugman) consider whether probation and social work are being deprofessionalized. In Chapters 10 and 11 issues are considered which cover the relationship between caring professionals and other occupational groups. In Chapter 10 Pamela Abbott explores the ways in which district nurses maintain and enhance their status by operating occupational closure against home helps. Davina Allen, in Chapter 11, explores the relationships between nursing and medical staff. In Chapter 12 John Clarke considers the way in which the 'New Managerialism', with its emphasis on private-sector management techniques, impinges on the work of caring professionals. Finally, Liz Meerabeau and Pamela Abbott reflect on what sociological analysis can tell us about the status and role of the caring professions.

Chapter 1

Professionals, Professionalization and the Caring Professions

Pamela Abbott and Liz Meerabeau

Introduction

The concept of 'profession' was largely taken for granted in sociology until the 1960s. Sociologists were concerned with defining what a profession was – what occupational groups could claim professional status – rather than with analyzing the role of professionals in society.

Subsequently, considerable debate has developed about professions' role and status, and attention has shifted from attempting to define 'profession' to analyzing professionalizing strategies – the steps taken by occupational groups aspiring to be recognized as professions. Much of this more recent literature has taken a critical stance, challenging the motivation of professionals and suggesting that they control clients and are concerned primarily with their own status and economic rewards. However, the work that professionals do is, arguably, both necessary and desirable, and more recent contributions to the debate have suggested that emphasis needs to be placed on the service professionals provide for clients (Freidson, 1994), while Meg Stacey (1992) has suggested that it is necessary to distinguish professionalism (behaviour) from professionalization (status and monetary reward).

The terms 'profession' and 'professional' are confusing and are used in a number of different and potentially contradictory ways. In everyday language 'professional' is often used to mean the opposite of 'amateur': someone who is paid to do a job – for example, a professional footballer. It is also used to denote a job that is well or properly done, as opposed to badly done or done in a slipshod manner, regardless of whether the work was paid or not. 'Professional behaviour' is used as a term of approval for what is perceived as ethical/moral behaviour, and 'a professional judgement' is generally seen as a sound or expert one. However, the most frequent use of 'profession' is to define occupational groups – occupations that are recognized as being professions. These are generally of high status with high financial rewards, but there is some ambiguity and dispute as to which occupations are professions, in terms both of everyday recognition by members of society and of sociological definitions. However, many white-collar occupational groups lay claim to professional status or develop strategies for achieving it. Both social work and nursing, for example, have been concerned to establish their professional status, to develop professionalizing strategies, and both have been divided internally as to whether or not professional status is something desirable and to be strived for. Some commentators have suggested that a distinction can be made between 'true' professions – the paradigm case often cited being medicine – and semi-professions such as nursing and social work. (An alternative term is 'bureau professionals', taking cognizance of the bureaucratic organization of their work – see the chapters by Hugman and Clarke in this volume.)

The class position of professionals has also been debated. While Marxists have argued that they act on behalf of the ruling class as agents of social control, others have suggested that professionals are an emergent new class (Bell, 1973), that societies are professionalizing and that career hierarchies are replacing social classes. Knowledge and skill are becoming, it is argued, increasingly important in post-industrial society, and old class and sectional interests of diminishing importance. In contradiction to this it is suggested that middle-class occupations, including professions, are being proletarianized, that knowledge and skill are being routinized and that these occupational groups are increasingly using 'trade union' tactics to maintain their relatively privileged position *vis-à-vis* other occupational groups. More recently it has been suggested that managerialism is increasingly controlling professional autonomy and judgement (see Clarke, and May and Annison, in this volume).

Defining a Profession

The idea of a 'profession' emerged from the mediaeval university, but until the eighteenth century 'profession' and 'occupation' were not separate terms. The prefix 'liberal' or 'learned' was used to distinguish occupational groups such as doctors and lawyers – occupations which were free and self-regulating and/or required an elite education. In 1711 Addison referred to 'the three great professions of divinity, law and physic' (quoted by Carr-Saunders, 1928, p. 4). During the nineteenth century 'professions' came to be used to refer to superior occupations, requiring intellectual training, a body of expert knowledge, a degree of self-regulation by a professional body and, often, a royal charter or establishment by statute. The aim was to exclude the unskilled and the unqualified, to establish a monopoly of practice and to regulate the labour market.

Sociologists have attempted to develop definitions of 'professions'. The earliest of these, generally referred to as 'trait' approaches, attempted to develop a set of criteria, an ideal type against which an occupation could be measured. A review of the literature indicates that a number of traits have been suggested by different commentators, but that the key ones are that the profession was based on a body of knowledge, that the members had specialized skills and competence in the application of this knowledge, and that professional conduct was guided by a code of ethics, the focus of which is service to the client (Goode, 1960). Carr-Saunders (1955), writing in this tradition, suggested that there were four types of profession:

1 the established professions – for example, law, medicine and the church – where practice is based on theoretical study and the members of the profession follow a certain moral code of behaviour;
2 the new professions, which are based on fundamental studies – for example, engineering, chemistry, and the natural and social sciences;
3 the semi-professions, which are based on the acquisition of technical skills – for example nursing, pharmacy and social work;
4 would-be professions – occupations which require neither theoretical study nor the acquisition of exact technical skills, but may require facility with modern practices in business administration – for example, hospital managers.

According to trait theories, then, professions are characterized by the monopolization of particular forms of expertise, the erection of social boundaries around themselves through entrance qualifications and extended training, and an ideology of public service and altruism – that is, they claim to serve higher goals than mere economic self-interest. This professional autonomy is justified by the self-policing mechanisms constructed through their own internal criteria of standards maintained by the profession itself. Thus, to enter medicine requires a lengthy period of study, a pledge to save life and adherence to standards of practice set by the teaching hospitals and by the professional associations of the medical profession itself. One consequence of these mechanisms is that they provide the basis for political power in the labour market, allowing the members of the profession to command higher status and high rewards for their services. However, critics have pointed out that the professions cannot necessarily be relied upon to police themselves effectively, nor to act in the public interest. Moreover, almost no occupation calling itself a 'profession' can meet all of these criteria.

On the whole, this approach of listing the characteristics of professions to measure how far different occupations meet them has been rejected as unhelpful. This is because the traits generally seen as delineating a profession are mostly based on an idealized conception of the characteristics of the archetypical professions – medicine and law. Trait theories thereby give tacit support to the view of themselves which these professions project to the public. They tend to obscure the middle-class nature of codes of ethics, and the ways in which the professions also act as agents of social control. Furthermore, they do not explain how and why an occupation became a profession, and they emphasize altruism rather than highlighting the economic and social rewards of being a professional (Ben-David, 1963). The approach is ultimately unhelpful because it tells us only what professionals claim to do. The German sociologist Max Weber pointed out that

> When we hear from all sides the demand for an introduction of regular curricula and special examinations, the reason behind it is, of course, not a suddenly awakened thirst for education but the desire for restricting the supply of these positions and their monopolisation by the owners of educational certificates. (quoted in Parry *et al.*, 1979, p. 73)

Freidson (1986) has suggested that it is more useful to consider the idea of 'professionalism' as used in practice. Becker (1971) suggested that 'profession' is a social symbol which people attach to some occupations but not to others, while Parry and Parry (1976) argue that the key question is how occupational groups achieve the status of profession and in the process gain ascendancy over other occupational groups.

Developing this analysis, feminists have argued that in the process of upward mobility the male-dominated professions gained control over and subordinated female-dominated occupations. This is most clearly illustrated in medicine, where the medical profession is male-dominated and where in the process of achieving its dominant professional status the female occupations of nursing, midwifery and health visiting were subordinated (Abbott and Wallace, Chapter 2 in this volume). Indeed, nurses are still fighting to gain recognition of the right to control their own work. Larson (1977) suggests that professions are occupations that by market strategies have gained dominance over areas of social concern, while Abbott (1988) suggests that there is a *system* of professions, with inter-professional contestation and the subordination of some occupational groups by others. He suggests that professions serve their own interests as much as those of others. Traditional professions have achieved high status and a high remuneration for their members. These professions have developed powerful councils which define the profession, control access to it and police its standards.

However, the problem of definition remains, even if it is recognized that it is problematic. Freidson (1994) has indicated that

> I use the word 'profession' to refer to an occupation that controls its own work, organised by a special set of institutions sustained in part by a particular ideology of expertise and service. I use the word 'professionalism' to refer to that ideology and special set of institutions. (p. 10)

The Role of the Professions

Functionalist accounts of the professions emphasized the functions they played for society and for their own members. Carr-Saunders and Wilson (1933) stressed the stabilizing effect for society, Marshall (1963) the importance of altruism and Parsons (1954) the collective orientation. In the case of medicine, for example, Parsons pointed to the crucial role of medical doctors in defining who is legitimately sick and can therefore be excused normal role obligations. Hughes (1963) pointed out that professions provide a service for clients – they solve problems that clients cannot solve for themselves – but on a more critical note also highlighted the ways in which they exploit their monopolistic dominance. Larson (1977) has also deawn attention to the privileges that accrue to professionals. Johnson (1972) argues from a Marxist perspective that professions form a particular, institutionalized form of client control. Their professional status stems from the assumed ignorance of the client as against the claims of professional specialist knowledge, thereby rendering clients relatively helpless. Professionals are accepted as specialists, and they often have legal backing for this, making their clients socially and economically dependent. In addition, clients are often socially distanced from their advisers in other ways – by social class, ethnicity, educational background and gender, for example.

While the Marxist critique sees professionals as acting as the agents of the capitalist state, the Right and feminists have also been critical of the way in which professionals exercise power. Illich *et al.* (1977), for example, have argued that professions are disabling – that is, they take away individuals' ability to care for themselves. While the New Right has attacked monopolistic practices and the political power of the professions, it has tended not to question their ability to provide a necessary service. However, the New Right has questioned the role of welfare professionals, especially social workers, arguing that individuals come to rely on them rather than solving their own problems (Minford, 1987). Feminists have been critical of the ways in which professionals use patriarchal ideology to reinforce the subordinate status of women, for example, by the assumption (often unstated) that women should prioritize the needs of their husbands and children over their own (Abbott and Wallace, 1996).

It is easy, however, to be critical of the interventionist work with clients that professionals undertake and to point to the ways in which they themselves benefit from their occupational role and act as agents of social control. At the same time, it is necessary to acknowledge that clients can and do benefit from intervention. As Sue Wise writes of her own attempt to integrate her feminism with her social work practice,

> I came to believe that I had set myself the wrong problem and that feminist social work . . . was a fantasy based on a fundamental misunderstanding . . . That is, I see 'social work' now as the policing of minimum standards of care for, and the protection of the rights of, the most vulnerable members of our society . . . my starting point is this: social work is about social control and especially the protection of children and other 'vulnerables' – and this is a morally proper function. (Wise, 1985, p. 71)

while Freidson (1994) says that his collection of essays

> . . . represent my considered response to the torrent of criticism to which professions in the United States have been subject over the past two decades by both radical and free-market ideologies. My past work on the medical profession has been cited often to support both positions, but I believe that both are ill-considered, especially in the light of the practical question, 'What are the alternatives to professionalism?' . . . The evaluative tradition of Tawney, Carr-Saunders and Marshall is reborn in my argument that professionalism is both necessary and desirable for a decent society. (p. 9)

However, he makes it quite clear that what he is primarily concerned with is the ethic of professionalism. Referring to skilled creative work that is performed without remuneration, he suggests that

> In such circumstances we find a professionalism that is, by choice or necessity, stripped of the compromising institutions that assure workers a living, a professionalism expressed purely as dedication to the committed practice of a complex craft that is of value to

> others. To liberate it from material self-interest is the most radical way by which professionalism could be reborn. (1994, p. 10)

Stacey (1992), similarly, has argued for a 'new professionalism'. Referring to the medical profession, she argues that doctors acting collectively have put their interests before those of the public, by their insistence on an exclusive cluster of knowledge, professional unity and the promotion and enhancement of their own status. She indicates that professions should build on the other nineteenth-century ideal of service: doctors must recognize, she insists, the centrality of others, including patients, to health and healing, and, accordingly, adjust their idea of clinical autonomy, their control of the 'professions allied to medicine', and their claim to the exclusive right of doctors to sit in judgement over other doctors. Hugman (1991) argues for democratic professionalism – a partnership between users and professionals. Jan Williams (1993) suggests that

> Instead of a one-way transmission of knowledge from professional to client, there is a two-way transaction, building on existing knowledge and experience of the client, according to the client's perceived needs and the professional's response to these . . .

and

> [the professional's] role has changed from one of controlling to one of supporting and enabling, helping the client to address and think through his own experiences and sharing her expert knowledge to help him develop his understanding. (pp. 11–12)

Celia Davies (1995) proposes a new professionalism for nursing; the new professionals, she suggests, should be engaged with patients, work with patients and other health care professionals and make reflexive use of their experience and expertise (pp. 149–50). Dominelli (1997) points to the potential for a sociological social work whose practitioners work with clients, recognize the structural problems the client experiences and redefine professionalism so as not to add to clients' oppression.

The Caring Professionals

Etzioni (1969) suggested that occupational groups such as nurses and social workers should be categorized as 'semi-professions' because

> Their training is shorter, their status is less legitimated, their right to privileged communication less established, there is less of a

> specialised body of knowledge and they have less autonomy from supervision or control than 'the' professions. (p. v)

Considerable scepticism has been expressed as to whether nurses and social workers require specialized training, knowledge and skills (e.g. Brewer and Lait, 1980). The work carried out by the caring professionals is often seen as an extension of work that women are expected to carry out in the domestic sphere, and therefore as work that they can do 'naturally'. This is exacerbated by the tendency of basic grade workers to be women, and managers to be (white) men (Abbott and Wallace, 1996; Dominelli, 1997). Men are in managerial posts in nursing, social work and primary teaching out of all proportion to their numbers in these occupations.

> . . . there is a sense in which nursing is not a profession but an adjunct to a gendered concept of profession. Nursing is the activity, in other words, that enables medicine to present itself as masculine/rational and to gain the power and the privilege of so doing. It has clearly not had first bite of the cherry in defining its work and . . . we get closer to the . . . matter in recognising that it is trying to put a conceptual framework around just those aspects of the work of health and healing that are 'left over' after medicine has imposed an essentially masculine vision. (Davies, 1995, p. 61)

Salvage (1985), however, has raised the issue of whether 'the question we should ask is not "Is nursing a profession?" but "Should nursing want to be a profession, and, if so, what do we mean by it?"' (p. 92). Similarly the question of whether or not social workers should aspire to professional status (and what that means) has been raised (Bamford, 1990; Dominelli, 1997). However, there have been professionalizing strategies within the caring professions and the use of trait models to argue that nursing and social work are moving towards professional status even if they have not already achieved it (Bamford, 1990; Lodd and Pepper, 1993; Payne, 1981; Schur and Turner, 1982).

We would suggest that a more fruitful approach is to examine the ways in which occupational groups make claims to be professions and to examine the extent to which they are successful. Nursing, midwifery, health visiting and social work have all made such claims: these occupational groups are still striving to demonstrate that caring is work and to find ways of caring that do not make them subservient, but which demonstrate that they have professional expertise. (See Robinson, and Meerabeau, in this volume.) A critical examination of the ways in which these occupations have developed since the nineteenth century shows clearly that a major aspect has been the attempts to achieve professional status (Abbott and

Wallace, and Kirkham, in this volume). These occupational strategies are often themselves based implicitly on a 'trait model' of what a profession is. Also, an examination of the history of nursing, midwifery, health visiting and social work challenges a passive interpretation of women's subordination. Women have challenged male domination and developed strategies to achieve professional status, and these have been resisted by men and by some women. Rather than rejecting claims to professionals status, it may be more relevant to recognize that this model of a profession is based upon man-made criteria in the first place. However, not all aspects of professionalization can be reduced to gender alone. Pamela Abbott (Chapter 10) indicates that the conflict between the occupational groups she describes is not a struggle between the sexes but resistance by district nurses to home helps taking on personal care work. Relations of domination and exclusionary tactics are not confined to class and gender.

Key elements in any claim to professional status seem to be autonomy or control over work, a clearly defined monopoly over an area of work and a knowledge base. It is in these areas that both social work and nursing have attempted to demonstrate that they are professions, and in which they have also been challenged. Neither social workers nor nurses have autonomous control as practitioners over their work. (Midwifery does have a clear area of control, but the interface with medicine remains a problem.) Not only are they supervised by their superiors in their day-to-day tasks, but those who supervise them may not even be qualified in their discipline (C. Davies, 1982). Nor do they necessarily have a monopoly over an area of work: caring work is often seen as women's work and closely identified with what women are supposed to be doing for their families without payment. The Nurses Act 1918 established the General Nursing Council which supervises the training and examination of nurses, but the title 'nurse' is not reserved exclusively for those on the register of qualified nurses. The Central Council for the Education and Training of Social Work[1] approves courses of training, but no qualification is necessary to practise as a social worker. Furthermore, CCETSW is a quango and training is determined by government policy.

These 'female' occupational groups have aspired to professional status by claiming an area of expertise and by extending the education and training required to become qualified. During the course of the twentieth century teaching, social work and nursing, for example, have all raised the entry qualifications for training, developed first-level training courses at university level and argued for in-service training and continuing professional development. However, considerable influence remains with employers: in social work, for example, the restructuring of social work education and training by CCETSW in the 1980s enhanced the influence of employers in curriculum design and implementation. The DipSW which replaced the CQSW and CSS follows the model established by the CSS, with consortia of employers working with university departments to ensure that curricula focus on equipping practitioners with relevant skills:

> . . . CCETSW is . . . enforcing a competency-based approach which favours the employers' and government's interests over those of the professionals and users. (Dominelli, 1997, pp. 122–3).

However, the perception of the close association between women's natural caring skills and abilities and the control exercised by managers or members of male-dominated professions has made it difficult for these occupational groups to claim a distinct, professional knowledge base and a unique expertise. They are also employed, usually, within state bureaucracies and subject to the constraints of managerial power. Their employer is the state (or a voluntary organization) rather than 'the client', and they have to 'fit' the client's 'needs' to the services and resources available. Indeed, despite the current rhetoric of consumerism, problems are often defined by the state rather than the client, and workers are accountable to managers, not clients. However, a gendered pattern has also developed within the caring professions – (white) men tend to be promoted and occupy the managerial roles, so that women work with clients and are managed by men (Witz, 1992; Grimwood and Popplestone, 1993; Abbott and Wallace, 1996; Dominelli, 1997).

While the aim to be recognized as a professional occupation of equal status with medicine and the law may not yet have been achieved by nursing and social work, both occupations strive to differentiate themselves from the unqualified carer. In claiming to be *professional* carers, nurses and social workers are marking out a boundary between themselves (as trained and qualified) and the untrained carers, whether paid or informal – they are claiming an occupational monopoly over defined areas of work (see Abbott, Chapter 10 in this volume). However, the introduction of National Vocational Qualifications (NVQs) has meant that jobs once undertaken by qualified workers are now being done by people, generally women, with the lower-level NVQ qualification (Dominelli, 1997). 'Caring' is generally seen as the positive experience of an inner emotional state. However, it is necessary to distinguish between 'caring about' (the cognitive/emotional aspect) and 'caring for' (the practical and physical aspect). Most practical care is undertaken by unqualified and/or informal carers – auxiliaries, care assistants, classroom assistants, mothers, daughters, husbands and wives. Furthermore, caring is seen as a natural attribute of women and is, therefore, downgraded and devalued – not recognized or rewarded for its skills. The concept of 'emotional work' – supporting, dealing with and necessarily controlling the emotional state of the cared-for person – has been used to refer to this form of labour (Hochschild, 1983).

Those who provide practical care, including informal carers, have to carry out the daily grind irrespective of affectional ties or emotions, and they often have their lives controlled by professionals – by the cared-for, by the wider society and by the state. Their work may be – and generally is – supervised by qualified workers: nurses, teachers, youth and community workers or social workers. Indeed, supervising unqualified workers may be seen as an important element of status for the qualified worker (see Abbott, Chapter 10 of this volume).

'Caring about' is seen as 'being concerned for' – being interested in the welfare of – rather than undertaking practical care (except in the case of female informal carers, where 'caring *about*' is seen as necessarily involving 'caring *for*'). It can involve organizing, supervising or paying for practical care. Qualified workers may undertake care work, but they are primarily responsible for managing/organizing it (Melia, 1987). However, caring professionals are employed within bureaucratic organizations and are responsible to the organization for the care they provide or administrate. Welfare provision tends to be service-led rather than needs-led. Furthermore, the extent to which it is 'care' or 'control' that is being provided is also open to debate. As Dominelli (1997) points out, there are situations where control over others is desirable – for example, protecting women from domestic violence, children from child abuse, and so on. Furthermore, social control may not be obvious, and indeed social work is often as much about controlling access to scarce resources as it is about primary care.

Nursing is seen as a traditional female role and, in the popular image at least, as subordinated to medical control. Nurses are seen as carrying out the instructions of doctors. The possibilities of nurses achieving professional status are limited as a consequence of its association in popular ideology with mundane bedside drudgery that is seen as 'women's work' (Gamarnikow, 1978; Rafferty, 1996). The characteristic features of nursing are low pay, low prestige, unsocial hours, high turnover and lack of job security (see Mackay in this volume). The development of educational programmes for nurses has not superficially improved their status in the medical hierarchy either in the hospital or in the community context. Indeed, Marie Anne Rafferty (1996) has suggested that nursing has been more concerned with moral values than intellectual knowledge, and midwifery is uneasy about its close proximity to nursing in higher education. Social work, similarly, has been associated with female roles (Dominelli, 1997). While it has not been dominated in the same way as nursing by other occupations in the division of labour, social workers have, nonetheless, not established themselves as autonomous practitioners.

While strategies of occupational closure result in the exclusion or marginalization of women by the male-dominated professions (Witz, 1992), or occupational segregation as in the case of midwifery (Donnison, 1977; Ehrenreich and English, 1979), the female-dominated professions have also exercised occupational closure, erecting barriers between themselves and care workers – mainly working-class females – and informal carers. Black people are also underrepresented in the caring professions, although overrepresented as clients. After the Second World War black people from the 'new commonwealth' countries were encouraged to come to Britain to fill the low-status personal service jobs that were vacant. In the health services, for example, black women are employed as domestics and care assistants. Trained black nurses were much more likely to have trained as state enrolled than as state registered nurses – the former not being eligible for promotion into supervisory and managerial posts (Hugman, 1991). If the caring professions have employed professionalizing strategies – enhanced educational qualifications for entry to training and barriers to in-service promotional opportunities – these will have discriminated disproportionately against black and working-class people, who are disadvantaged by racism and 'classism' in the educational system and in British society generally.

However, in developing a knowledge base, nursing and social work have relied heavily on the social as opposed to the natural sciences – the latter often seen as having a higher status. Both occupations have found it difficult to develop a unique knowledge base to underpin professional practice. Both have come increasingly to stress the importance of evidence-based practice – practice based on sound research. However, this has been slow to develop, and often practitioners continue to work on the basis of previous routine.

Furthermore, research is generally based on the methodologies, including qualitative ones, of the social sciences. The scientificity of these methodologies is challenged by a profession such as medicine, whose knowledge base is grounded in conclusions developed using natural science methods, including the randomized controlled trial. Nurses and social workers have to challenge not only the argument that their work is based on common sense and skills naturally possessed by women but also the claim that the knowledge base they have developed is derived from other disciplines, and/or developed using 'non-scientific' research techniques. Anne Marie Rafferty has suggested that nursing and social work have had to occupy a space left by medicine. However, in developing a knowledge base, they have used the possession of this as the basis for excluding other workers, in the same way as they themselves have been excluded. Knowledge and access to knowledge are central to the ability to put up occupational boundaries, but knowledge itself is organized hierarchically and some knowledge is seen as superior to other knowledge. Those who possess 'superior' knowledge can construct occupational boundaries. Knowledge status also relates to class, gender and race, and those occupations which possess high-status knowledge are powerful.

Professionalized caring work, then, is work undertaken predominantly by middle-class white women, employed within state bureaucracies. The work is seen in relation to natural female abilities – women's ability to care and natural altruism – and as an extension of women's natural role as nurturers in the family.

However, there is a contradiction in the nature of these professions. 'Care' is their core activity and justification, but it has been argued from a variety of perspectives that their expert knowledge is not used primarily to meet the needs of clients but to 'police' and monitor them. The caring professions are exercising social control over their clients – who are in general poor and working-class and include a disproportionate number of black people, women, people with disabilities, children and the elderly. Social work, for example, has been referred to as 'the iron fist in the velvet glove' (Open University, 1978) and health visitors as 'soft policemen' (Abbott and Sapsford, 1990). The issue, then, is whose interests the caring professions serve and who benefits from the work they do. The power of these occupations tends to rest on their occupational position, the legitimacy accorded them as a result of this, and the power they exercise based on their claims to knowledge (see the chapter by David McCallum in this volume). The caring professions are powerful because they not only aim to change and control behaviour but also help to structure the context of social and cultural life in a more general sense – through their power to command definitions of reality by which the lives of their clients are shaped. In other words, they both create the object of their intervention – the neglectful mother, the wayward teenager, the bad patient – and at the same time make these the targets of their intervention. Intervention is designed to normalize, to make subjects conform to the defined norms. In this model people are seen as having, or being, problems, and experts as having solutions – the knowledge to solve the problems. Nurses and social workers claim the right (power) to instruct, to tell people what they need to know and how they ought to act. To define someone as a client is to determine that they have a need and that the need can be met by the expertise of the social worker or nurse. The professional, not the client, defines the problem, and the solution is seen to come out of the professional knowledge of the social worker or nurse.

Welfare professionals have been challenged from a number of perspectives – from the political Left for being 'agents of the capitalist state', from feminists for working within patriarchal ideologies and reinforcing the subordinate status of women, from black perspectives for using racist ideologies and discriminatory practices, from people with disabilities for assuming that the 'problem' is an individual trait, from older people for being ageist, from gay and lesbian people for heterosexism and homophobia, and from the political Right for creating dependency. What is common to all these challenges is their dissent from the view that professionals can define problems and solutions to them, that professional practice is disinterested and client-centred, and that the caring professionals have a scientific knowledge base that enables them to be objective and value-free.

These concerns about the role that the caring professionals play have developed as much from within as outside the professions themselves. In the 1970s Marxist and 'political economy' critiques of, in particular, social and community work (see, e.g., Loney, 1983; Mayo, 1975; Gough, 1979) were developed. Two major arguments mere made. First, it was argued that existing social work theory and practice in effect blamed the victim rather than recognizing that the major causes of social problems were outside the control of the individual – for example, poverty and unemployment. In other words, the clients of social workers *had* problems rather than *being* problems. The second argument was that professionals, including caring professionals, acted as agents of social control on behalf of a capitalist state by individualizing social problems – by intervening in ways that suggested that the victims were to blame for their plight. Loney (1983), for example, has described the way in which Community Development Projects were established in the 1960s, underpinned by a 'community pathology' model of poverty – that is, that people were poor because of community or individual pathology, not structural inequalities – the 'cycle of deprivation' view of poverty (Joseph, 1972). Community Development Workers came quickly to develop a radical critique and demonstrated the structural basis of poverty, which was perpetuated by social and economic structures, and which created an unequal distribution of resources and power throughout society. The Community Development Workers worked with client groups to empower them to improve their situation collectively, by, for example, forming Claimants' Unions, Tenants' Associations and so on. The response of successive governments to this analysis and response was negative, and eventually funding was withdrawn.

Radical social work subsequently came to be criticized from black and feminist perspectives. These indicated that the radical critique did not question the ways in which professional interactions controlled and subordinated women and black people (see, e.g., Mayo, 1977; Hanmer and Statham, 1988; Dominelli, 1990, 1997; Dominelli and McLeod, 1989; John, 1981). The voices of disabled people, people with mental health problems, people with learning disabilities and gay men and lesbian women have been added to the concerns expressed about the ways in which the practice of caring professionals often does not meet their needs, but subordinates and controls them (Taylor, 1993).

Conclusions

We have argued that it is more profitable to examine what an occupational group does, what expertise its practitioners claim to have, how it intersects with other occupational groups in the division of labour and the strategies it adopts to improve its status *vis-à-vis* other groups, than merely to categorize occupations. In this way we can raise questions about the relationships with the clients of those in client-centred occupations, the division of labour between occupations that share clients, and the strategies occupational groups use to maintain dominance over both clients and other occupational groups. In this respect it is important to note that social workers and nurses, in attempting to be upwardly mobile as professions, exclude and marginalize other groups: in the case of social workers – social service workers and, in the case of nurses – care assistants.

Social workers and nurses have used a variety of strategies to lay claim to the status of 'professional'. In Western societies 'professional' is generally a term of approval, and one that implies payment for special skills and proficiency. To claim to be a profession is to suggest independence, autonomy and control over work, but neither social workers nor nurses have achieved recognition as professional occupations in terms of financial reward or autonomy over work. Both groups have justified their strategies for achieving professional status by arguing that this would improve client/patient care. However, it is not clear that achieving professional status would necessarily do this. The strategies successfully used to achieve professional status by the medical profession seem as much about protecting and enhancing the status of doctors as about protecting the public and providing a higher level of service. Jane Salvage (1985) has argued that, if nursing became professionalized, this would lead to nurses identifying with doctors rather than with care assistants and ancillary staff, relatives and the friends of the patients. This, she suggests, could strengthen barriers between nurses and patients and also create barriers between workers, rather than encouraging them to work as a team to meet the needs of patients. She concludes by arguing that strategies of professionalization are less about meeting the needs of patients/clients than about an occupational group pursuing its own narrow interests.

Finally, we want to point to a key element, one often ignored in sociological texts on the professions, namely, the ways in which the words 'profession' and 'professionalism' are used in everyday language to *control* those who use or lay claim to the title. Social workers and nurses, as well as other professional and semi-professional groups, are often accused of 'acting unprofessionally' – that is, failing to put their patients or clients first (e.g. when they threaten industrial action in pursuit of higher wages or better conditions of work). To be 'professional', the caring professions are expected to be selfless, putting the needs of others before their own. In part this is not surprising, given that many of the workers in the semi-professions are female, and given also the power of family ideology to circumscribe and define the occupations in the 'female sector' of the division of labour. Beyond this, however, another discourse comes into play: the idea of professionalism is used to police the actions of those who lay claim to professional status. Certain standards of performance and behaviour are expected of them, standards set in essence from outside the control of the profession itself. Groups who aspire to professional status are laying themselves open to being controlled by externally-defined standards – a 'professional discourse' which both defines what is to be counted as professional behaviour and targets those who are perceived not to conform to it. The power of the discourse is used to control the behaviour of the aspiring profession. One of the outcomes of this is that a sector of the middle class – including caring 'professionals' – is prepared, indeed in some cases eager, to accept the historical constraints of professional status in order to acquire what it sees as its freedom of action. In turn, the discourse that defines professions has developed in tandem with male specialisms such as medicine and the law and incorporates a range of essentially patriarchal assumptions and definitions which then become incorporated into the new professions, whether or not they may be appropriate. Hence the idea of 'professionalism' serves contradictory functions in the case of the caring professions. On the one hand, it defines and enhances the nature of these occupational groups. On the other, given the uncertain nature of the knowledge bases to which the groups lay claim, it constrains the ways in which they are able to define their tasks, and lays them open to attack on the grounds of structurally unprofessional conduct.

Note

1 Superseded by the National Board for Nursing, Midwifery and Health Visiting, and the United Kingdom Central Council for Nursing, Midwifery and Health Visiting in the mid-1980s.

References

Abbott, A. (1988) *The System of Professions: An Essay on the Division of Expert Labor*, Chicago: University of Chicago Press.

Abbott, P. and Sapsford, R.J. (1990) 'Health visiting: Policing the family?', in Abbott, P. and Wallace, C. (Eds) *The Sociology of the Caring Professions* (1st edn), Basingstoke: Falmer.

Abbott, P. and Wallace, C. (1996) *An Introduction to Sociology: Feminist Perspectives* (2nd edn), London: Routledge.

BAINES, C.T., EVANS, R. and WEYSMITH, S. (Eds) (1991) *Women's Caring: Feminist Perspectives on Social Welfare,* Toronto: McClelland.

BAMFORD, T. (1990) *The Future of Social Work,* Basingstoke: Macmillan.

BECKER, H. (1971) *Sociological Work,* Chicago: Aldine.

BELL, O. (1973) *The Coming of Post-Industrial Society,* New York: Basic Books.

BEN-DAVID, S. (1963–4) 'Professions in the class system of present-day societies', *Current Sociology,* **12**, pp. 296–9.

BOWLES, S. and GINTIS, H. (1976) *Schooling in Capitalist America,* London: Routledge & Kegan Paul.

BREWER, C. and LAIT, J. (1980) *Can Social Work Survive?,* London: Temple Smith.

CAMPBELL, B. (1998) *Sweet Secrets,* London: Virago.

CARR-SAUNDERS, A.M. (1928) *Professions – Their Organisation and Place in Society: The Herbert Spencer Lecture,* Oxford: Clarendon Press.

CARR-SAUNDERS, A.M. (1955) 'Metropolitan conditions and traditional professional relationships', in FISHER, A.M. (Ed.) *The Metropolis in Modern Life,* Garden City (NY): Rooksbury.

CARR-SAUNDERS, A.M. and WILSON, P.M. (1933) *The Professions,* London: Oxford University Press.

DAVIES, A. (1987) 'Hazardous lives – social work in the 1980s: A view from the Left', in LONEY, M., BOCOCK, B., CLARKE, J., COCHRANE, A., GRAHAM, P. and WILSON, M. (Eds) *The State or the Market,* London: Sage.

DAVIES, C. (1982) 'The regulation of nursing: An historical comparison of Britain and the USA', *Research in the Sociology of Health Care,* **2**, pp. 121–60.

DAVIES, C. (1995) *Gender and the Professional Predicament in Nursing,* Buckingham: Open University Press.

DAVIS, K. and MOORE, W.E. (1967) 'Some principles of stratification', in BENDIX, R. and LIPPSET, S.M. (Eds) *Class, Status and Power,* London: Routledge & Kegan Paul.

DOMINELLI, L. (1990) *Women and Community Action,* Birmingham: Venture Press.

DOMINELLI, L. (1997) *Sociology for Social Work,* London: Macmillan.

DOMINELLI, L. and MCLEOD, E. (1989) *Feminist Social Work,* London: Macmillan.

DONNISON, J. (1977) *Midwives and Medical Men,* London: Heinemann.

EHRENREICH, B. and ENGLISH, D. (1979) *For Her Own Good: A Hundred Years of the Experts' Advice to Women,* London: Pluto Press.

ETZIONI, A. (1969) *The Semi-Professions and their Organisation,* New York: Free Press.

FREIDSON, E. (1970) *Professional Dominance: The Social Structure of Medical Care,* New York: Atherton Press.

FREIDSON, E. (1986) *Professional Powers: A Study of the Institutionalisation of Formal Knowledge,* Chicago: University of Chicago Press.

FREIDSON, E. (1994) *Professionalism Reborn: Theory, Prophecy and Policy,* Cambridge: Polity.

GAMARNIKOW, E. (1978) 'Sexual division of labour: The case of nursing', in KUHN, A. and WOLPE, A. (Eds) *Feminism and Materialism,* London: Routledge & Kegan Paul.

GOODE, W.J. (1960) 'Encroachment, charlatanism and the emergent professions', *American Sociological Review*, **25**, pp. 902–14.

GOUGH, I. (1979) *The Political Economy of the Welfare State*, London: Macmillan.

GRIMWOOD, C. and POPPLESTONE, R. (1993) *Women, Management and Care*, London: Macmillan.

HANMER, J. and STATHAM, D. (1988) *Women and Social Work: Towards a Woman-Centred Practice*, Basingstoke: Macmillan.

HOCHSCHILD, A.R. (1983) *The Managed Heart*, Berkeley (CA): University of California Press.

HUGHES, E. (1963) *Men and Their Work*, New York: Free Press.

HUGMAN, R. (1991) *Power in the Caring Professions*, London: Macmillan.

ILLICH, I. *et al.* (1977) *Disabling Professions*, London: Boyars.

JOHN, G. (1981) *In the Service of Black Youth*, Leicester: National Association of Youth Clubs.

JOHNSON, T. (1972) *Professions and Power*, London: Macmillan.

JOSEPH, K. (1972) 'The next ten years', *New Society*, 5 October.

LARSON, M. (1977) *The Rise of Professionalism: A Sociological Analysis*, Berkeley (CA): University of California Press.

LODD, S. and PEPPER, J.M. (1993) *Conceptual Bases of Professional Nursing* (3rd edn), Philadelphia: Lippincott.

LONEY, M. (1983) *Community against Government: The British Community Development Project 1968–1978*, London: Heinemann.

MARSHALL, T.H. (1963) *Sociology at the Crossroads*, London: Heinemann.

MAYO, M. (1975) 'The history and early development of CDP', in LEES, R. and SMITH, G. (Eds) *Action Research in Community Development*, London: Routledge & Kegan Paul.

MAYO, M. (Ed.) (1977) *Women in the Community*, London: Routledge & Kegan Paul.

MELIA, K. (1987) *Learning and Working: The Occupational Socialisation of Nurses*, London: Tavistock.

MINFORD, P. (1987) 'The role of the social services: A view from the New Right', in LONEY, M., BOCOCK, B., CLARKE, J., COCHRANE, A., GRAHAM, P. and WILSON, M. (Eds) *The State or the Market*, London: Sage.

OPEN UNIVERSITY (1978) *DE206 Social Work, Community Work and Society*, Milton Keynes: Open University.

ORR, J. (1986) 'Feminism and health visiting', in WEBB, C. (Ed.) *Feminist Practice in Women's Health Care*, Chichester: Wiley.

PARRY, N. and PARRY, J. (1976) *The Rise of the Medical Profession*, London: Croom Helm.

PARRY, N., RUSTIN, M. and SATYAMURTI, J. (1979) *Social Work, Welfare and the State*, London: Edward Arnold.

PARSONS, T. (1954) *Essays in Sociological Theory*, Glencoe (IL): Free Press.

PAYNE, R.H. (1981) *Professional Discipline in Nursing*, Oxford: Blackwell.

RAFFERTY, A.M. (1996) *The Politics of Nursing Knowledge*, London: Routledge.

SALVAGE, J. (1985) *The Politics of Nursing*, London: Heinemann.

SCHUR, M.C. and TURNER, J. (1982) *Nursing Image or Reality?* London: Hodder & Stoughton.

STACEY, M. (1992) *Regulating British Medicine: The General Medical Council*, Chichester: Wiley.

TAYLOR, G. (1993) 'Challenges from the margins', in CLARKE, J. (Ed.) *A Crisis in Care? Challenges to Social Work*, London: Sage.

WILLIAMS, J. (1993) 'What is a profession? Experience versus expertise', in WALMSELY, J., REYNOLDS, J., SHAKESPEARE, P. and WOOLFE, R. (Eds) *Health, Welfare and Practice: Reflecting on Roles and Relationships*, London: Sage.

WISE, S. (1985) *Becoming a Feminist Social Worker. Studies in Sexual Politics 6*, Department of Sociology, University of Manchester.

WITZ, A. (1992) *Professions and Patriarchy*, London: Routledge.

Chapter 2

Health Visiting, Social Work, Nursing and Midwifery: a History

Pamela Abbott and Claire Wallace

In this chapter we intend to examine the development of nursing, midwifery, health visiting and social work as caring professions. In doing so, we are presenting a *reading* of the processes involved in the transformation of nursing and social work from predominantly philanthropic work undertaken by unpaid ladies into modern occupational groups. Our argument is that there is no such thing as a 'factual' history, but, rather, accounts or readings of history that are influenced by the theoretical position of the authors and the purpose for which the history is written. In our reading of the history of nursing and social work we are heavily influenced by feminist and Foucauldian theories. Foucault was concerned to explore the ways in which modern Western society has become increasingly disciplined, regulated and kept under surveillance. We consider how the essentially female occupations of nursing and social work came to exercise power and regulate social life through the development of knowledge bases, which are in turn embedded in discourses emerging at different points in time within a patriarchal setting. The claim to these knowledge bases as 'truth' – as operating beyond everyday common sense – leads to the legitimizing of particular spheres of professional expertise; and, similarly, the weakness or ambiguity in these knowledge claims can lead to the challenging of professional expertise – resistance. Consequently, it is important to look at the historical emergence of different discourses as they relate to the various caring professions and the way in which they were institutionalized through welfare bureaucracies. The Foucauldian approach differs from other approaches in that it takes a non-essentialist view of these claims to knowledge or 'truth'. Thus, we can examine how discourses surrounding the idea of the family, crime, the nature of deviance, poverty and health emerged, the ways in which they structured the conceptual world and their effects on professional practice, without having to concern ourselves with their 'truth' or 'falsehood'.

Foucault has analyzed the relationship between certain medical and social science discourses and the exercise of power in modern Western societies. He was concerned to examine the relationship between discourses, practice and professional groups. He suggests that power/knowledge has become organized around enquiries into the body (of the individual) and bodies (of the population). The body has become both the object and the target of power. The techniques of disciplinary power are the means by which bodies are observed and analyzed. 'Biopolitics' is his term for the development of concern about the health and welfare of individuals and populations, and the power strategies used to normalize individuals and populations in this respect. Scientific/medical discourses and the associated exercise of professional power were involved in the growth of surveillance of societies through the exercise of discipline over the body and the population. From the eighteenth century onwards medical men, philanthropists, social workers, health visitors, etc. become the new receivers of confession – the collectors of the inner thoughts, attitudes and assumptions of private citizens. The bureaucratic questionnaire became the link between the individual citizen and the public world of politics and administration. The regulating state regulates the individual citizen. As mind is assimilated to body with the development of a discourse of psychological regulation in the twentieth century (Rose, 1985; 1989), the emphasis has shifted from physical and moral health to mental health, and surveillance has become correspondingly more detailed and intrusive (Sapsford, 1993). Furthermore, the technologies of discipline, hierarchical observation and normalizing judgement rely increasingly on the patients/clients assessing themselves – monitoring their own lifestyle.

For Foucault power resides in the claim to truth, and what is understood by 'truth' in medicine and the social sciences has played a large part as justification for the exercise of social control. Medicine and the social sciences, including their psychological/psychoanalytic branches, claim the arbitration of truth because of their scientific nature (as branches of the overall 'discourse of positivism' which has won the battle for truth in the modern world), and, to the extent that these new discourses became established as 'having truth', they acquired power. Thus, the advances in social medicine, the social sciences, biology and psychiatry provided a power/knowledge base for a large group of professions which intervened in the lives of individuals and populations. This led to, and its growth was stimulated by, new methods of surveying the population and the routine collection of statistical information about population growth – making it possible, for example, to monitor the birth rate. Thus, the population was created as an object of government and as a subject of needs, through the creation of the means to measure and monitor it. The concern with the health of the population arose out of new discourses, and gave rise to a range of new tactics and techniques of power, concerned with the health and wellbeing of individuals and of the population as a whole. The tactics of intervention are seldom direct and coercive; more often they involve teaching people (e.g. mothers) how to achieve goals which they and the experts 'agree' are desirable. In accepting the goals and the advice, however, mothers accept the expert's definition of the situation, and so the expert comes to determine the nature of the mother's social world. 'Pastoral' power – the power entailed in advising, counselling and facilitating – is no less effective than coercive power in determining how people shall understand and live in the social world.

Health Visiting

Health visitors were one group of the agents of pastoral power that became established in late-nineteenth- and early-twentieth-century Britain. The origins of health visiting and the conditions for the existence of health visitors can be located in biopolitics and the medical and hygiene discourse that developed in nineteenth-century England. By deploying techniques of surveillance, health visitors played an important role in normalizing the working-class family, and especially the mother, in the early twentieth century (see Davin, 1978; Rowan, 1985), and the practices of health promotion (preventing ill-health), through its techniques of surveillance, produced health visiting as we know it today. The basis of health visitors' power at that time was the medical discourse on infant care, diet and hygiene. Subsequently they have extended their knowledge base to include material on the psychological and biological growth of the normal child. While the focus of attention was the infant and child, the major target of normalization was the working-class mother. Health visitors used their power/knowledge to create a certain type of mother – the modern mother whose major focus of concern is the health and wellbeing of her family and specifically her child(ren). With the increased influence of psychology/psychiatry and the consequent growth in the complexity of the mother's task, what was in origin a form of control of working-class mothers has become applied to all mothers, and a movement that in origin tried to impose middle-class norms on working-class mothers has now come to exercise control over middle-class mothers as well (Sapsford, 1993).

Health visiting, like social work, has its historical roots in the nineteenth-century visiting movements (Prockoska, 1980), with their concern about the condition of the poor and the regulation of the population (Bland

and Mort, 1984). Part of this concern was with the conditions in which the poor lived, which were seen as a potential source of contagious diseases as well as of social and moral corruption. These movements were influenced by a number of different motivations and interests, however. Evangelicalism, with its emphasis on personal salvation and the need to save the immoral and prevent immorality, was one clear influence. Banks (1981) has argued that the involvement of middle-class women was an outcome of growing feminism in Victorian England: philanthropic good works were an outlet for upper-middle-class women who were no longer satisfied with their roles as wives and mothers but who continued to share Victorian values as to the appropriate roles for women. These Visiting Societies were often made up of male committees using (unpaid) female visitors, although some were set up and run by women. Often the major motivation for visiting the poor was religion, but the visitors frequently undertook nursing duties and gave advice on hygiene, childcare, cooking, etc. These societies were philanthropic – that is, they were concerned with personal conduct and morality. They aimed to correct and reform the poor by the giving of advice. Their philosophy was based on ideas of self-reliance and self-help rather than of charity (see Donzelot, 1977, for an extended discussion).

At the same time there was a growing concern about the health of the poor and a realization that a healthy workforce was a more efficient one (see, e.g., Chadwick, 1842). Specific concern was focused on hygiene, urged on by the cholera epidemics and the fears of the middle class that contagion would spread from the working-class areas of the towns (Wohl, 1986). A medical discourse centering on cleanliness developed, arguing not only for social reform but also for the working class to be instructed in matters of cleanliness (see Dowling, 1963; Wohl, 1986). Medical men played an important role both in advocating public health reforms and in the Health of Towns Association, established in 1844.

The discourses surrounding hygiene and cleanliness became articulated with the growing social science discourses with the founding of the Ladies' National Association for the Diffusion of Sanitary Knowledge in 1857, a sub-group of the Association for the Promotion of Social Science. This Association expressed concern about the hygienic circumstances in which the working class lived and about the ignorance of mothers. Attention was particularly drawn to the fatal effects in poor districts of childhood and infant diarrhoea, whooping cough, measles and bronchitis, illnesses that were seldom fatal among middle- and upper-class children. It tended to be suggested that the excessive infant mortality rate was mainly due to the poor management of children by their parents.

The Ladies' Sanitary Association set up branches around the country. Like the Visiting Societies they visited the homes of the poor on a systematic basis, but they were specifically concerned to distribute information on matters of health. There is some dispute as to when the first 'health visitors' (as they were later called) were employed. Many accounts (e.g. Dingwall, 1979; McCleary, 1933) argue that it was in Manchester in 1867; however, Dowling (1963) suggests that when the Manchester Ladies' Sanitary Association was formed there were already 134 woman Bible/sanitary missionaries employed in London. Certainly Mrs Raynor, a founding member of the Association in London, was the first person to employ a working-class woman to visit the homes of the poor, disseminating religious tracts and giving advice on matters of hygiene. However, the title 'health (sanitary) visitor' was first used in Manchester, and in 1890 Manchester Corporation was the first to take on the responsibility for paying salaries to health visitors – although by that time some local authorities were employing lady sanitary inspectors (Dowling, 1963). During the second half of the nineteenth century a number of branches of the Ladies' Sanitary Association were founded, mainly in large towns. Generally working-class women were paid from charitable monies to visit the homes of the poor, but they were supervised by unpaid middle-class women. Initially the working-class visitors had been untrained, but by the end of the nineteenth century there were some moves towards providing training. (For a detailed history see Dowling, 1963.)

By the end of the nineteenth century, then, we have a relatively small number of employed working-class women visiting the homes of the poor. The work of these women was supervised by middle-class female volunteers. Although the Sanitary Reform Movement and the sanitary reform legislation demonstrated some recognition that health and hygiene were at the mercy of factors beyond the control of individuals, the sanitary visiting movement clearly had an individualistic approach. The problem was seen as the neglect by the working class of matters of hygiene and cleanliness, and the solution as the instruction of the poor (and especially poor women). The movement was heavily dominated by *laissez-faire* ideas and much constrained by the reluctance of the state to tax citizens to pay for reforms and improve the conditions of the poor.

In the early twentieth century, however, in response to what were perceived as 'new' dangers to the health of the British population, health visiting began to develop more rapidly, and health visitors became agents in the construction of the 'new' working-class mother.[1] The new concerns provided the space to justify intervention in the family and to overcome the view that children were the property of their parents alone; medical discourses and the developing discourses of psychology provided the 'knowledge' with which to justify and on which to base the form that the interventions took.

In the first decade of the twentieth century there developed a growing concern about the health and fitness of the population; Weeks (1981) has suggested that it amounted to a moral panic. This concern was informed by the two scientific discourses of eugenics and neo-hygienism; that is, these discourses identified/created the problem, targeted certain groups or individuals as the 'cause' of it and suggested strategies of intervention to 'solve' it. One of the key figures created and targeted in the debate was 'the neglectful mother', and of specific concern was the working-class mother who did not provide a hygienic environment for her children, and who was seen as even more neglectful if she went out to work. The neglect was seen as the outcome of poor domestic management rather than of poverty or the conditions in which the poor lived. These assumptions about working and neglectful mothers shaped the early infant welfare services. Furthermore, it became accepted that the regulation of the quality of the population was a proper concern of the state, that the conditions of urban life were deleterious to the health and wellbeing of the working class, that pathological physical and moral states were hereditable, and that there was evidence of the progressive degeneration of the population (see Abbott, 1982; Abbott and Sapsford, 1988). The population became seen as something to be valued, known and categorized, with the recognition that the state could and should play a key role in surveying and monitoring its health.

These developments occurred at a point of transition from nineteenth-century *laissez-faire* attitudes to poverty, where the individual was seen as responsible for his or her own poverty and unfitness. Pauperism was seen as the result of individual failure, and the pauper as needing to be regulated and controlled – i.e. the problem was the poor, not poverty. While there had been some concern over the conditions created by urbanization, resulting in the reform of insanitary conditions as a means of improving the health of the (working-class) population, it was the surveys of Booth (1890) and Rowntree (1901) into urban poverty and pauperism that had the most substantial impact on thinking about poverty and its causes. Booth argued that it was necessary to make a clear distinction between the employable and unemployable poor. Not all poverty could be blamed on the moral and physical characteristics of those living in it. Unemployment could then be seen as both the cause of poverty (for the employable) and the outcome of their own nature (for the unemployable). This enabled a distinction to be drawn between members of society (the employable), who should be helped to become self-dependent, and those considered unemployable, who should therefore be excluded from society – that is, admitted to the workhouse.

At the same time the science of eugenics (influenced by social Darwinism) argued that anti-social behaviour was an inherited characteristic – that there was a scientific basis for explaining the degeneration of the British race and for planning programmes to remedy it. Racial progress would come from the scientific control of nature – from preventing tainted stock from propagating. This meant that the norm had to be established scientifically, and scientific methods of singling out the unfit developed. This led to the development and use of tests to separate the fit from the unfit.

The discourse of eugenics articulated with imperialist discourses. Concern grew that the population was deteriorating physically and psychologically at the same time as it seemed that Britain was declining as a military, industrial and commercial nation. The economic recession of the 1870s, the defeat of Gordon at Khartoum at the hands of 'natives', the debates surrounding the Contagious Diseases Act, the military and industrial growth of Germany and the United States, and the poor physical condition of men enlisting to fight in the Boer War all fanned the fires of concern.

At the same time a different concern about the health of the population was being articulated. During the last decade of the nineteenth century concern grew about the infant mortality rate, which had not only not declined along with the general mortality rate but in some years actually went up. Although a number of causes of infant death were acknowledged, attention focused on summer diarrhoea, for two main reasons: it was seen as preventable, and it attacked and killed healthy as well as sickly children and could therefore not be seen as eugenic in the way that, for example, wasting diseases might be. Neo-hygienists focused on hygiene in the home and methods of infant care, including feeding. Mothers were seen as the main cause of infant death and, by implication, of poor health in children and adults (see, e.g., Black, 1915; Rathbone, 1924; Bell, 1907).[2]

As a consequence of the fears about the health of the population, an Interdepartmental Committee on Physical Deterioration was set up, and it reported in 1904. The Committee heard from a wide range of experts, but carried out no original research. It rejected the eugenicist arguments and accepted environmentalist and hygienist ones. It agreed that there was a need to improve the health of children and accepted the evidence put to it that one of the major problems was neglectful and employed working-class mothers. Among a large number of recommendations, it suggested the employment of health visitors. Probably this recommendation was taken up because health visiting was seen as an inexpensive way of dealing with the problem, as opposed to the high cost of improving the housing, environment and wages of the poor. The household was seen as a machine for the raising of children, and mothers were seen as having the main responsibility for rearing a physically, mentally and morally efficient population.

The neo-hygienists had a considerable impact on welfare measures in the early twentieth century and on the health education directed at mothers. They translated concern about public health into individualistic preventive medicine which targeted especially the working-class mother. While in the first decade of the century attention was focused on the neglectful mother and especially on infant feeding practices – contamination being seen as a major cause of infantile diarrhoea – by the end of the First World War the concern had widened to include the health of the mother as well as that of the child (Rowan, 1985).

Nevertheless, while health was seen as something positive and to be sought, its achievement was thought to be brought about by scrutinizing individuals and the relationships between them at the level of the family. The key figure was the mother, who, it was argued, was responsible for the health of her family. The target of intervention was therefore the mother: effort was directed at training her as a mother and inspecting the home, at the inspection of infants and schoolchildren, and at the provision of school meals for needy children. While families and especially mothers, it was argued, were to bring up their children on behalf of the nation, and the state had a right and a duty to ascertain that they were doing this, it was the family that remained responsible for providing for the medical and other needs of their children.

The bulwark of the infant welfare movement was the health visitor. The title used to refer to these workers was itself important. Many of the early workers in the field had been employed as sanitary inspectors, but the term 'health visitor' was preferred because it did not carry overtones of inspection. Florence Nightingale described the health visitor's role as helping the mother and making no judgements, and Sir Thomas Barlow stressed that the health visitor was not to be regarded as a policeman or sanitary inspector (see Greenwood, 1913). The importance of being non-judgemental was also reinforced by health visitors themselves in the evidence they gave to the 1904 Interdepartmental Committee. Whether employed by a local authority or a voluntary organization, health visitors visited the working-class mother in her home to advise on hygiene and infant care management as well as to inspect the home. They were also employed by the milk kitchens and schools for mothers and by the infant welfare clinics. In this period not only did their numbers grow, but the occupation was transformed. The state became increasingly involved with the work of health visiting. An increasing number of local authorities began to employ health visitors (who worked under the direction of the medical officer of health); the Notification of Births Act 1909 (made mandatory in 1915) was designed so that health visitors could visit all newborn babies as soon after birth as possible, and central government not only suggested that local authorities should employ them but also assisted with funds. In 1917 the Local Government Board stated that all sanitary authorities should employ them, and that it had money for grants to aid expenditure in respect of maternity and child welfare services (Local Government Board, 1917).

In its 1917 Report the Local Government Board stressed that the main responsibility of health visitors was to advise mothers on matters of hygiene and infant care. It was suggested that they should visit all mothers as soon after the birth of the baby as possible, and certainly by the tenth day. They should also visit cases of *ophthalmia neonatorum* and young children with certain infectious diseases. In the summer, they should pay calls on all homes with young children to warn against the dangers of epidemic diarrhoea, to ensure that any child suffering from it was being properly cared for, and to look into the death of any child to ascertain the cause of death. It noted that health visitors' duties were being extended to include visiting expectant mothers and continuing the visitation of infants until they reached school age. Additionally, health visitors were being used at infant welfare clinics. Health visiting was no longer seen as middle-class women teaching working-class ones how to 'care' for their babies and young children, but as a service directed at all mothers. Mothers were seen as needing to come under state surveillance – to be monitored by the state to ensure that they were carrying out their duties – and to be 'trained' when they were deemed to be failing. The state had taken on responsibility for ensuring that mothers were carrying out 'good enough mothering'. The agents of the state were women – women policing other women – but the discourses were patriarchal.

During the period when the state was taking over responsibility for health visiting, the type of person becoming a health visitor also changed. While its status remained low, health visiting became seen as a suitable vocation for middle-class women rather than just a philanthropic endeavour. In the late nineteenth century it had begun to be argued that some training should be provided. In 1892 Buckingham County Council was the first local authority to provide a training course, but it was in the early twentieth century that permanent formal courses as a recognized route to qualification were established, that it became compulsory for employed health visitors to be so qualified, and that health visitors were required to have nursing and midwifery qualifications. In 1907 Bedford College for Women and Battersea Polytechnic started a two-year course for educated women (and a six-month course for trained nurses), so the link between health visiting and nursing was not yet a necessary one. In 1908 the Royal Sanitary Institute started to set a health visiting examination. (It remained the examining body until the establishment of the Council for the Education and Training of Health Visitors in 1965, now itself replaced by the National Boards for Nursing, Midwifery and Health Visiting and the United Kingdom Central Council for Nursing, Midwifery and Health Visiting.) In 1909 London County Council laid down that in future all its health visitors should have a medical degree, full nurse training or a certificate of the Central Board of Midwives, have been previously employed as a health visitor, or else have some nurse training and a Health Visitor's Certificate. In 1916 the Local Government Board recommended that health visitors should have two of three qualifications: nurse training; a Sanitary Inspector's Certificate; or a Certificate of the Central Midwives' Board. In 1919 the Ministry of Health and the Board of Education recommended three modes of entry: a one-year post-nursing course; a different one-year course for university graduates; or a two-year course for others. In 1925 the Ministry of Health required that all new entrants should have midwifery training, and in 1928 that they should have a Health Visitor's Certificate.

Subsequently the period of training was reduced to six months for state registered nurses (but increased again to a year in 1965), and the courses for people other than nurses died out because they failed to attract students. (However, it was not until 1962 that SRN certification became a requirement for entry to training.)

By the 1920s health visiting had become firmly established as a state service employing low-status semi-professional female workers, working under the direction of doctors (medical officers of health). The health visitor's main role was educating mothers in the care of young children, monitoring child development and inspecting the homes of the working class. By the 1930s, with the infant mortality rate declining, there was a move towards greater emphasis on child care – improving the health of surviving children (McCleary, 1933). Health visitors came increasingly to be seen as 'well-baby' nurses. Their knowledge/power was based on neo-hygienic/medical discourses on the causes of ill-health and especially infant diarrhoea, but underpinned by eugenic ideas of separating the fit from the unfit. In this role they played a largely symbolic part in constructing and policing the 'new mother' – the woman whose main responsibility was ensuring the physical, mental and moral health of her children (and husband) on behalf of the nation. The intervention of the state's representatives in the family was legitimized by concern about national efficiency. Child protection was justified while health visitors could claim to be helping mothers to achieve what they wanted – the best for their children. Health visitors played a role in creating and identifying the 'inadequate mother'. They then became involved in programmes of reform to transform her, to shape her behaviour so that she becomes an adequate, a 'good enough' mother.

While advice on hygiene continues to be one of the functions of the health visitor, work with families has widened to include advice on the mental, emotional and cognitive development of children. Health visitors have also become more aware of the societal causes of social problems, although their interventions still tend to be individualistic. Events in the 1930s and the experience of widespread unemployment dissolved, if only temporarily, the link between personal characteristics and unemployment and between personal habits and social problems. It was recognized that social problems were located in society rather than in the individual. This resulted in the acceptance of the right of citizenship – that everyone should enjoy fundamental basic rights – and the acceptance also of the idea that the state should intervene to plan economic activity and social services. In the same period doctors and nutritionists began to show the relationship between income, diet and health, and this gave further impetus to the campaign for the endowment of motherhood.

Thus, the space was created for discourses that saw material differences as the main problem to be solved. The welfare legislation after the Second World War was designed to eradicate poverty and provide adequate health care for all citizens, while the associated management of the economy was to ensure full employment. Social workers were to pick up the casualties of the welfare state – those who could not cope without additional support. Health visiting, however, became a universal service, concerned with monitoring the health of the whole population, but with a major responsibility still for the pre-school child and his or her family. A need was still seen to reduce infant and child mortality further and to improve the health of children. In this period, as after the First World War, there was concern about a decline in the size of the population. As we have noted already, while the discourses may have emphasized the importance of the family as a unit, in practice, health visiting intervention continued to target the mother and to be concerned with the health and development of young children.

Health visitors continued to play a major role in the surveillance of the family and in 'creating' mothers, especially in a period when the 'need' for mothers to work full time in the home was being stressed (Riley, 1983). Their knowledge had come to incorporate new discourses on mental health which argued that major mental disturbances were preventable by early recognition and treatment. Part of the health visitors' role became the surveillance of *mental* hygiene, to pick up minor problems before they developed into major ones. They also incorporated new ideological propositions influenced by Freudian theory – propositions which stressed that the natural family was a biological necessity for the healthy development of the children, that it provided the right environment for the development of a harmonious and well-rounded character. Increasingly mothers began to be held responsible not just for the health of their children but for their emotional and cognitive development, which gave them responsibility for (and the experts a legitimate concern with) children's day-to-day thoughts and feelings. Thus health visitors began to work with the 'knowledge' that particular familial relations were correct/desirable. After the Second World War the work of Bowlby and Winnicott came to dominate ideas on children, and especially ideas on the role of the mother as the key figure in the normal development of children. Bonding became a key concept in the work of health visitors, who stressed the important role that mothers played in the development of their children and the young child's need for mothering by a loving, natural mother. (Thus mothers became responsible to health visitors and other experts for the nature of their feelings towards their children.) The Jameson Report emphasized that health visitors were likely to be increasingly concerned with the mental aspects of health, especially as the need for advice on physical aspects was declining. Especially important would be advice on the importance of a normal and happy family life for the mental health of the child. (So the mother was responsible to the health visitor even for whether the child was happy or not.) This change in emphasis was reflected in the new syllabus for health visitor training introduced in 1965.

A history of health visiting enables us to see that a number of discourses have informed it and continue to inform it – medical/sanitary, philanthropic, psychological/psychiatric – and it is shaped by, and plays its role as agent of social control through, a number of not always compatible ideological positions. With the reduction in infant mortality rates and the improvement in the diet, housing and environment of a majority of the population, the need for them to advise mothers on how to keep their children alive has decreased. They have moved into the 'child development business', where they have become the main workers because they see every child at an early age, but this is an area already well colonized by people with better claims on paper to expertise, such as psychologists, psychiatrists and paediatricians. However, health visitors' individualistic mode of intervention, parallelling that of medicine and social work, has been challenged by cultural and political/economic explanations for health inequalities, as well as by the feminist movement. The low status of health visiting and the medical dominance over its practice is clearly rooted in the importance of medical discourse in its foundation and development. Like nurses, health visitors were in part established to work on behalf of and under the direction of medical men (or, in the very early years, under lady volunteers who themselves accepted the advice and direction of medical men). The problems they experience in extricating themselves from this dominance and establishing an independent professional status relate to the development of health visiting as a female occupation, based on medical knowledge at a time when medical knowledge was a male preserve.

Social Work

Social work, like health visiting, developed out of a number of disparate voluntary, charitable and paid nineteenth-century endeavours associated with Victorian philanthropy. Like health visiting it provided a role for middle-class women. While both middle- and upper-class men and women worked as volunteers, for the men this was either an interval before entry to paid full-time work or an occupation taken up on retirement. For middle-class women it provided the opportunity to develop a career. The Charity

Organisation Society (COS), founded in London in 1869, is credited with developing the social work method of individualized casework. (In addition to the trend within the COS that led towards individualization, however, there was another that led towards community organization and the aim of mobilizing the resources of the community to meet human need – see e.g. Woodroofe, 1962.) At the same time, the National Society for the Prevention of Cruelty to Children was established, and its officers began to develop child protection work. The Settlement Movement and Youth Club Movement that developed in late-nineteenth-century Britain can be see as the precursors of social group work. Hospital almoners, the forerunners of medical (hospital) social workers, were originally employed in the voluntary hospitals, initially at the suggestion of the COS (the first being appointed in 1895, at the Royal Free Hospital), to determine which patients could afford to pay for treatment and which needed charitable help. Along with probation officers, an occupation that developed from the court missionaries first appointed in London in 1876 (see May and Annison in this volume), they were amongst the first social work groups to develop formal training and a professional vocation. During the First World War both groups established professional associations. Residential social work developed out of the work of voluntary bodies such as Dr Barnardo's Waifs and Strays, the Church of England Children's Society and the National Children's Homes. These bodies were set up to care for abandoned and neglected children. Psychiatric social work, by contrast, was 'imported' from the United States, a training course being introduced by the London School of Economics and Political Science (LSE) in 1929.

Social work developed to deal with various problem groups – groups such as the sick, the old, the poor, the workless and the criminal. In the nineteenth century there was a general fear of the 'dangerous' classes and it was thought that if left uncontrolled they would contaminate the respectable and healthy members of society. A response to this was the monitoring and surveillance of the lower-class groups in society, although the concept of institutionalization – the poor in the workhouse, the mentally ill in asylums – dominated nineteenth-century thinking about social problems (see, for example, Scull, 1977). This, however, was not a complete answer – it was attacked by some reformers, and in any case the majority of those perceived as 'problems' were not incarcerated. Many of the mentally ill, for example, were left to be 'cared for' by their families, and some workhouse unions provided outdoor relief for able-bodied paupers. Increasingly, the view was taken that at least some of the 'problem' groups – the deserving poor – could be normalized; that is, they could become respectable self-supporting members of society if given the right kind of assistance and guidance. At the same time evangelical Christians with a strong religious commitment to charity began to argue that charity *per se* demoralized the poor. They argued that the deserving poor should be trained in thrift and self-help. They further suggested that the administration of the Poor Law needed to be tightened up so that it had the intended deterrent effect: that is, that the undeserving poor should *not* be given outdoor relief, but should be admitted to the workhouse. Finally, they argued that there needed to be rationalization of private charity in order to find ways of coping with the 'clever' paupers – the paupers who abused the system and encouraged the corruption and demoralization of the 'honest poor'. Indeed, it was argued that indiscriminate charity could pauperize the poor. Lord Derby, in his speech at the opening meeting of the Charity Organisation Society in 1870, said that

> By want of proper supervision and control, by excessive laxity and abuse of discrimination between the deserving and the undeserving, we are pauperising, year by year, an increasing number of our people. (Derby, 1870, pp. 5–6)

Octavia Hill, in 1889, speaks in the same vein of

> families, learning to sing like beggars in the streets – all because we give pennies. (Hill, 1889, p. 25)

The Charity Organisation Society was concerned to ensure that a clear distinction was drawn between the undeserving and the deserving poor. It was underpinned by moral values that were used to determine which individuals were 'in real need' and which were 'playing the system'. The dominant *laissez-faire* ideology that underpinned its moral values saw two causes of poverty: those who were poor because of natural disasters (such as widowhood) and those who were poor due to their own 'moral failing' – that is, being unwilling to work, or spending money on drink and gambling. It thus linked with an individualistic explanation for the causes of poverty. The deserving poor, those whose poverty was no fault of their own and who displayed willingness to help themselves and exhibited the moral virtues of thrift, sobriety and self-discipline, were to be assisted. The 'clever' paupers, however, were to be admitted to the workhouse.

Social casework developed out of the work of the Charity Organisation Society. The officers of this organization were concerned to assess and classify different kinds of applicants – and, therefore, different kinds of poverty – to ensure that the 'clever paupers', who were undeserving, did not take advantage of the system. The religious orientation of the organization meant that they were also concerned with moral regulation and inculcating habits of thrift, providence and industry in their clients. This concern was embodied in the 'casework' approach to individual applicants whereby their families were investigated and they were encouraged to conform to particular 'virtuous' middle-class models of what the family life of the poor should consist of, in order to qualify. Those given assistance were followed up so that it could be seen how the money was spent, and the officers kept 'case notes' for all those who were assisted. The aim of giving charity was not only to alleviate poverty, but to raise the moral status of the individual and society – to encourage independence and strength of character and to strengthen the family as the basic unit of society. The work of the COS was based on five principles (see Lock 1895, pp. 698–9):

1 that the recipient of relief should become independent;
2 that Society's workers should help or even force those receiving help to fear destitution and the shame of having to seek Poor Relief;
3 that the family should be considered as a unit – that families should as far as possible care for their own members;
4 that full enquiry into the circumstances of those seeking relief was essential;
5 that the amount of help given should be sufficient in kind and quality to enable the recipient to become independent.

This casework approach also identified the family as a particular site of intervention, the place where social problems arose and where they could be prevented or overcome. The family was, therefore, a subject of moral regulation and surveillance in these instances (Clarke, 1988). However, in becoming this, the family was constituted in particular ways. First, there was the separation of the public and private spheres, the family being located in the private sphere and its members being seen as 'naturally' subject to patriarchal authority: what a man did to his wife, or parents to their children, was their own concern, not that of the state. Furthermore it was seen as the responsibility of the father to control his family. For this reason, it was at first the concern of welfare organizations to ensure the proper conformity of family members to this model of the patriarchal nuclear family. However, by the end of the nineteenth century it was recognized that the individuals could also be abused by their own family members. Campaigns by the National Society for the Prevention of Cruelty to Children (NSPCC) and Dr Barnardo's Children's Homes – assisted by the evolving ideology of childhood as a stage of individual development when people could be saved from vice by an improved environment – led to the intervention of welfare officers in the private sphere by taking children away from homes deemed to be unsuitable.

If patriarchal authority was the means for regulating the family, women were supposed to be the *moral* guides for the household. They had to be more temperate, more religious and more sexually pure than men, and their main role in life was seen as serving others dutifully. The officers of the COS thus targeted mothers particularly, since they were seen as being responsible for improving the morals of their husbands and children. This image of Victorian femininity also provided a model for the women who ran the Charity Organisation Society and for other welfare professions, as we saw in the case of health visiting.

An attempt to set up formal training for COS social workers was made through the initiation of a 'School for Sociology' in 1903 which was later incorporated into the London School of Economics in 1912. (The pressure for professional training came mainly from women, for whom social work provided a career opportunity. The high proportion of women entering both voluntary and paid social work established it from the outset as a female profession.) The COS argued that social workers should be regarded as social practitioners tending the ills of society. Lock suggested in 1906 that

> doctors have to be educated methodically, registered and certified . . . Charity work is the work of the social physician. It is to the interests of the community that it should not be entrusted to novices, or to *dilettanti*, or to quacks. (p. xix)

Helen Bosanquet (1902) had indicated

> that scientific principles are as much involved [in social work] as chemistry in architecture or any other of the arts of life. (p. 138)

The development of formal training coincided with the decline of the COS view of poverty and the change to a more 'scientific' and professional model. Paid workers were employed by the COS and other voluntary societies to work alongside the volunteers and, once a body of paid workers was established, they began to develop a career structure. As the century progressed, social workers accumulated more specialized functions – child care, adoption and fostering, the elderly, and so on. Each of these involved the further elaboration of classifications and theories of disadvantage and in the process more secular models emerged. The decline of moral theories of poverty and the advent of trained and paid workers resulted in a demand for a systematic body of knowledge on which social work practice could be based – a basis for *professional* social work. The training that emerged had three key elements: social studies; the theory of casework; and supervised practical experience. Of these, the theory of casework was the key to the theory and practice of social work, providing the foundation for social work theory (see McCallum in this volume). Psychology replaced religious morality as the 'science' which legitimized intervention and served to classify different forms of deprivation. Rose (1985) referred to this as 'the psychological complex'. From this perspective human society is seen as intrinsically individualized, with individuals possessing qualities – physical and mental – which are measurable. Psychology argued for the existence of a set of developmental stages – childhood, adolescence, normal adulthood and old age – through which people passed and during which they had particular needs. The family was seen as central to 'normal' psycho-social development. Psychology prescribes the 'norms' of behaviour and this 'knowledge' became the basis of professional social work intervention in families. By defining the normal, psychology also defined the abnormal, and this provided the knowledge for targeting individuals and families as objects of intervention. Childhood was a period of special care and nurture during which the child must not be allowed to fall into vicious ways, and old age was a period of dependency and decrepitude.

Likewise, sociology stressed the social origins and context of particular social problems. However, psychology legitimized the role of individual casework, and the family as the site of intervention. Social workers learned about the normative models of family life (often derived from middle-class families) which enabled them to classify families according to whether they were 'deviant' or 'normal' – deviant families included all those without conventional male household heads, or those from ethnic minorities or different class cultures which did not conform to the models of the normal family held by those who taught or practised social work. Social work claimed to have replaced the morality of the COS by scientific theories. Corner (1959) suggests that

> Slowly but surely, a change of emphasis has taken place. We speak no longer of the immoral but the immature; the lazy good-for-nothing of those days is the inadequate of today; the harlot and fallen woman have been transformed into call-girls; the pervert has become a deviant; the drunkard an alcoholic whom we try to help by psychiatric treatment . . . I suggest in fact that moral values are no longer at the core of things in the practice of casework.

In the period before the Second World War the dominant model was that of the 'problem' family – families which increased the numbers in the 'social problem' groups by passing on physical and mental deficiencies from one generation to the next. This model focused attention on children as victims of physical neglect and deprivation. The blame was usually placed upon the mother for failing to care adequately for her children. Children came to provide the main justification for the entry of social workers into families and thus gave impetus for the imagery of the neglected child during the Second World War. The Report of the Committee on Care of Children, published in 1946, recommended a specialized social work service for children. The 1948 Children's Act established local authority children's departments which were to employ specialist trained social workers: child care officers responsible for working with families and children in need of care. (A division of labour was thereby established between health visitors who were to work with all families – providing advice on and monitoring infant and child development – and social workers who were to intervene in 'problem' families.)

These developments provided the foundations for the development of professional social work after the Second World War in Britain. At the same time, separate services were provided for the physically and mentally sick, the handicapped and the elderly. The child care officers appointed by the local authorities were the main group of qualified social workers existing at the end of the Second World War. Psychology continued to dominate the theory and practice of social work, and casework was likewise the main paradigm used.

However, the paradigm changed and the theories of Bowlby (e.g. 1954) and others stressed the importance of maternal bonding and the problems associated with maternal deprivation and 'latchkey' children. As the childcare services developed, the trained workers began to advocate preventative work. Hence, the Children and Young Persons Act of 1963 provided children's departments with the power to give financial or other help to prevent the reception of children into care. The emphasis was on keeping families, particularly mothers and children, together. Social problems were blamed upon ignorance rather than poverty, and the problem family characterized as lacking in social skills, so that the social worker should interpret their problems on their behalf and act as intermediary between them and the state. By the 1960s poverty was not thought to be the main problem facing 'problem families'. Rather, it was their inability to cope with an increasingly complex society:

> The service that is needed must set out by concentrating on the few families that get into serious difficulties but would be available from the beginning to all those who wish to make use of it (it would be a 'family casework service', not a 'problem families service'). It must be manned by workers with a sensitive understanding of family relationships, and special skills in mobilising the will and the energy of the bewildered, anxious and aggressive people (thus it would be based primarily on the skilled use of personal relationships, rather then the provision of material help and expert advice). (Donnison and Stewart, 1958, p. 7)

It was not until the early 1970s, following the Seebohm Committee Report (1968), that state social work was reorganized into unified local authority departments charged with providing statutory and non-statutory services for those in need. This established the form that social work took in Britain until the 1990s – generic departments with generic social work training and methods based on psychological theories of interpersonal relations within the family. The childcare workers exerted the strongest influence on the work of the new departments with their emphasis on casework, and the main focus of work is still seen as being with families and young children. Social workers were divided into two categories: field and residential. The former generally had a professional qualification (CQSW) validated by the Central Council for Education and Training in Social Work and awarded after study at an institution of higher education. The latter staff received less training and were less well qualified, being seen generally as social service staff rather than as professional social workers (see Sibeon, 1990), those with a qualification generally having the lower-status and more practically-based CSS.

Although social work has developed from voluntary work based on values into an occupation consisting of paid workers basing their interventions on 'scientific' knowledge, it is not securely established as a profession and its areas of expertise remain vague and ill-defined. Over the last twenty years social work has been attacked by the Left – for exercising social control and for failing to tackle the root causes of social problems – and by the Right for being naive 'do-gooders' trying to take away people's sense of responsibility. Furthermore, successive scandals in child abuse have helped to vilify social workers in the papers, especially after the much-publicized deaths of Maria Colwell and Jasmine Beckford. Social workers are vilified for leaving 'at risk' children with their families as in these cases, and for unjustified interference or breaking up families, as in the much-publicized Cleveland scandal (see Campbell, 1988). This has led to a further crisis in confidence for a fragile profession. Cuts in welfare benefits, and the burgeoning numbers of social work clients with rising unemployment, rising numbers of elderly and the recent discovery of child sexual abuse, have meant that social workers are mainly concerned with responding to crises rather than preventing crises from occurring (if they ever did that), and their role has been one of rationing increasingly scarce resources (see the Barclay Committee Report, 1982). The situation was exacerbated in 1993 when the community care provisions of the National Health Service and Community Care Act 1990 came into force, giving Social Service departments the responsibility for assessing clients for services and 'purchasing' services on their behalf.

These criticisms have led some to challenge the whole basis of social work's professional practice – that is, to challenge the truth of the scientific discourses (mainly psychology) on which social workers base their practice. However, the various scandals have led to calls within the profession for more broadly-based and extended training as the basis of professional expertise, and the need for social workers to enter the profession as mature entrants with some experience of voluntary work – that is, the solution is seen as better training and better selection. There exists, nevertheless, a large penumbra of untrained and semi-trained volunteers who undertake much social service work, and this would seem to undermine the claims of social work to professional expertise and knowledge, as does their apparent inability to carry out diagnostic and preventative work in the area of child abuse.

However, it is essential to recognize the role that social workers can and do play in helping to protect the least powerful and most vulnerable members of society, while at the same time acknowledging the role they play as agents of social control.

Adult Nursing

The origins of nursing also lie in the nature of nineteenth-century philanthropy and in discourses of the family. Modern nursing was originally established in the voluntary hospitals, and subsequently the elite nurses from these hospitals took over nursing in the Poor Law hospitals and asylums (see Carpenter, 1977). While doctors and medical specialists amongst the plethora of other professional paid healers were known from the Middle Ages, their activities were fairly narrowly defined, and many people could not afford to see them. Much healing work was undertaken by women and was seen as part of their domestic routine. By the nineteenth century, however, allopathic medicine had successfully come to claim a monopoly of medical expertise and in Britain this was given state recognition in the 1852 Medical Act which gave medical doctors monopolistic rights (see Stacey, 1989). Independent nurses and midwives continued to practise but were condemned by social reformers such as Florence Nightingale for being inexpert, unprofessional and uninformed by recent medical theories.

In the late nineteenth century, at the same time as modern scientific medicine was gaining its hegemonic position and female health workers were being condemned by reformers, there emerged a concern for the health of the poor and with public health generally. This took the form of efforts to prevent the spread of epidemics such as cholera and a concern with eugenics – breeding the right sort of people fit to rule, work and fight for the Empire. We have already demonstrated how health visitors were used to 'police' poor families and educate working-class mothers in these hygienic pursuits. It is evident from this that medical and moral discourses were aligned. Nursing was established as a profession supplementary to medicine (Gamarnikow, 1978) but also heavily influenced by the hygiene discourse; the 'sanitary discourse' formed the basis of early nursing knowledge.

Nursing emerged in the late nineteenth century as a distinct occupational category in a form recognizable today. However, it is important to recognize that the origins of contemporary nursing are diverse, and are reflected in the nursing specialisms that exist today – adult nursing, children's nursing, mental health nursing, learning disability nursing and community nursing. Here we are going to look in detail at adult nursing, which exemplifies the development of an occupational group to meet the needs of doctors for assistants as medical practice changed in the late eighteenth and nineteenth centuries. We shall also consider midwifery, as an example of an occupation that became subordinated to medicine in the process of medical men striving to achieve a dominant role in the medical division of labour.

Hearn (1982) has argued that the process of professionalization is a process of male assumption of control over female tasks. Thus as male doctors acquire the status of a profession they not only exclude female healers from practising but also gain control over female workers, who take on a subordinate role in the medical division of labour. Part of the process of gaining control lies in the ability to claim scientific superiority for the knowledge that underpins intervention. Medical science became dominant, and nurses were seen as working to support doctors – to carry out orders. Nurses were to have responsibility for the day-to-day surveillance of patients, but were exercising power only on behalf of doctors. They conformed, and were to ensure that patients conformed, to the instructions of doctors. Nursing, like the other female-dominated occupations that developed in the late nineteenth century – schoolteaching, health visiting, midwifery and social work – did provide a career for middle-class women. The development of these occupations in the twentieth century, with recognized training courses and state employment, opened up the possibility for middle-class women to have secure, high-status employment. On the one hand, however, they remained subordinate to male occupations (in terms of status, remuneration and jurisdiction) and generally controlled, in the case of nurses, health visitors and midwives, by male doctors, and by male managers in the case of teaching and social work. On the other hand, they controlled unqualified or less well qualified working-class women (increasingly, after the Second World War, from ethnic minority groups) – auxiliaries, classroom assistants and care assistants (see Abbott, in this volume). The development of training and recognized paid careers did not provide opportunities (at least, initially) for the paid working-class woman but rather for the middle-class female volunteer to become trained.

Nurses play a subordinate role in the medical division of labour, although there has been resistance to this subordination ever since the establishment of nursing as a recognized occupation in the nineteenth century. Mrs Bedford Fenwick identified the nurse question – the fight for government recognition of nursing as a profession with its own knowledge base and its own state examinations – as identical with the woman question (Dock and Stewart, 1931). Anne Witz points out that changes taking place in nursing that seek to challenge the power of medicine must be seen within the historical context (Witz, 1992). Nursing has always been, and continues to be, a predominantly female province. Most nursing is, of course, done by women as unpaid carers in the domestic sphere; this has been, and still is, a major barrier to nurses' contention that they have specialized knowledge and expertise necessitating a long theoretical, as well as practical, training and justifying a claim to professional status. However, nursing in the public sphere is also a predominantly female occupation. While caring for the sick was undertaken in a variety of institutions in the past, it was not until the middle of the nineteenth century that nursing emerged as a separate occupation. Prior to that nursing in voluntary hospitals was seen as a form of domestic work that required little specific training, and was usually undertaken by married women doing work for their patients that was litte different from what they did for their families at home. The demarcation between nurses and patients was blurred – the able-bodied convalescent patients were expected to help the nurses with the domestic work on the wards. Paid helpers were also employed in private households to assist with nursing the sick. The poor would have used handywomen who often acted as midwives, while the better off would have employed private nurses who might or might not have had some experience of hospital nursing.

The reform of the nursing profession is often attributed to Florence Nightingale, who claimed that nursing was done mainly at home by those 'who were too old, too weak, too drunken, too dirty, too sordid or too bad to do anything else' (quoted in Abel-Smith, 1960, p. 53). The argument that nurses needed training, and the recognition by doctors that bedside medicine meant that patients needed monitoring, developed before Florence Nightingale's reforms were put into practice at St Thomas's Hospital in London in 1860, and thereafter taken elsewhere by the graduates of the Nightingale Training School. From the 1830s doctors had begun to develop new ways of practising medicine and to argue that they needed a new type of assistant who could monitor the patients. At the same time the sister model (based on the model of religious orders) begin to develop in the voluntary hospitals – working-class women did the nursing work and were supervised by middle-class women using household managerial skills which they had learned from supervising servants. Many of the sisters were motivated by religion, undertaking nursing as a calling – a vocation. However, Florence Nightingale did attempt to develop nursing as an occupation and to recruit middle-class women who would receive training – a training based on one year's organized, practical experience. However, not only did other hospitals set up training schools, but other training opportunities developed rapidly (Davies, 1988). These reforms took place in the voluntary hospitals, and from that time it began to be argued that workhouse infirmaries should employ skilled nurses rather than use pauper women. The model developed in both the voluntary and the poor law hospitals of a small number of trained nurses (sisters) supervising the work of strictly-disciplined trainees and untrained staff.

While Florence Nightingale recognized the need for trained nurses, she trained them in obedience, so that in the division of labour between nurses and doctors, nurses were seen and saw themselves as subordinates of the doctors and as under medical control. Furthermore, she stressed that nursing was a vocation, not a profession, and accepted the prevailing ideas of a nursing hierarchy with a stress on strict obedience and control over moral behaviour both in and out of work. Both nurses and probationers were expected to 'live in' at the hospital, were strictly controlled in their behaviour both at work and during non-working hours, and had no set hours of work, emphasizing the cloistered separateness of the nursing community. This model was reinforced by the idea of a vocation – the selfless sacrifice of the nurse to the needs of the patient. Nor did Nightingale challenge the link between womanhood and nursing. The notion of women being trained to develop their 'natural' skills did not, for example, challenge the Victorian view, used to exclude women from medical training, that they were too weak to undertake a university education. Gamarnikow (1978) has pointed out that, in the Nightingale model, nurses were still responsible for the cleaning of wards as well as the care of patients. She suggests that the relationship between doctor and nurse parallelled the relationship between the Victorian husband and the wife in the family. The nurse looked after the physical and emotional environment, while he, the doctor, decided what the really important work was and how it should be done. Thus the good nurse was the good mother, concerned with caring for her patients. Indeed, as Carpenter (1977) points out, nurses were responsible for 'controlling rather than indulging patients in the interests of hygiene' (p. 167). This reflected Victorian models of dutiful femininity and the family already described. Because nursing was a female profession, it was its characteristics of duty and subservience that were stressed, rather than status or rewards. The subservience of nurses to doctors was given 'scientific' legitimacy because of the basis of nursing knowledge. Nursing did not develop an autonomous body of knowledge, but the nursing tasks emerged out of the 'sanitary idea', and this gave coherence to the disparate tasks undertaken by nurses – medical tasks delegated by doctors, plus care for the patient's physical needs and the maintenance of the cleanliness of the wards (Davies, 1976). Cure functions were seen as primarily male (and upper-class), and care functions as primarily female (and lower-class but supervised by middle/upper-class women). As a consequence of this, the only role left available for the trained nurse was not that of autonomous practitioner but the management of trainee nurses and untrained helpers.

In the twentieth century, while nurses no longer see themselves as handmaidens of doctors, they have remained trapped in their status as subordinate to doctors (see Allen in this volume). In 1919 the Nursing Register was introduced, and the Nurses Act 1943 established the lower grade of State Enrolled Nurses as well as State Registered Nurses, but neither kind were recognized as independent practitioners.

The main struggle in the twentieth century has been between those who want nursing to become an autonomous profession and those who see nursing as more of a vocation and are more concerned with practice than with developing theories to underpin practice. This struggle started in the nineteenth century between the professionalizers led by Mrs Fenwick and the vocationalists led by Florence Nightingale. Giving evidence to the Parliamentary Select Committee on Registration in 1904, Sydney Hallard, Head of the London Hospital, argued that

> We want to stop nurses thinking themselves anything more than they are, namely, the faithful carriers out of doctors' orders. (quoted by Abel-Smith, 1960, p. 66)

Mrs Fenwick was concerned that there should be a national standard of nurse education and qualification, that nurses should be technically qualified and that they should have parity of esteem with the medical profession. Florence Nightingale argued that the personal qualities (as opposed to the technical knowledge) of the nurse were the main criteria, and that nurse training should be concerned with learning practical skills, not technical knowledge. The Nurses Registration Act of 1919 was a compromise between these groups. It resulted in the establishment of a register of trained nurses and, in 1920, of the General Nursing Council, which was charged in 1923 with maintaining a register and determining the conditions of entry to that register – that is, what examinations had to be passed in order to be placed on the register. Only nurses on the register could call themselves State Registered. However, while the 'registered nurse' title was protected, this was *not* a prerequisite for employment as a nurse. The Act did not give nurses the power to control entry to the profession or to oversee training, or the monopoly of practice that, for example, the 1852 Medical Act had given medical doctors.

Nurses had not made a move towards a particular role, nor had they gained autonomous control over their work. The outcome of this was that nursing continued to be an occupation that was based on a predominantly practical training and one where the qualified supervised the unqualified trainees. The situation has not fundamentally changed since for either hospital or community nurses. Indeed, it could be argued that subsequent changes have removed the managerial role of nurses rather than enabling them to gain fundamental autonomy and a particular role. The Salmon Report (1966) reflected the views of the nursing elite that trained nurses should be concerned predominantly with managerial and clinical aspects of nursing work and that routine 'dirty' work should be done by other groups under their control – state enrolled nurses, trainees and auxiliaries. This would enable the establishment of a career (managerial) status for nurses. This was based on an industrial model of line management and of professional managers. Emphasizing managerial aspects of promoted posts and the need for specific managerial skills as criteria for promotion has downgraded the need for the caring (female) qualities for nursing. In their search for a career ladder and higher status, nurses adopted a managerial solution that resulted in the tighter control of nursing staff and militated against the development of nurses as autonomous practitioners. Indeed it continued and developed the process by which most nursing work is done by the untrained and the trainee. Furthermore, the changes in management hierarchies in the 1980s, following the Griffiths enquiry, mean that nurses can now be managed by non-nurses.

The fight between the managerialist faction and the professionalizers has, however, continued. Those who emphasize a professional model for nursing have tended to be concentrated in schools of nursing and they advocate a more theoretical training for nursing, the development of nursing theory, evidence-based practice and a nursing-process methodology. This view influenced the Briggs Report (1972) and more recently Project 2000. While the Nurses, Midwives and Health Visitors Act of 1979 did not reflect the aspirations of the professionalizers, it is possible that Project 2000 succeeded in doing so. There has been an increased emphasis on theory as the basis of nursing practice and on the need for evidence-based practice. Grades of nursing (State Enrolled Nurse and Auxiliary Nurse) other than Registered Nurse have been abolished and a new assistant grade introduced, but without the title 'nurse'. There is an increased emphasis on the nurse as an autonomous practitioner – a 'knowledgeable doer' able to marshal information, make an assessment of needs, devise a plan of care and monitor and evaluate it (UKCC, 1987, p. 2). The UKCC's 1992 Code of Practice emphasizes professional competence and the individual nurse's judgement in applying principles to practice – as opposed to merely delivering patient care on terms dominated by medicine (see Meerabeau, in this volume).

However, a number of factors militate against the new diploma nurse gaining professional status. It is unclear what the 'new' nurse will do that is different from what existing qualified nurses do – that is, managing the work of non-qualified nurses. (See Allen in this volume, however, for a discussion of the expanded and the extended nursing roles.) The tight managerial structure of nursing has not been modified. Furthermore, developments such as the nursing process, which is seen as the basis for autonomous nursing work, will enable both qualified (supervisory) nurses and those whose work they are directing to be more strictly monitored and evaluated.

Additionally, as the research of Kath Melia (1987) demonstrates, staff numbers make the implementation of the nursing process problematic, and ward culture continues to emphasize 'getting the job done' and the routinization of nursing tasks rather than the diagnostic care, planning and implementation approach of the nursing process. Nursing, like social work, is still developing its own body of knowledge to provide the theoretical basis for practice. It seems unlikely that doctors will, on the basis of diploma training, come to see nurses as equal but different in the health care division of labour, and it is more likely that they will continue to see them as inferior to medical practitioners. Nor are patients going to change their view of nurses as doctors' aides. Patients value what nurses do for them, but they are unlikely to accord them the status of knowledgeable expert that they accord to doctors. The lack of power of nurses can be seen to be related to their inability to develop an autonomous knowledge base, to underpin an area of work where they are perceived as experts. Nurses have failed to gain the necessary autonomy, prestige or power accorded to the status of professional.

Nursing in the late twentieth century is seen as a predominantly low-paid, female occupation, but there are clear ethnic and class divisions in nursing. Women from ethnic minorities were concentrated in the auxiliary and state enrolled grades and are likely in future to be care assistants rather than registered nurses, and white middle-class women in the registered grade in the prestigious teaching hospitals. Furthermore, more men are entering nursing, and a disproportionately large number of men have been appointed to management posts. Although men have been able to become general nurses only since 1943, they have moved increasingly into senior posts in what was once, as far as the nursing of physical illness was concerned, an all-woman and woman-managed occupation.

More recently, the reorganization of nursing suggested by the Griffiths Report (1983) emphasized the role of managerial control through financial constraints and the breaking down of nursing tasks. Griffiths himself was imported from J. Sainsbury plc, a highly successful private retail company, to provide new models and ideas in public service (see Clarke in this volume).

Midwives

Women healers retained control over childbirth for a much longer period than they did over healing generally (but see Versluysen, 1988), but even in midwifery they began from the 1660s to have their dominant role challenged by male midwives (obstetricians), the latter claiming to have scientific knowledge and technical expertise not possessed by female midwives. It is possible that the origins of male midwifery relate to the invention of the obstetrics forceps, or more simply that it was just another example of males attempting to take over a field previously dominated by females. However, there was opposition to male midwifery, first, from the general public (who thought it was indecent), secondly, from female midwives (on account of the threat to their livelihood) and, finally, from established medical men (who saw this as degrading women's work and not part of medicine at all).

It is not evident why male midwives were gradually able to usurp the role of the female midwives. Although the invention of obstetric forceps was certainly a breakthrough, and their use was restricted to members of the guild of barber-surgeons from which women were excluded, the number of cases where they helped was small, and the risk of infection and death as a result of their use was enormous. Women were also excluded from practising in the lying-in hospitals, but these hospitals only took in low-risk cases and risk of infection and death was much higher than for home delivery. Probably the key factor was the claim of medical men to have access to scientific (and therefore true) knowledge which female midwives lacked, and the way support was given for this claim by the trend for wealthy people to employ male midwives from the seventeenth century onwards.

However, it was not until the late nineteenth century that medical doctors accepted that midwifery should be undertaken and controlled by men. During the nineteenth century the Colleges of Physicians and Surgeons both argued against doctors' involvement in midwifery, but by 1850 lectures in midwifery were being given in British medical schools, and by 1866 proficiency in it was necessary for qualification as a medical practitioner. The claim by doctors to control childbirth was made on the basis that medical men had superior knowledge, a claim that had been generally accepted, as medical men successfully excluded or marginalized other forms of healing and other practitioners:

> By 1880 a great advance had been made in the science and art of midwifery. This was due chiefly to the introduction of male practitioners, many of whom were men of learning and devoted to anatomy, the groundwork of obstetrics. (Spicer, 1927, quoted in Oakley, 1980, p. 11)

This claim was not justified on medical grounds. In the nineteenth century a quarter of all women giving birth in hospital died of puerperal fever, and those delivered at home were more likely to be infected if they were attended by a male doctor rather than a female midwife. Puerperal fever was particularly a risk from male doctors because they moved between the sick, the dead and parturient women. Nevertheless, medical men were determined to gain control of midwifery and to determine the role of female midwives – to establish a division of labour between them and the female midwives. Thus they set out to demarcate what areas were rightfully theirs, at the same time as defending medical prerogative. The struggle between medical men and female midwives since the seventeenth century had begun to establish a distinction between *assistance at* childbirth and *intervention in* childbirth, a distinction between 'normal' and 'abnormal' childbirth. Only male doctors (qualified medical practitioners) were allowed to use forceps and to intervene surgically. The Midwifery Registration Act of 1902 resulted in the registration and education of midwives coming under the control of medical men, and a doctor had to be called if anything went wrong with a delivery. A major reason why doctors did not usurp the role of midwives was that they realized that there was no way in which they could meet the demand – in the late nineteenth century seven out of every nine births were attended by female midwives. Also, many doctors did not want to attend poor women. Doctors thus deskilled and deprofessionalized midwives, and while female midwives continued to attend poor women in childbirth, doctors attended the wealthy. Medical domination of childbirth continues in the late twentieth century, and indeed it could be argued that it has increased because the majority of births take place in hospital under the (official) control of a consultant, and because of the increased use of medical technology. Whilst most women are actually delivered by a (female) midwife, the ultimate control remains in the hands of the (generally male) obstetrician – although this may be changing (see Department of Health, 1993). The consequence of this is that midwives are not seen as playing a different role from doctors, but as being subordinate to doctors. In order to free themselves from this control and establish themselves as an autonomous profession, they have not only to challenge the need for medical supervision of their work, but to establish that theirs is a particular kind of work, distinct from medical work, and that they have a unique knowledge and expertise which underlies their practice. The medicalization of childbirth has not only brought women under the control of medical men, but also denied an autonomous area of work for midwifery – midwives are now seen to work with medical knowledge, rather than with a distinct body of knowledge over which they have exclusive rights (see Kirkham, in this volume, for an extended account).

Problems of Professionalization

Gender ideologies are an important factor in all the caring professions. First of all, the idea of 'care' itself and the growth of this work from women's activities means that it is seen as an extension of female roles and therefore less privileged in status. Secondly, the clients, too, are often women and the caring professions impose certain gender ideologies upon them – ideologies embedded in the (patriarchal) scientific discourse that underpins practice. In social work and health visiting the professionals tend to impose norms of motherhood and gender division of labour upon their clients in terms of the 'normal' family and the role of mothers, reinforced by psychological and sociological knowledge. In nursing, midwifery and health visiting, women clients are expected to demonstrate adherence to social norms of femininity in order to exhibit 'correct' health attitudes. Thirdly, many of the workers within those professions are women. Nursing is an almost exclusively female profession and constituted in the most obviously feminine way. However, many social workers, too, are women, especially those in basic rather than managerial grades. When professions become feminized they tend to suffer a lowering of rewards, prestige and status as has been well documented in the case of clerical workers. The caring professions were created as female occupations from the outset, with the drive for professionalization coming from middle-class women themselves. The transformation of nursing, social work, and primary-school teaching into paid occupations with a requirement for credentials was part of the struggle of (predominantly) middle-class women to enter the public sphere. Middle-class women wanted to develop for themselves occupations that would have the same status as those developed by middle-class men and from which they had been excluded in the course of the nineteenth century. However, the conditions under which these female occupations were allowed to develop meant that women entered the public sphere on terms defined by men and exchanged private patriarchy for public patriarchy (Walby, 1990). Caring professionals are generally employed by the patriarchal state and controlled by men. Training is seen as developing and building on skills that women already have, informed by, rather than based on, scientific knowledge – the knowledge base itself being more heavily reliant on the social than the natural sciences.

All the professions have been affected by the policies of the New Right Conservative government that was in power from 1979 until April, 1997. The government was antagonistic towards professionals and attacked their basis of power where possible, either by removing their monopoly – as in the legal profession – or by financial controls – as in the medical profession. For those employed by the state there was a lowering of rewards and increased managerial control – as in the introduction of the national curriculum and new conditions of service for teachers. In addition, the use of managerial models of control and financial constraints imported from private industry would appear to be antithetical to professional autonomy. Managerialism, the introduction of general managers into the health and social services, has been seen by nurses and social workers as an attack on their professionalism. The former argued that there was a need for professionals to make decisions and use their professional expertise, as against the claim of general managers to be able to improve efficiency. However, the process has been contradictory. During the same period there has been a demand for the extension of training for caring professionals, and comprehensive plans for reorganization such as that introduced for social work and nursing have led to the increased division of labour in those services between the qualified and the unqualified. Nurses have adopted the new managerialism, seeing it as a way of upgrading the professional and managerial role of trained nurses, especially with the introduction of the new Care Assistant grade. The Children Act 1989 and the National Health Service and Community Health Care Act 1990 have increased the power of social workers. However, the reforms were more concerned with controlling the professional power of social work, increasing managerial control and reducing the role of Local Authority social services in the delivery of services. In particular, a major aim of the 1990 National Health Service and Community Care Act was to replace professional by user-led services. Indeed, the key grade of Care Manager was not reserved as a social-worker task, despite its responsibility for assessment and the purchasing of services which could include social work.

To conclude, it is evident that the development of the caring professions of social work and nursing since the nineteenth century have a lot in common with other welfare occupations such as teaching and probation work. However, the way in which 'caring' has come to be understood and its implications for professional status today need to be seen in terms of the historical development of ideologies surrounding it and its position in the social division of labour more generally. In particular, a Foucauldian perspective enables us to understand how 'care' exercises power and at the same time controls those who offer it.

Notes

1 Familial ideology in the nineteenth century had already established the idea that women and children should be dependent on men and that men should be paid a 'family wage'. Certainly, by the beginning of the twentieth century this idea was firmly established (see, e.g. Roberts, 1984). Also, in the nineteenth century middle-class women had become identified principally as wives and mothers responsible for the care of their children (but see Helterine, 1980). What was new about the early twentieth century was that women came to be seen as guardians of their children on behalf of the nation. (This of course enabled women to fight back and demand some payment for carrying out this responsibility.)

2 While these feminist accounts clearly document the dominant identification of the neglectful mother, they also clearly argue that the major problem was poverty. They demonstrate vividly how women managed to raise large families in constant poverty, while themselves suffering poor health. Although they recognize that some women were better managers than others, they document that these were 'superwomen', not a norm which other women should be 'fired' to imitate. Indeed, reading these accounts one is left to marvel at how anyone could manage to feed and care for a family on the incomes of many households. There are also indications, though not much firm evidence, that working-class women resented the advice and interference of health visitors (see, e.g. Thane, 1982).

References

ABBOTT, P. (1982) *Towards a Social Theory of Mental Handicap*, PhD Thesis, London: Thames Polytechnic.

ABBOTT, P. and SAPSFORD, R.J. (1987) *'Community Care' for Mentally Handicapped Children: The Origins and Consequences of a Social Policy*, Milton Keynes, Open University Press.

ABBOTT, P. and SAPSFORD, R.J. (1988) 'The body politic: health, family and society', Unit 11 of Open University Course D211, *Social Problems and Social Welfare*, Milton Keynes: the Open University.

ABEL-SMITH, B. (1960) *A History of the Nursing Profession*, London: Heinemann.

BANKS, O. (1981) *Faces of Feminism*, Oxford: Martin Robertson.

BARCLAY REPORT (1982) *Social Workers: Their Role and Tasks*, London: Bedford Square Press.

BELL, LADY (1907) *At the Works* (Repub. with intro. by JOHNS, A.V. 1983), London: Virago.

BENNET, E.M. (1918) 'Babies in peril', *Maternity and Child Welfare*, **2**, November, pp. 370–6; and **2**, December, pp. 410–18.

BLACK, C. (Ed.) (1915) *Married Women's Work* (Repub. with intro. by MAPPEN, E. 1983), London: Virago.

BLAND, L. and MORT, C. (1984) 'Look out for the "good time" girl', in *Formation of Nation and People*, London: Routledge & Kegan Paul.

BOOTH, W. (1890) *In Darkest England and the Way Out*, London.

BOSANQUET, H. (1902) *The Strength of the People*, London: Macmillan.

BOWLBY, J. (1954) *Child Care and the Growth of Love*, Harmondsworth: Penguin.

BRIGGS REPORT (1972) *Report of the Committee on Nursing*, London: HMSO.

CAMPBELL, B. (1988) *Unofficial Secrets*, London: Virago.

CARPENTER, M. (1977) 'The New Managerialism and professionalism in nursing', in STACEY, M. *et al.* (Eds) *Health Care and the Division of Labour*, Beckenham: Croom Helm.

CHADWICK, E. (1842) *Report on the Sanitary Conditions of the Labouring Population of Great Britain* (Repub. with intro. by FLEIN, M.W. 1965), Edinburgh: Edinburgh University Press.

CLARKE, J. (1988) 'Social Work: The personal and the political', Unit 13 of Open University Course D211, *Social Problems and Social Welfare*, Milton Keynes: the Open University.

CORNER, E.P. (1959) 'Morals and the social worker', in *Report of the Conference, September 1959*, London: Association of Social Workers.

DAVIES, A. (1987) 'Hazardous lives – social work in the 1980s. A view from the left', in LONEY, M., BOCOCK, B., CLARKE, J., COCHRANE, A., GRAHAM, P. and WILLSON, M. (Eds) *The State or the Market?*, London: Sage.

DAVIES, C. (1976) 'Experience of dependency and control in work: the case of nurses', *Journal of Advanced Nursing Studies*, **1**, pp. 273–81.

DAVIES, C. (1982) 'The regulation of nursing: An historical comparison of Britain and the USA', in ROTH, J. (Ed.) *Research in the Sociology of Health Care*, **2**, pp. 121–60.

DAVIES, C. (1988) 'A constant casualty: nurse education in Britain and the USA to 1939', in DAVIES, C. (Ed.) *Rewriting Nursing History*, Beckenham: Croom Helm.

DAVIN, A. (1978) 'Imperialism and motherhood', *History Workshop*, **5**, pp. 9–63.

DEPARTMENT OF HEALTH (1993) *Changing Childbirth: Report of the Expert Maternity Group*, London: HMSO.

DERBY, LORD (1870) *Speech at the inaugural meeting of the Society for Organizing Charitable Relief and Repressing Mendicity, held at Wallis Rooms on 30 March.* Reprinted for the Society. London: COS.

DINGWALL, R. (1979) *The Social Organization of Health Visiting*, Beckenham: Croom Helm.

DINGWALL, R. and LEWIS, P. (Eds) (1983) *The Sociology of the Professions*, London: Macmillan.

DOCK, L.L. and STEWART, I.M. (1931) *A Short History of Nursing* (3rd edn – original edn pub. 1920), New York and London: G.P. Putnam's Sons.

DONNISON, D. and M. STEWART (1958) *The Child and the Social Services*, London: Fabian Society.

DONZELOT, J. (1977) *The Policing of Families* (Eng. edn 1980), London: Hutchinson.

DOWLING, W.G. (1963) *The Ladies' Sanitary Association and the Origins of the Health Visiting Service*, MA Thesis, University of London.

FOUCAULT, M. (1975) *Discipline and Punish: The Birth of the Prison* (Eng. edn 1977), Harmondsworth: Allen Lane.

FOUCAULT, M. (1976) *The History of Sexuality Vol. I: An Introduction* (Eng. edn 1979), Harmondsworth: Allen Lane.

GAMARNIKOW, E. (1978) 'Sexual division of labour: The case of nursing', in KUHN, A. and WOLPE, A. (Eds) *Feminism and Materialism*, London: Routledge & Kegan Paul.

GREENWOOD, F.J. (1913) 'The evolution of the health visitor', *Journal of the Royal Sanitary Institute*, **34**, pp. 174–82.

GRIFFITHS REPORT (1983) *NHS Inquiry Report*, House of Commons Social Services Committee.

HEARN, J. (1982) 'Notes on patriarchy, professionalism and the semi-professionals', *Sociology*, **16**, pp. 184–202.

HELTERINE, M. (1980) 'The emergence of modern motherhood: motherhood in England 1899–1959', *Insternational Journal of Women's Studies*, **3**, pp. 590–614.

HEWITT, M. (1983) 'Biopolitics and social policy: Foucault's account of welfare', *Theory, Culture* and *Society*, **2**, pp. 67–84.

HILL, O. (1889) *The COS*, paper read at a meeting of the Fulham and Hammersmith COS Committee on 1st February and reprinted as COS Occasional Paper, First Series, No. 15, London: COS.

LOCAL GOVERNMENT BOARD (1917) *Maternity and Child Welfare*, London: HMSO.

LOCK, C.S. (1895) 'Manufacturing a new pauperism', *The Nineteenth Century*, **37**, p. 218.

LOCK, C.S. (1906) 'Introduction' to *Annual Charities Register and Digest* (15th edn), London: Longmans.

MCCLEARY, G.P. (1933) *The Early History of the Infant Welfare Movement*, London: H.K. Lewis.

MCKEOWN, T. (1976) *The Role of Medicine: Dream, Mirage or Nemesis?* London: Nuffield Hospital Trust.

MELIA, K. (1987) *Learning and Working: The Occupational Socialization of Nurses*, London: Tavistock.

OAKLEY, A. (1980) *Subject Women*, London: Fontana.

ORR, J. (1986) 'Feminism and health visiting', in WEBB, C. (Ed.) *Feminist Practice in Women's Health Care*, Chichester: Wiley.

PROCKOSKA, F.K. (1980) *Women and Philanthropy in Nineteenth Century England*, Oxford: Clarendon.

RATHBONE, E. (1924) *The Disinherited Family* (Repub. with intro. by FLEMING, S. 1986), London: Falling Wall.

RILEY, D. (1983) *War in the Nursery: Theories of the Child and Mother*, London: Virago.

ROBERTS, E. (1984) *Women in England: Sexual Divisions and Social Change 1870–1950*, Brighton: Wheatsheaf.

ROBINSON, G. (1849) *On Education as Connected with the Sanitary Movement in Newcastle*, London: Longman.

ROSE, N. (1985) *The Psychology Complex: Psychology, Politics and Society in England 1869–1939*, London: Routledge & Kegan Paul.

ROSE, N. (1989) 'Individualising psychology', in SHOTTER, J. and GERGEN, K.J. (Eds) *Texts of Identity*, London: Sage.

ROWAN, C. (1984) 'For the duration only: motherhood and nation in the First World War', in SCHWARZ, B. (Ed.) *Formation of Nation and People*, London: Routledge & Kegan Paul.

ROWAN, C. (1985) 'Child welfare and the working-class family', in LANGAN, M. and SCHWARZ, B. (Eds) *Crisis in the British State 1880–1930*, London: Hutchinson.

ROWNTREE, B.S. (1901) *Poverty: A Study of Town Life*, London: Macmillan.

SALMON REPORT (1966) *Report of the Committee on Senior Nursing Staff Structure*, London: HMSO.

SAPSFORD, R.J. (1993) 'Understanding people: The growth of an expertise', in CLARKE, J. (Ed.) *A Crisis in Care? Challenges to Social Work*, London: Sage.

SCULL, A.T. (1977) *Decarceration, Community Treatment and the Deviant: A Radical View*, Englewood Cliffs (NJ): Prentice Hall.

SEEBOHM COMMITTEE (1968) *Report of the Committee on Local Authority and Allied Personal Social Services, Cmnd. 3703*, London: HMSO.

SHAKLADY SMITH, L. (1978) 'Sexist assumptions and female delinquency', in SMART, C. and SMART, B. (Eds) *Women, Sexuality and Social Control*, London: Routledge & Kegan Paul.

SIBEON, R. (1990) 'Social work knowledge, social actors and deprofessionalisation', in ABBOTT, P. and WALLACE, C. (Eds) *The Sociology of the Caring Professions* (1st edn), Basingstoke: Falmer.

SMART, B. (1985) *Michel Foucault*, London: Tavistock.

STACEY, M. (1989) *A Sociology of Health and Healing*, London: Unwin Hyman.

THANE, P. (1982) *Foundations of the Welfare State*, London: Longman.

UKCC (UNITED KINGDOM CENTRAL COUNCIL FOR NURSING, MIDWIFERY AND HEALTH VISITING) (1987) *Project 2000: The Final Proposals*, London: UKCC.

UKCC (1992) *The Scope of Professional Practice*, London: UKCC.

VERSLUYSEN, M.C. (1988). 'Old wives' tales? Women healers in English history', in DAVIES, C. (Ed.) *Rewriting Nursing History*, Beckenham: Croom Helm.

WALBY, S. (1990) *Theorising Patriarchy*, Oxford: Blackwell.

WEEKS, J. (1981) *Sex, Politics and Society: The Regulation of Sexuality Since 1800*, London: Longman.

WILLIAMS, A. (1987) 'Making sense of feminist contributions to women's health', in ORR, J. (Ed.) *Women's Health in the Community*, Chichester: Wiley.

WITZ, A. (1992) *Professions and Patriarchy*, London: Routledge.

WOHL, A.S. (1986) *Endangered Lives: Public Health in Victorian England*, London, Dent.

WOODROOFE, K. (1962) *From Charity to Social Work*, London: Routledge & Kegan Paul.

Chapter 3

Nursing: will the Idea of Vocation Survive?

Lesley Mackay

Introduction

'Attracting and keeping a nursing workforce has been, and will continue to be, a major concern for health service managers.' It is rather salutary to find that, since I first wrote these words in the late 1980s (Mackay, 1990), and despite so much happening in the health service and in nursing in the intervening years, so little appears to have been done to improve the situation in which nurses find themselves (Seccombe and Smith, 1996; Land, 1994). Suggestions that consideration needs to be given to flexible working, annualized hours, childcare facilities and in-house development opportunities in order to meet the needs of the nursing workforce are still having to be made (Newton, 1996). The morale of nurses is not high (Ackroyd, 1993) and the dissatisfactions of nurses appear to be growing (Seccombe and Smith, 1996). Why has there been a lack of concerted effort to retain the nursing workforce? In part this is due to the continuing perception that the nursing workforce is relatively easy and cheap to replace (Davies, 1995). However, it will be argued here that it may also be a reflection of the vocational ethos which is held within nursing. It is suggested that the numerous changes within nursing, nurse training and the NHS may be acting to reduce the salience of the idea of vocation amongst nurses.

The Demand and Supply of Nurses

There have been continuing alarms regarding the supply of, and demand for, nurses. The recurring nature of these alarms may be connected with what Davies (1995, Ch. 4) has described as the 'male model' of manpower planning adopted in the NHS, since managing a female labour force is more difficult than managing a male one. In the late 1970s there was concern that nurses would remain too long in one post and there would not be enough movement (Redfern, 1978). By the mid-1980s the concern was reversed, as rates of turnover amongst nurses were rising rapidly.

The prediction that there would be too few potential recruits to nursing in the late 1980s was followed by a period in which there was a dearth of jobs for newly qualified nurses (Buchan, 1994; Humphreys, 1993). While there appears to be no great shortage of recruits to nursing today (there are apparently two applicants for each Project 2000 training place), wastage amongst student nurses continues to average out at around 15 per cent per annum (Newton, 1996). Another nursing shortage is apparently looming (Hancock, 1996) and a nationwide campaign was started in early 1997 to try to attract more recruits into nursing. How effective it will be is open to debate (Williams *et al.*, 1991a). Although the number of nurses in the NHS has gone down in the 1990s (Seccombe and Smith, 1996), there has been a corresponding increase of 6 per cent in the number of nurses working in the private sector (Newton, 1996). It has been acknowledged that little is known about the supply of and demand for nurses (Maynard, 1994), yet few efforts appear to have been made to overcome the uncertainties of this through active management policies to retain the nursing workforce (see also Audit Commission, 1997).

A Changing Health Service

The changes which have taken place in the NHS in the last few years have been fundamental. These include the introduction of competition, internal markets and the split between purchasers and providers, together with the creation of self-governing trusts and the redefinition of the patient as the customer. The recent change of government is also likely to have substantial repercussions on the organization and management of the NHS. Nursing was given little more than passing attention in the reforms of the last few years (Davies, 1995, p. 163), yet substantial changes within nursing have been taking place. Most important was the acceptance of the recommendations of the UKCC regarding nurse training in Project 2000 (UKCC, 1987). Within some ranks of nurse educators there had been growing concern to establish nursing as a profession in its own right and to break the link between service delivery and nurse training. The Project 2000 proposals recommended that students should no longer be counted in the staffing complement of a ward, but were to be supernumerary, receiving a more theoretically-based training with less emphasis on the experience of day-to-day nursing work. In *Nursing a Problem*, I predicted that the greater cost of training nurses under Project 2000 would mean that they were less likely to be treated as a disposable workforce (Mackay, 1989, p. 180). As mentioned above, this does not appear to have happened. I also suggested that the removal of nurse training from the practical to the academic setting might weaken the sense of vocation which our research had identified amongst nurses and learners (Mackay, 1989; Francis *et al.*, 1992). Recent research suggests this has not yet happened (Winson, 1995). However, there continues to be a growing emphasis on the professional nature of nursing (see Davies, 1995) which may, in time, act to undermine its vocational ethos.

Since the late 1980s there has also been a change in the work which qualified nurses do: in the staffing structure on the wards and in the organization of nursing work. The reduction in junior doctors' hours (see Dowie, 1989) and the reappraisal of the work of junior doctors (NHSME, 1991; SCOPME, 1991) has meant that

> In many hospitals nurses and other professionals are now working in areas which were traditionally regarded as the province of doctors. (Audit Commission, 1995, p. 18)

In effect, nurses have been encouraged to take on a number of tasks previously within the remit of junior doctors, such as giving intravenous injections.

The phasing-out of the enrolled nurse and the introduction of the health care assistant (HCA) to replace the nursing auxiliary accompanied the Project 2000 changes. Rigorous scrutiny of nurse staffing levels on the wards with a growing emphasis on 'skill mix' has meant tighter staffing levels on the wards. Today, it appears that qualified nurses are less likely to be involved in the routine hands-on care, or what has been termed the 'lower skilled areas of traditional nursing work', which is being picked up by HCAs (Newton, 1996). Also, the qualified nurse is more likely to be involved in managerial and supervisory duties than before (Hurst, 1992).

There has also been a widespread adoption of primary nursing and the named nurse (for a discussion of this, see Wright, 1992; Hancock, 1992). With primary nursing a patient is allocated a named nurse, the primary nurse, who will be supported by an associate nurse in caring for that patient. The intention has been to move from a task-centred to a patient-centred organization of nursing, although research has shown that these aims are not always realized (Procter, 1989, p. 185). The introduction of primary nursing also reflected a wish for nurses to move to a professional, one-to-one relationship with the individual patient, in a manner similar to that of the doctor. It was thus another strand in the professionalizing process of nursing.

It seems likely that all these changes – Project 2000 training, taking on tasks previously done by junior doctors, the tighter skill mix, the introduction of health care assistants together with primary nursing – will have affected the sustaining occupational ideologies within nursing.

Occupational Ideologies

Occupational ideologies are a resource which shape the way in which people feel, think and act at work (Fox, 1971). They present a view of an occupation to society as a whole, to the public and to patients, as well as to individual members of the occupational group. Occupational ideologies are, thus, both 'parochial' and 'ecumenic' (Dibble, 1962), and aimed at, and informing, the perceptions of nursing within both groups. Within any occupational group there are likely to be a number of ideologies, overlapping and competing, which reflect the range of interests and experiences of the members. Occupational ideologies are, therefore, not necessarily, or even usually, unitary (Beattie, 1995), and they change over time (Chua and Clegg, 1989). In Australia, researchers have looked at the differences in perspective among nurses (Gardner and McCoppin, 1986), and the shifting of nursing education to the tertiary sector has resulted in role models being found within the educational institution rather than the practice setting, presenting students with new values (Du Toit, 1995).

Within nursing in the UK different groups have been identified with different views of nursing (Williams, 1987; Carpenter, 1977; Melia, 1987; Francis *et al.*, 1992). For the most part, a broad dichotomy has been described within nursing between those who adopt a vocational view and those who adopt a professional view of their occupation (Melia, 1987; Mackay, 1989) based respectively in the area of practice and the educational sector (Chua and Clegg, 1989). The presence of these competing world views within nursing has been recognized by many commentators (such as Kramer, 1974; Benner, 1984). A third view of nursing has recently been identified by Francis *et al.* (1992), who found that a substantial minority of nurses see nursing as 'just a job', little different from any other. This may reflect the impact of wider societal changes, in that it has been argued that nursing is becoming less likely to offer a job for life (Buchan, 1994; Humphreys, 1993).

There are questions which pose themselves regarding occupational ideologies in nursing today. For example, can an occupational ideology which stresses the value of public service survive in a materialist and consumerist society? Or are the moves towards increasing the professional status of nursing affecting the adherence to the belief that 'good nurses' need to have a vocation for nursing?

The Research

Prior to recent changes in the NHS, our research into some of the issues relating to 'nurse recruitment and wastage' in a health authority in the North of England (Mackay, 1989) resulted in the need to ask some fundamental questions about nursing. Data had been obtained through questionnaires and interviews in a variety of hospital specialities with nurses who had left (154 questionnaires and 50 interviews) or who had stayed in (435 questionnaires and 50 interviews) one health authority. (Detailed findings from the questionnaire are presented in Bagguley, 1988.) A series of interviews with 21 learners were conducted during the first year of their training (7 individual interviews were also conducted with nurse tutors and nursing officers). It is with these, and the interviews with 50 nurses who left and 50 nurses in a range of specialities who continued working in the health authority, that this chapter is primarily concerned. This health authority may not have been representative of the country as a whole. However, the issues and problems which emerged in our research were similar to those reported elsewhere in previous research. (For a brief overview of some of that previous research see Mackay, 1989, Appendix 2; also Soothill *et al.*, 1996.)

Our initial investigation of nurse recruitment and wastage demonstrated that the 'problem' was not why nurses left, but why, given the often extremely difficult conditions under which they worked, they stayed. The health authority's 'problem' was nurses' 'solution' to their demanding work environments. Thus, there were different ways of viewing the research question. As the research progressed, the original brief was broadened and other questions presented themselves: not only why nurses left, but why did they not leave? why did they stay? what did they get out of their work? and what changes would encourage them to stay or cause them to leave nursing? It soon became obvious that explanations of nurses' recruitment and retention could not simply be sought in individual differences, such as in particular satisfactions and dissatisfactions with work, but had to be situated within the systems in which nurses participate. Thus, we became concerned with the ideologies embedded in everyday working practices, professionalization, issues of gender and of power, systems of training and control, and many others.

The research was designed to unwrap nurses' perception of their work and themselves as nurses. Our pilot study enabled us to identify and develop the topics and themes which should inform the main study. The aim was to build our categories and interpretations from the discourses of the nurses and, in this way, develop theories which were 'grounded' in the everyday experiences of nurses (see Glaser and Strauss, 1968). With this perspective the explanations and accounts given by these nurses were used to develop concepts and theories of why things were the way they were. Although grounded theory can be potentially ahistorical, it became evident as the interviews progressed that it was imperative to take a broader and longer-term view of the situation in which nurses found themselves.

Our brief was to look at 'wastage' amongst nurses. Nurse wastage was the popular phrase in the 1980s and is both a pejorative and an emotive term suggesting that somehow nurses themselves should be blamed for leaving nursing (Soothill *et al.*, 1996, pp. 268–9). In looking at 'wastage' amongst nurses, we reported that movement by nurses from one nursing job to another appeared to be both necessary and expected within the system, whether for purposes of training, gaining wider experience or promotion (Mackay, 1989). Indeed, for a nurse to stay on one ward for many years could be viewed as a sign of stagnation or a lack of ability to move elsewhere. Nurses who wished to train further often had to move to another health authority which offered the specific course they wanted. The need for movement was built into the system. In complaining about the high level of wastage amongst nurses, the management in the health authority was in effect, although they didn't recognize it, complaining about the system within which nurses had to work.

Nurses as a Disposable Workforce

From our research it appeared that nurses had effectively been treated as a disposable workforce, because they were seen as young, female and easily replaced. Evidence in support of this 'disposable workforce' explanation emerged from other research (see, for example, Waite and Hutt, 1987). Thus, nurses' demands for further training were largely unmet. Promotion and career opportunities had not been developed to meet the aspirations and needs of nurses (Mackay, 1989), now recognized as changing throughout women's working life cycle (Shindul-Rothschild, 1995). (In the absence of systems of career development in which nurses had expressed interest (Mackay, 1989) action has now been taken within the nursing profession. Nurses are now required by the UKCC to monitor and record their own career and professional development through professional profiling in order to be able to re-register (see Kaur and Hamer, 1995).) There was a dearth of childcare facilities, and the demand for flexible working hours had gone largely unheeded: this still appears to be the case (Land, 1994). Given the cost implications of increases in nurses' pay for the National Health Service as a whole, demands for substantial increases in pay have largely not been met. Today, dissatisfaction about levels of pay appear to be growing. Considerable anger has been expressed amongst nurses about the introduction of local pay bargaining (Seccombe and Smith, 1996), to which the RCN has made clear its opposition (Hancock, 1996). More recently, there appears to have been a move away from local pay bargaining towards national pay bargaining, but this has also coincided with a period of fiscal restraint.

In short, during the 1980s there was a continuing failure to offer career and promotion opportunities, training opportunities were limited, there was a lack of childcare facilities or flexible working hours, and there appeared to be little attempt to retain the nursing workforce. In spite of the widely-publicized shortage of nurses facing health service managers, little or nothing was done, or indeed has been done since to meet the needs and explicit demands of the nursing workforce (Mackay, 1988 a and b).

A Follow-up Study of Leavers

A three-year follow-up study of nurses who left the same Health Authority was undertaken (Williams *et al.*, 1991, b–e). Of those leavers who were traced and who answered the questionnaire (90 nurses, a response rate of 49 per cent), two-thirds remained in nursing. In the follow-up study it was found that two-thirds of these 'leavers' were working elsewhere within the NHS, while a substantial minority had moved to the private health care sector (Soothill *et al.*, 1996). The authors commented that the recurring themes in the questionnaires focused on staff shortages, lack of resources, the workload getting in the way of doing the work properly, the lack of personal development opportunities in their own training and careers, the management of the NHS, non-existent childcare facilities and difficulties for parents in coping with shift work, together with an overall feeling of not being appreciated and being devalued both financially and by their managers and government. These same themes were to recur in interviews conducted with a sub-sample of these leavers (Soothill *et al.*, 1996).

To talk of a 'nursing workforce' is simplistic and also, in seeking to understand issues relating to recruitment and retention, misleading. Nurses come from a broad range of backgrounds and work in a wide variety of settings and in a range of specialities, calling for differing skills and aptitudes. Nursing is certainly not an homogenous workforce. Around 90 per cent of nurses are women, and women's careers are different from those of men (Davies, 1995; Hakim, 1996). Women take breaks in their careers and, contrary to received opinion, these breaks are often temporary (Waite *et al.*, 1990) perhaps reflecting different stages in their life cycle (Shindul-Rothschild, 1995).

Our research with nurses in one region in the UK revealed that there were substantial differences between nurses as to why they worked as nurses, how they saw their careers in relation to their home lives, their participation in the nursing workforce and their orientations to nursing work.

Table 3.1 The attitudes of 435 nurses towards nursing

	%	Sample (n)
Nursing, come what may	18	79
Nursing, but for how much longer?	18	77
Battling it out	19	82
Just a job	28	123
Other views of nursing	17	74
Total	100	435

Data taken from Francis *et al.*, 1992

Nurses' Views of Their Nursing Careers

In the questionnaire survey (Francis *et al.*, 1992) a range of views of nursing were given by the respondents (see Table 3.1). One group of nurses (18 per cent) gave replies which suggested they saw their work in terms of a vocation and the problems of pay, career opportunities, etc., which were reported by others in nursing were least evident to this group. These were the 'nursing, come what may' group. Whatever the trials and tribulations of the job, these nurses would continue to nurse (Francis *et al.*, 1992, p. 66). They have a commitment which has brought them into nursing and will help ensure their return after a break (Williams *et al.*, 1991b).

Two groups of nurses saw nursing in terms of a career. The first of these groups of career-oriented nurses (18 per cent) sought a well-paid career, whether in nursing or elsewhere. These were the 'nursing, but for how much longer?' group. The other group wanted their career to be in nursing. They were the 'battling it out' group (19 per cent) who were particularly concerned with levels of pay and 'all the trappings which transform a mundane job into a career (e.g. training opportunities, promotion possibilities, special responsibility pay, more auxiliary help)' (Francis *et al.*, 1992, p. 66). Nurses in this group would be unlikely to sacrifice their careers for their children, and it was from this group that there was the greatest demand for improvements regarding childcare facilities. The fourth and largest group (28 per cent) of nurses saw nursing simply as just another job. They did not feel particularly attached to nursing and might leave if and when the opportunity arose. Their pay needed to be good, and many within this group indicated that they would be attracted by the private sector in health care. A further 17 per cent of the nurses were not included in any of these groups, displaying a range of orientations (Francis *et al.*, 1992). Clearly, the nursing workforce is diverse.

Having a Vocation?

Only 18 per cent of nurses displayed a vocational attitude to nursing. However, the belief that nursing is a vocation is reflected in a variety of attitudes expressed within nursing, whether in relation to the practice of nursing or the character of the good nurse. The dictionary definition of vocation is 'a divine call to, sense of fitness for, a career or occupation' (Concise Oxford Dictionary). It is a term which has long been associated with nursing (see Pavey, 1951). The word 'vocation' is commonly used about those who enter the ministry or a religious order. It is no coincidence that both nuns and nurses use the title of sister, evoking the notion of familial and non-sexual love, and there is a notable overlap and common interest between nuns and nurses in the hospice movement. Losing the familial title of sister for the more distant and hierarchical title of ward manager has come at a time when there appears to be a growing interest in professional status amongst nurses (Davies, 1995). The nurses were not asked about their religious beliefs in our study, but it would have been interesting to see if there was any relationship between such beliefs and the idea of vocation. However, during the interviews there were continuing references to sentiments which suggested that quite a number of nurses felt they had 'a calling' for nursing, and to staying in nursing despite themselves: 'This is definitely my vocation – I should have seen it sooner'; 'I've always wanted to be a nurse. I wouldn't do anything else'; 'it's not just a job, it gets to be a way of life'; 'it's my life'; 'I feel that it's something worthwhile'; 'it's the satisfaction of helping people'; and patients 'can't demand for themselves, they can't be vocal and somebody has to make sure that they get what they deserve' (Mackay, 1989, pp. 134–8).

Within nursing there has been an acknowledged tension between a vocational and a professional view of the nurse (see Salvage, 1985). The professionalizing group within nursing, like doctors, would wish to emphasize the skills and training of nurses rather than their personal characteristics. (For an extended discussion of the idea of profession within nursing, see Davies, 1995.) The professionalizing group has had its base in nurse education (Melia, 1987) and particularly at national level (Salvage, 1985). This group wants nurses to be seen and treated as professionals, establishing closer links and equivalence with the medical profession. It was hoped that this would, in part, result from situating nurse training in institutions of higher education rather than in schools of nursing, and this has been accomplished with the adoption of the recommendations of Project 2000 about nurse training (see Chapter 5). Thus the professionalizing group within nursing has gained the ascendancy, despite opposition to the professionalizing agenda from commentators such as Salvage (1985). As mentioned earlier and in part due to the various changes within nursing and the health service, vocational views and sentiments may become a thing of the past. The idea of vocation is also likely to be further weakened, as it sits uneasily with the tenets of the marketplace being followed in the NHS. So it seems that the occupational ideologies of nurses are facing a period of substantial challenge (Du Toit, 1995; Elzubeir and Sherman, 1995).

Although most of the nurses interviewed did not feel that nurses needed to have a vocation, the concept of vocation is embedded in many of the accepted practices and attitudes within nursing, such as being of service to others and putting others first. Such sentiments were voiced by many nurses, even those who felt that pay was the most important element in their work. There was, for example, considerable emphasis both in the school of nursing and by those working on the wards on the character of potential recruits to nursing. In the somewhat closed world of nursing education and practice in the 1980s and prior to the introduction of Project 2000, where the school of nursing was often situated within the hospital grounds, where it was nurses who predominantly taught other nurses and there was an absence of systematic contact with other students, there was arguably more affinity between the views of tutors, nurses and students than is likely to be the case today. Although aspirations for professional status may primarily have been held in the world of nurse education as Melia (1987) argues, such aspirations tended not be expressed in the interviews with nurse tutors in my research in the North of England.

It is around the qualities that constitute the good nurse that the way in which a notion of vocation is embedded in nurses' perceptions of nursing becomes evident. For example, a nursing student reflecting on her idea of the good nurse said 'I think they have to give part of themselves when necessary, like to their dying patients – they have got to give an extra bit of love really' (Mackay, 1989, p. 153). In descriptions of the good nurse, great stress was laid on the importance of the personal qualities of the nurse, with a curious lack of emphasis on their academic abilities and training (Mackay, 1989; 1993). This view of the good nurse has a long history, owing much to the views of Florence Nightingale (Baly, 1986; *pace* Whittaker and Olesen, 1978). The female nature of the qualities of the good nurse have been noted by Gamarnikow (1978). Caring, nurturing, kind, loving and supportive, the 'good nurse' looks suspiciously like the 'good woman' (Oakley, 1984) and, while her attributes can be developed, they cannot be learnt (Gamarnikow, 1978). It is interesting to note that, in comparison, doctors' views of what constitutes the good nurse tend to focus on competence, knowledge and skill and not on the belief that the good nurse is 'born, not made' (Mackay, 1993, pp. 164–5).

The influence of the vocational perspective of nursing can also be found in nurses' views of academic qualifications and the growing emphasis on theory rather than practice in nurse training. Thus, the lack of reference to expertise or skill in the comments about the 'good nurse' was accompanied by a distrust of the academically 'clever' nurse. Repeatedly it was said that what the patients wanted was someone caring and kind, rather than someone who was, as one sister put it, 'very, very clever and had all the degrees in the world' (Mackay, 1989, p. 48). It seems likely, therefore, that there will be some discomfort within the ranks of nurses as increasing numbers of Project 2000-trained nurses enter the wards.

The ramifications for nurses in subscribing to the idea of vocation seem to have been extensive. For example, in the questionnaire survey, pay emerged as a cause of considerable dissatisfaction (Mackay, 1989). However, in response to a question in the interviews as to what improvements were required within nursing to make more nurses stay, nurses' comments about pay were seldom made regarding themselves but in respect of colleagues – nursing assistants, learners, enrolled nurses – and their need for improved pay. An acceptance of the notion of vocation leads to the 'I-will-always-manage' sentiment which in turn could result in less overt anger about tangible benefits (Mackay, 1989, pp. 74–7). Salvage has noted that the view of nurses as 'angels' almost precludes them from taking 'their destiny into their own hands' (1985, p. 20). It also helps explain the remarkably low salary levels in nursing, compared, say, with the police (see Mackay, 1989). Thus, by subscribing to some extent to an idea of vocation, nurses' demands for more pay may be muted. However, this may be in the process of changing (see below).

Having a vocation also appears to have affected the nature of trade union membership and activity. Being unable to put oneself forward, or being scorned for doing so, means that one is less likely to complain, particularly through 'self-seeking' organizations such as trade unions. Nurses prefer to join associations like the RCN, which combine professional association with trade union roles, than trade unions themselves, attitudes to which were often lukewarm (Bagguley, 1992; Mackay, 1989). Similarly, there was a reluctance to go on strike, although nurses expressed considerable anger about the way in which they and the NHS were treated by the government (Mackay, 1989). Partly, the anger expressed was on behalf of patients, but many nurses were angry on their own behalf as well. Yet nurses appeared to be reluctant to give full expression to that anger by, for example, taking industrial action, since they said they were unwilling to leave their patients (Mackay, 1989, pp. 121–2). At the time of the research, there seemed to be a belief amongst nurses that because they eschewed speaking out for themselves ('the good nurse doesn't complain'), others must speak out for them, whether this be nursing leaders, the government or the general public; it is reminiscent of being unable to ask for the salt at the dinner table in the nunnery and having to wait until it is offered to you.

The idea of vocation may be useful in sustaining nurses in performing some of the very unsavoury tasks which they are called upon to do. In other words, 'having a vocation for nursing' can act as a protection against the realities of nursing work. It is noteworthy that many of the learners who were interviewed talked about the need for a vocation, while older and more experienced nurses referred to it less often (Mackay, 1989). It is, after all, the learners who were having (at the time the data was collected which was before the formalization of student nurses' supernumerary status) to do battle with many of the unsavoury basic tasks of nursing (Pavey, 1951, p. 485; Lawler, 1991). Nevertheless, in the interviews with nurses of all grades the need for, or the importance of, vocation was mentioned frequently (Mackay, 1989). Little reference to this aspect was made in the questionnaires.

The idea of vocation was often accompanied by a repeated emphasis on the need for discipline and obedience (Mackay, 1989). An emphasis on these during training, both in the school of nursing and on the wards, was mentioned in the interviews with the learners (Mackay, 1989). There is, of course, an undoubted need for discipline, even obedience, in nursing, as situations occur in which directions are issued by medical colleagues and which have to be responded to quickly and effectively. However, this combination of obedience and discipline may have helped produce a quiescent and relatively unquestioning nursing workforce. Thus, a workforce which has learned its place in the health care team may have failed to question the *status quo*, especially the relationship with the medical profession, in a way that the professionalizers might do. A vocationally-oriented workforce is arguably more easily manipulated and contained than one which is professionally oriented.

The Impact of the Vocational Ideology

It appears that the idea of vocation is deeply embedded in the views and actions of nurses: in the way they see and practice nursing; in the way they express their needs and demands; in their views of trade unions and industrial action; as a sustaining ideology buttressing the realities of performing basic and often unsavoury tasks for patients; and, perhaps as part of this, in the need for discipline and obedience. The idea of vocation may be an aspect of the anticipatory socialization of recruits to nursing, in the playing of doctors-and-nurses games and the solicitous attitudes of the players, as well as during the occupational socialization of nursing students. These are all aspects of the origins and content of ideologies in nursing which it would be particularly interesting to investigate further.

For the moment, I would like to argue that adherence to the idea of vocation may help explain why the expressed needs of the nursing workforce have been ignored by health service managers. Under pressure to recognize the needs of patients and services within the health services, nurses back down from pursuing their own claims. In evincing an 'I-will-always-manage' sentiment, nurses can be seen as potentially more malleable and less demanding than more vociferous NHS employees, such as some ancillary workers, who espouse a more instrumental view of work. In this way, nurses' sense of vocation and their accompanying commitment to patients may be used against them.

Similarly, the dislike of the academically clever nurse and the belief that being a 'good nurse' reflects personal characteristics and cannot be taught (Mackay, 1993, pp. 162–3; Allen, 1997), combine to downgrade the intellectual requirements of nursing. Within nursing the emphasis on practical skills may mean that the learned skills and techniques as well as the levels of responsibility taken by nurses may not be sufficiently recognized or rewarded. In addition, the past failure of those within management, both inside and outside nursing, to listen to the demands of nurses may have acted to inhibit nurses giving louder voice to their demands for improvements in their employment conditions. In effect, some of the occupational ideologies held within nursing may have been used against them. Of course, other factors such as the gender of the nursing workforce and the perception that many nurses, as women, do not want a career, are likely to have affected the way the nursing workforce has been treated, both within the health service and by successive governments (Mackay, 1989; Davies, 1995).

Nurses are one of the largest and, therefore, one of the most expensive components in NHS expenditure, yet can be seen as having been viewed as a 'soft touch' amongst the other groups of health care workers. As Davies (1995) points out, nursing issues have been given little attention in many of the recent reforms in the NHS, despite the key contribution which nurses make to patient care. However, long-needed attention has been directed to the workings of the medical profession. Thus, challenging, as well as responding to, the demands of the medical profession has been a major focus in the changes which are taking place, whether in the number of consultants, their contracts, or in the tasks and hours of junior doctors. Perhaps it is reasonable, given the tremendous upheavals which have taken place in nursing in the last few years, to let nursing and nurses settle down again, and wait to see what results – and what sort of occupational ideology– emerge from these upheavals.

What is the Future for the Idea of Vocation?

In the past nurses have enjoyed considerable public sympathy. Nurses were often referred to as 'angels' (see Salvage, 1985) and were seen as, in some way, different from other health care workers. Perhaps this public view of nursing was an echo of the vocational idea to which nurses were seen to subscribe. There was a popular television series entitled *Angels*, whose demise in the early 1980s may have resulted in the epithet being less often applied to nurses. There have been many changes within the NHS and the wider society, which may have affected the way in which nurses are seen by their patients and the public at large.

Considerable media attention has been given to the embattled state of the NHS, whether to the rising numbers of patients on waiting lists or the reduction in the number of hospital beds. The introduction of the *Patient's Charter* (Department of Health, 1991) setting out the rights of patients implicitly suggests that, prior to this, the treatment of patients by health care staff was not always of the best. The grateful patient of the past may have been replaced by the righteous patient who demands attention rather than waiting for it to be offered. Following the emphasis on the market within health care, the patient has also come to be redefined as the customer. The workload of nurses is seen to have increased substantially, reducing the time for patient care (Nolan *et al.*, 1995). The shorter stay and faster throughput of patients means that patients' contact and relationships with nurses are also changing. It becomes more and more difficult for nurses to get to know their patients or for their patients to get to know them, when patients are in the ward for only a couple of days. The longer-stay patient who helped set the dinner table or who did little jobs in the ward is not to be found today. Patients may be less aware of, perhaps even less sympathetic to, the situation in which nurses find themselves. Thus, the relationship between nurses and patients is likely to be changing. In turn, this may well affect the sort of satisfaction nurses obtain from their jobs which, in the past, has come from helping patients, and from being given appreciation for a job well done. The occupational ideologies within nursing appear to be in the process of being challenged.

There may be evidence of changing occupational ideologies in the way that the previous reluctance to take industrial action has been overcome, so that nurses have given overt expression to anger about their levels of pay in one-day strikes (Healy, 1997). It would be interesting to know in the light of all these changes how nurses are seen by their patients, and whether the introduction of the Patient's Charter has affected the way in which nurses now view their patients.

Today, using the word vocation may not be fashionable in an occupation which is clearly seeking professional status (Salter and Snee, 1997). Yet vocation and profession are not necessarily mutually exclusive perceptions of nursing. It is possible to maintain that it takes a special kind of person to be a nurse, and yet to acknowledge the need for advanced training and skills in nursing. How are the occupational ideologies held within nursing adapting to the changing environment? Is the idea of vocation still held amongst nurses, and how salient is it? Has it been integrated in some way with the professional view of nursing, encouraged by siting nurse training in higher education? Will contact with students in other disciplines affect the views of nurses towards their chosen occupation? How have the predicted tensions in nursing resolved themselves?

The frequently expressed rejection of the 'academic' and the scorn aimed at the 'clever' nurse (Mackay, 1989, p. 151; see also Davies, 1995, p. 109) were themes which were to be repeated in later research (Mackay, 1993). Nurses are 'born not made' was the clarion call which acted to give graduate nurses and other high-fliers a poor reception. How have Project 2000 nurses been greeted in nursing, given the considerable antipathy to the proposals (Mackay, 1989; 1993)? There has been a continuing and heated correspondence in the columns of the *Nursing Times* during the 1990s regarding the perceived lack of practical preparation of today's nursing student. What, if any, changes have taken place in the practice of nurses? Davies, for example, suggests that, while nursing education may have been put on a new footing through Project 2000, nursing practice remains much as it has always been (1995, p. 12). Does that mean that the idea of vocation will survive? Also, how are nurses from the two different types of training adjusting to one another as they work together? Tensions, if they exist, may be in the perceived antithesis between the good nurse and the academically clever nurse.

Recent research suggests that the idea of vocation might not have gone away, at least among recruits to nursing. Winson (1995) has reported from her sample of nearly 500 students that three-fifths of new student nurses expressed some sort of vocational reason for entering nursing. Whether this is to be found more generally amongst recruits to nursing, and whether it can be sustained through the training years and the contact with the culture of higher education, would be interesting to investigate.

The confounding element in the occupational ideologies of nurses is the substantial number who saw nursing as 'just a job' like any other (Francis *et al.*, 1992), even though some of their views may reflect vocational ideas. The increasing number of job opportunities in private health care and the decreasing number in the health service (*Nursing Standard*, 1995) may act to erode a public service ethos. Can an occupational ideology which stresses the value of public service survive in this consumerist society? When jobs are scarce, nurses' thoughts might reasonably turn to survival rather than to sentiments of self-denial. And perhaps contact with the financial realities of working in the National Health Service, and the additional loads placed on staff through these realities, will have an impact on the survival of the vocational ideology. Is this 'just a job' view of nursing set to increase?

Finally, I would like to argue that the idea of vocation has given a special quality to nurses and nursing work – one of putting patients first.

The attractions of being 'a professional' and establishing nursing on an equal footing with medicine cannot be denied, but something intrinsic to nursing practice would be lost if the vocational element were extinguished. It is, after all, an occupational ideology which has informed nurses and nursing practice for the last hundred years.

Note

This chapter is based on a study, 'Nurse Recruitment and Wastage', conducted under the general direction of Professor Keith Soothill and supported by the Leverhulme Trust.

References

ACKROYD, S. (1993) 'Towards an understanding of nurses' attachments to their work: morale amongst nurses in an acute hospital', *Journal of Advances in Health and Nursing Care*, **2**, pp. 23–45.

ALLEN, D. (1997) 'Nursing, knowledge and practice', *Journal of Health Services Research Policy*, **2**, pp. 190–3.

AUDIT COMMISSION (1995) *The Doctor's Tale: The Work of Hospital Doctors in England and Wales*, London: HMSO.

AUDIT COMMISSION (1997) *Finders, Keepers: The Management of Staff Turnover in NHS Trusts*, Abingdon: Audit Commission Publications.

BAGGULEY, P. (1988) *A Report of a Study of Turnover and Work Dissatisfaction amongst UK Professional Nurses*, University of Lancaster: Department of Sociology.

BAGGULEY, P. (1992) 'Angels in red? Patterns of union membership amongst UK professional nurses', in SOOTHILL, K., HENRY, C. and KENDRICK, K. (Eds) *Themes and Perspectives in Nursing* (2nd edn), London: Chapman & Hall.

BALY, M.E. (1986) *Florence Nightingale and the Nursing Legacy*, London: Croom Helm.

BEATTIE, A. (1995) 'War and peace among the health tribes', in SOOTHILL, K., MACKAY, L. and WEBB, C. (Eds) *Interprofessional Relations in Health Care*, London: Edward Arnold.

BENNER, P. (1984) *From Novice to Expert*, Menlo Park (CA): Addison-Wesley.

BUCHAN, J. (1994) 'Employment of newly registered nurses', *Nursing Standard*, **9**, (19 October), p. 31.

CARPENTER, M. (1977) 'The New Managerialism and Professionalism in Nursing', in STACEY, M. and REID, M. (Eds) *Health and the Division of Labour*, London: Croom Helm.

CHUA, W.F. and CLEGG, S.R. (1989) 'Contradictory couplings: occupational ideology in the organisational locales of nurse training', *Journal of Management Studies*, **26**, pp. 103–28.

DAVIES, C. (1995) *Gender and the Professional Predicament in Nursing*, Buckingham: Open University Press.

DEPARTMENT OF HEALTH (1991) *The Patient's Charter*, London: Department of Health.

DIBBLE, V.K. (1962) 'Occupations and ideologies', *American Journal of Sociology*, **63**, pp. 220–41.

DOWIE, R. (1989) *Junior Doctors' Hours: Interim Report*, London: British Postgraduate Medical Federation.

DU TOIT, D. (1995) 'A sociological analysis of the extent and influence of professional socialisation on the development of a nursing identity among nursing students at two universities in Brisbane, Australia', *Journal of Advanced Nursing*, **21**, pp. 164–71.

ELLIOTT, P. (1973) 'Professional Ideology and Social Science', *Sociological Review*, **21**, pp. 211–18.

ELZUBEIR, M. and SHERMAN, M. (1995) 'Nursing Skills and Practice', *British Journal of Nursing*, **4**, pp. 1087–92.

FOX, A. (1971) *A Sociology of Work in Industry*, London: Collier-Macmillan.

FRANCIS, B., PEELO, M. and SOOTHILL, K. (1992) 'NHS nursing: vocation, career or just a job', in SOOTHILL, K., HENRY, C. and KENDRICK, K. (Eds) *Themes and Perspectives in Nursing*, London: Chapman & Hall.

GAMARNIKOW, E. (1978) 'Sexual division of labour: the case of nursing', in KUHN, A. and WOLPE, A. (Eds) *Feminism and Materialism*, London: Routledge & Kegan Paul.

GARDNER, H. and MCCOPPIN, B. (1986) 'Vocation, career or both', *Australian Journal of Advanced Nursing*, **4**, pp. 25–35.

GLASER, B.G. and STRAUSS, A.L. (1968) *The Discovery of Grounded Theory*, London: Weidenfeld & Nicolson.

HAKIM, C. (1996) *Key Issues in Women's Work: Female Heterogeneity and the Polarisation of Women's Employment*, London: Athlone Press.

HANCOCK, C. (1992) 'The named nurse in perspective', *Nursing Standard*, **7**, pp. 39–42.

HANCOCK, C. (1996) 'Where have all the nurses gone?', *The Independent* (25 September), p. 15.

HEALY, P. (1997) 'The pay issue', *Nursing Standard*, **11**, pp. 14–16.

HUMPHREYS, J. (1993) 'An insecure future', *Nursing Standard*, **7**, pp. 26–27.

HURST, K. (1992) 'Changes in nursing practice 1984–1992', *Nursing Times*, **88**, p. 54.

KAUR, S. and HAMER, S. (1995) 'Implementing professional profiling', *British Journal of Nursing*, **4**, pp. 226–9.

KRAMER, B. (1974) *Reality Shock and Why Nurses Leave Nursing*, St. Louis: C.V. Mosby.

LAND, L.M. (1994) 'The student nurse selection experience – a qualitative study', *Journal of Advanced Nursing*, **20**, pp. 1030–7.

LAWLER, J. (1991) *Behind the Screens: Nursing, Somology and the Problem of Body*, Edinburgh: Churchill Livingstone.

MACKAY, L. (1988a) 'The nurses nearest the door', *The Guardian*, (18 January), p. 18.

MACKAY, L. (1988b) 'Career Women', *Nursing Times*, **84**, pp. 42–4.

MACKAY, L. (1989) *Nursing a Problem*, Milton Keynes: Open University Press.

MACKAY, L. (1990) 'Nursing: just another job', in ABBOTT, P. and WALLACE, C. (Eds) *The Sociology of the Caring Professions* (1st edn), Basingstoke: Falmer Press.

MACKAY, L. (1993) *Conflicts in Care: Medicine and Nursing*, London: Chapman & Hall.

MAYNARD, A. (1994) 'Numbers nonsense', *Nursing Management*, **1** (6), p. 7.

MELIA, K. (1987) *Learning and Working: The Occupational Socialisation of Nurses*, London: Tavistock.

NATIONAL HEALTH SERVICE MANAGEMENT EXECUTIVE (1991) *Junior Doctors: The New Deal*, London: HMSO.

NEWTON, G. (1996) 'Talking up nursing', *Health Service Journal*, **11** (2).

NOLAN, M., NOLAN, J. and GRANT, G. (1995) 'Maintaining nurses' job satisfaction and morale', *British Journal of Nursing*, **4**, pp. 1149–54.

NURSING STANDARD (1995) Editorial, *Nursing Standard*, **9** (19), p. 12.

OAKLEY, A. (1984) 'The importance of being a nurse', *Nursing Times*, **80**, pp. 24–7.

PAVEY, A.E. (1951) *The Story of the Growth of Nursing: As an Art, a Vocation and Profession* (3rd edn), London: Faber & Faber.

PROCTOR, S. (1989) 'The functioning of nursing routines in the management of a transient workforce', *Journal of Advanced Nursing*, **14**, pp. 180–90.

REDFERN, S.J. (1978) 'Absence and wastage in trained nurses: a selective view of the literature', *Journal of Advanced Nursing*, **3**, pp. 231–49.

SALTER, B. and SNEE, N. (1997) 'Power dressing', *Health Service Journal*, **107**, pp. 30–1.

SALVAGE, J. (1985) *The Politics of Nursing*, London: Heinemann.

SECCOMBE, I. and SMITH, G. (1996) *In the Balance: Registered Nurse Supply and Demand 1996*, Brighton: Institute of Employment Studies/Royal College of Nursing.

SHINDUL-ROTHSCHILD, J. (1995) 'Life cycle influences on staff nurse career', *Nursing Management*, **26**, pp. 40–4.

SOOTHILL, K., MACKAY, L. and WEBB, C. (Eds) (1995) *Interprofessional Relations in Health Care*, London: Edward Arnold.

SOOTHILL, K., WILLIAMS, C. and BARRY, J. (1996) 'Understanding nurse turnover', in SOOTHILL, K., HENRY, C. and KENDRICK, K. (Eds) *Themes and Perspectives in Nursing* (2nd edn), London: Chapman & Hall.

STANDING COMMITTEE ON POSTGRADUATE MEDICAL EDUCATION (SCOPME) (1991) *Improving the Experience: Good Practice in Senior House Officer Training: A Report on Local Initiatives*, London: SCOPME.

UNITED KINGDOM CENTRAL COUNCIL (1987) *Project 2000: The Final Proposals*, London: UKCC, Project Paper 9.

WAITE, R. and HUTT, R. (1987) *Attitudes, Jobs and Mobility of Qualified Nurses: A Report for the Royal College of Nursing*, Falmer: University of Sussex, Institute of Manpower Studies, IMS Report No. 130.

WAITE, R., BUCHAN, J. and THOMAS, J. (1990) *Career Paths of Scotland's Qualified Nurses*, Brighton: Institute for Manpower Studies.

WHITTAKER, E. and OLESEN, V. (1978) 'The faces of Florence Nightingale: functions of the heroine legend in an occupational sub-culture', in DINGWALL, R. and MCINTOSH, J. (Eds) *Readings in the Sociology of Nursing*, Edinburgh: Churchill Livingstone.

WILLIAMS, C., SOOTHILL, K. and BARRY, J. (1991a) 'Love nursing, hate the job', *The Health Service Journal*, **101**, pp. 18–21.

WILLIAMS, C., SOOTHILL, K. and BARRY, J. (1991b) 'Targeting the discontented', *The Health Service Journal*, **101**, pp. 20–1.

WILLIAMS, C., SOOTHILL, K. and BARRY, J. (1991c) 'Why Nurses Leave the Profession Part 1', *Nursing Standard*, **5** (39), pp. 33–5.

WILLIAMS, C., SOOTHILL, K. and BARRY, J. (1991d) 'Why Nurses Leave the Profession Part 2', *Nursing Standard*, **5** (40), pp. 33–5.

WILLIAMS, C., SOOTHILL, K. and BARRY, J. (1991e) 'Why Nurses Leave the Profession Part 3', *Nursing Standard*, **5** (41), pp. 33–6.

WILLIAMS, K. (1987) 'Ideologies of nursing: their meanings and implications', in DINGWALL, R. and MCINTOSH, R. (Eds) *Readings in the Sociology of Nursing*, Edinburgh: Churchill Livingstone.

WINSON, S.K.G. (1995) 'Demographic differences between degree and diploma student nurses', *Nursing Standard*, **2** (23), pp. 35–8.

WRIGHT, S. (1992) 'The named nurse', *Nursing Times*, **88** (11), pp. 27–9.

Chapter 4

The Case in Social Work: Psychological Assessment and Social Regulation

David McCallum

In this chapter, I wish to show how particular methods of survey and investigation were productive of certain knowledges of the particular and psychological make-up of individuals, which in turn became the object of a new person-centred approach to social work practice. In the early twentieth century, a different type of subject of social work was being formulated. A space was created in which statistical and survey techniques produced particular conceptions of the reality and 'truth' of psychological knowledge. Two issues are explored: first, the population question and the histories of this question, as well as the 'biologizing' of the individual apparent at this time; secondly, I want to look at an example of a blueprint and manual for social workers as practitioners of a 'technology of the social' (Henriques *et al.*, 1984, p. 121) – Mary Richmond's *Social Diagnosis*, published in 1917 and reprinted 17 times before 1955, and recognized in social work history in the United States as a major informing text for training in social casework (Gordon, 1988, p. 65). Casework emerged also as the key feature of a reformist social work practice in the post-war period in Australia.

Social work's own understanding of its past is largely affirming and celebratory of a reconstitution of social work practice within the new frameworks of scientific, psychological and psychiatric knowledges formulated during the first half of this century. In Australia, these knowledges are understood to have produced a gradual transformation of the practices of a voluntary, untrained but well-meaning group of charity workers into those of a professional cadre of social workers, 'equipped with relevant knowledge about individuals and the community . . . [and] alive to the multiple causes of maladjustment' (Lawrence, 1965, pp. 30–2). Both in Australia and in Britain the incorporation of these new knowledges was seen as tardy and unenthusiastic, leaving practitioners too long at the mercy of 'unadulterated intuition and commonsense' (Younghusband, 1964, p. 19). The Americans, on the other hand

> took hold of what the scientific study of living human beings had to tell them about the development of children, about the way people behave in relation to each other, particularly in families, about the characteristics of different kinds of people, for example, the ill, the delinquent, the solitary, the aggressive, the uprooted . . . In short, they have used organizational method and applied scientific knowledge as the basis for developing the professional practice of social work. (p. 19)

Yet, it is not merely the characteristics of a technical expertise which are at stake here and found wanting among the Australian and British social workers compared with their counterparts in the United States (Lawrence, 1965, p. ix). There is also the prioritizing of a new type of relationship with the object of social work practice, which required the closest investigation and scrutiny of the individual's character, the laying bare of the facts of an individual's life and relationships, and the opening up of the individual to the gaze of psychological, medical and sociological enquiry. Again, in social work's view of its past, these are the hallmarks of a new, progressive, interpersonal, humanist and even radical approach to understanding social life. This approach shared a similar framework and emerged at the same historical moment as the child-centred pedagogy in education, person-centred management of occupational selection and the individualized assessment and treatment of the delinquent and the inmate. In social work a new terminology was to take the place of such moral categories as *deserving* and *undeserving*, in the form of the case and casework, process, social diagnosis and what came to be called *social network analysis.*

It is not the intention in this chapter to enter into a debate around the question of the origins of a specifically professional approach to social work in Australia (Kennedy, 1988, p. 237). Such debates and the histories they produce need to be understood as histories of the present in which the current 'truth' of social work practice is presented as legitimate, or as merely an effect of class and gender relations. Instead, I want to begin to examine the formation of the individual subject of social work practice and the way in which psychological knowledges of the individual can be linked to new modes of regulation in the twentieth century. This type of analysis draws especially on the work of Michel Foucault and others influenced by his work, particularly Nikolas Rose and Ian Hacking, and my own work on the history of psychological testing in Australia. Here, one of the main claims to be advanced is that psychology has played a major part in the production of modern forms of individuality, and that the meanings and assumptions by which we understand ourselves must be understood as historically specific products (Rose, 1985; 1990; 1996; Hacking, 1986; McCallum, 1990).

Like the extension of the medical gaze through the operation of the Dispensary in Great Britain in the early part of the twentieth century, as described by Armstrong (1983), the techniques of a new social work practice came to represent the Panopticon writ large, a whole community 'traversed throughout by hierarchy, surveillance, observation, writing' (M. Foucault, cited in Armstrong, 1983, p. 9). These techniques were another method of exercising power, requiring the social body to be monitored to include both the normal and the abnormal, and fixing the gaze on bodies that can be 'individualized by their relations'. So, like the Dispensary, these were techniques applied not so much on individual bodies as on the interstices of society, imposing on the spatial arrangement of bodies '. . . the social configuration of their relationships'.

Armstrong's analysis thus becomes a description of the mechanisms of power which order and constitute the social realm itself; it is a mode of analysis

> for making visible to constant surveillance the interaction between people, normal and abnormal, and thereby transforming the physical space between bodies into a social space traversed by power. At the beginning of the twentieth century the 'social' was born as an autonomous realm. (pp. 9–10)

Concern about the efficient and rational management of certain groups was part of what became known as the population question during the last quarter of the nineteenth century in Australia. In this period psychological reasoning broke away from philosophy to adopt the scientific mode, to claim jurisdiction in the selection of immigrants, the organization of public schooling, and the assessment of delinquents, prisoners, the feeble-minded and the insane. In alliance with medicine and psychiatry, psychology sought to extend and refine the purely physical examination of the population through its investigation of the mind and mental operations, although it is important to stress that these knowledges did not speak with one voice, and were often contradictory and specific to the location of their production. Compared with the weight of prevailing medical opinion, psychology asserted a progressive stand on questions concerning the abnormal and the management of a range of behaviours and conditions affecting the quality of the population and ultimately the 'survival of the race'. In this sense, the formation of the individual in the first instance was made problematic, not within the domain of speculative philosophy about 'man' or the individual in general, but in respect to a particular section of the population, and in regard to quite practical and even mundane problems of administration and management (Minson, 1985, p. 18).

Among others, Jeffrey Weeks (1985) in Britain and Carol Bacchi (1980) in Australia have drawn attention to an increasingly interventionist approach in the politics of the population question. The problem of population was able to be framed in the earliest census data on births and marriages at the beginning of the nineteenth century, in the tendency of the poor to reckless overbreeding, thus producing their own poverty and becoming what was called 'swamped in vice and misery'. Against the Malthusian conception of immutable laws of population due to 'inevitable moral degeneracy', a new approach towards control of the population became evident later in the century in line with demands to maintain the imperial race and industrial supremacy – conditions which could not be met in the nineteenth-century slum. Intervention emphasized public health, the notification of births and more careful statistics gathering, correct childrearing and the removal of children from unsuitable parents. Good mothering became a national duty (Weeks, 1985, pp. 190–2; Abbott and Wallace, Chapter 2 in this volume). In Australia, social efficiency and the defence of the Empire were linked to relatively progressive forms of population control and social programmes, reflecting the importance of a combination of eugenics and hereditarian theories, particularly as these were adopted in medical, educational and other professional circles (Bacchi, 1980; McCallum, 1990).

Histories of the rise of the population question and the so-called displacement of moralism by science have focused largely on the effects of Darwin's discovery of the theory of the 'survival of the fittest'. According to Richard Hofstadter, the theory of social selection adapted by Herbert Spencer during the last quarter of the nineteenth century was a representative translation of Darwin's ideas about natural selection on to people and human societies. For Spencer, the pressure of subsistence was '. . . the immediate and utmost cause of human progress'. The pressure of subsistence meant that a premium was placed on 'skill, intelligence, self-control and the power to adapt to technological innovation', which would sort out the best of each generation for survival (Hofstadter, 1945, p. 25). Another perspective implicates British imperialism in the extension of the 'survival of the fittest' idea on an international scale, that war, for example, as a natural law of history would proclaim the fittest of the 'races' (Semmel, 1960, p. 23). Again, in Gillis' history of youth, social Darwinism supposedly alerted an educated public to the danger of physical and moral degeneration, which justified the increased confinement of the young in schools and other asylums (Gillis, 1974, p. 156), the latter ensuring that the worst of the degenerate would not procreate.

These histories have also tended to focus on the problem of the legitimization of a social order, giving central place to the concept of ideology in the management of political consent. Russell Marks, for example, argues that in the event of the failure of the Protestant work ethic to be a plausible explanation for social differences in North America at the turn of the twentieth century, alternative means were sought to legitimize the grim realities of low-skilled, low-paid industrial work. According to Marks, ideas about natural selection and an 'aristocracy of ability' served to persuade employees to consider themselves less bright, and to adapt to their fate in a genial fashion (Marks, 1980, pp. 86–122; see also Fitzpatrick, 1949, p. 194).

Rather than seeing the conditions for the production of the knowledges and practices of social work as lying in some separate sphere such as the state or the class system, I would like to argue that we need to look for these conditions within the sphere of the production of scientific knowledges about particular types of individuals – in particular from medicine and psychology, and in the specific practices of population management. In the case of the child, the conditions arise from the convergence of mass schooling and biological discourses in the late nineteenth century: first, the gathering of children into classrooms as product and raw material of a scientific enquiry in the form of a sizable group of the population performing more-or-less regular and 'normalizing' tasks on an individual basis; secondly, the naturalization of the mind as an object of science, permitting the calibration of the individual pupil, to be carried out by appeals to individualism as a natural state. In this example, according to Couze Venn,

> it is nature itself which becomes the origin and foundation; all explanations have to find their basis in natural processes. Additionally, they are the processes *as described by science*, so that the question of how we know that the natural processes are as we think them to be is answered by an appeal to scientific authority. (Henriques *et al.*, 1984, pp. 144–5)

The purpose here is not to pronounce psychology to be wrong or to indicate its errors along the pathway to some final true knowledge of the individual. The point is rather to examine the insertion of psychology into everyday practices, the manner in which it produces individuals as objects of enquiry, and the effects of this process upon institutional practices. This assumes that the effects of psychology are not governed simply by rules and propositions internal to scientific discovery, but rather that they are at work in definite applications of social management – the effects of psychology as a 'technology of the social'. The power/knowledge relationship is thus crucial to understanding the way psychology 'works'. The individual produced by psychology, and the individualizing techniques of institutional practices, establish a system of mutual support and reinforcement.

Within this context and set of working assumptions, I now look briefly at Mary Richmond's book *Social Diagnosis*. I have described it as a manual for use in training social workers in the techniques of investigation, and

Lawrence's foundational work on the history of social work mentions it as signalling a turning-point in relations between social workers and their clients:

> . . . the clients' own ideas and feelings become the core of the diagnosis and treatment, and 'process' became one of the most used words in the social workers' vocabulary. (Lawrence, 1965, p. 11)

Social Diagnosis outlines the role of what is called 'social evidence' in social work practice: that is,

> all the facts as to personal or family history which, taken together, indicate the nature of a given client's social difficulties and the means to their solution. (Richmond, 1917, p. 50)

The book is, in effect, like a map showing where social workers would do best to go in order to obtain evidence on individuals and their relationships. There are chapters on the first interview with the client, then on other sources of evidence extending outward, so to speak, through family, relatives, medical sources, school sources, employers, documentary and neighbourhood sources, and social agencies, including other social workers as sources. There follow chapters on specific cases where variation in the collection of evidence may apply: the immigrant family, desertion and widowhood, the neglected child, the unmarried mother, the blind, the homeless and inebriate, the insane and the feeble-minded. The role of evidence in social work is made to correspond to evidence in legal terms – that is, its admissibility in constituting the individual as 'a case', and also in medical terms as constituting a case based on the accumulation of scientific facts. Its task is to provide 'the intimate understanding of character', as outlined by Octavia Hill as early as 1869 in an address to the London Social Science Association:

> By knowledge of character more is meant than whether a man is a drunkard or a woman is dishonest; it means knowledge of passions, hopes, and the history of people; whether the temptation will touch them, what is the little scheme they have made of their lives, or would make, if they had encouragement; what training long past phases of their lives may be afforded; how to move, touch, teach them. Our memories and our hopes are more truly factors of our lives than we often remember.

In the period of institutional transformation from a system of Charity Organisation Societies in Great Britain, North America and Australia, mechanisms of surveillance and measurement of the population begin to appear, breaking down the anonymous mass of the population into individual cases and regrouping these cases around certain statistical norms. James Donald has described this 'hierarchic surveillance' and 'normalizing judgment' in relation to the effects of schooling on the organization of social relations and subjectivity around the turn of the century (Donald, 1985, p. 233). Deborah Tyler in Australia has outlined a framework for understanding child psychology as imbricated in the arts of modern government, demonstrated by the early-twentieth-century shift of the kindergarten from a philanthropic institution to one whose function becomes a systematic psychological study of the child (Tyler, 1997). *Social Diagnosis* proposes an extension of the techniques already applied in the physical and mental examination of children in psychological clinics attached to the Children's Court in Chicago, and from 1917 at the Judge Baker Guidance Centre in Boston (Gordon, 1988, p. 68), techniques which also became a regular operation in Australian courts in the 1920s (Berry, 1929, p. 24). The measuring, individualizing and medicalizing practices of the psychiatrists and psychologists produced in this case a particular 'reality' of delinquency, formulated in textbooks by the Chicago-based William Healy entitled *The Individual Delinquent, Pathological Lying,* and *Honesty,* in which stealing was constructed as 'a symptom, not a disease, and that the physical, mental and social facts behind that symptom must be grasped and interpreted if we are to effect a cure'. This was to become the domain of 'the social'.

I want to conclude with the definition of the *self* announced by the psychologist James Baldwin, and cited in Richmond's book as the underlying philosophy of casework and social diagnosis. Baldwin writes:

> the thought of self arises directly out of certain given social relationships; indeed, it is the form which these actual relationships take on in the organization of a new personal experience. The ego of which he thinks at any time is not the isolated-and-in-his-body-alone situated abstraction which our theories of personality usually lead us to think. It is rather a sense of a network of relationships among you, we and the others, in which certain necessities of pungent feeling, active life, and concrete thought require that I throw the emphasis on one pole sometimes, calling it me; and on the other pole sometimes, calling it you or him. (Richmond, 1917)

The social was constructed in Richmond's book around the psychological theory of the 'wider self', located as a biological entity in the mind and produced through an organized system of connections, bonds and associations which was the sum total of the individual's life experiences. Richmond summarizes the theory in the phrase 'a man is the company he keeps'. This was to be the object of social work, the spatial arrangement of bodies, the multiple configurations wiring up the 'wider self'. According to psychologists like Baldwin and Edward Thorndike, their science would then be capable of predicting '. . . what any given situation or stimulus will connect with, or evoke, in the way of thought, feeling, word or deed'.

In summary, then, Richmond's *Social Diagnosis* announced the inauguration of a 'discipline' of social work which reflected a 'disciplining' and fixing of bodies according to a psychological mapping. The problematic 'case' which became the object of a newly-theorized social work practice was produced through the mapping of the individual within a social field. Rather than having a general prior existence whose essence or truth is then subject to the historically repressive forces of eugenics or imperialism, 'the social' was formed for the discrete administrative objectives of 'social diagnosis' – in this instance an extension in ever-widening concentric circles of the spaces between individuals. In the context of more recent pronouncements on 'the end of the social', it might be possible to consider critically the varying ways in which the domain of the social is constructed, such as those which derive from the conceptual terrain of 'community', for example, which seek to map out a space for the further administration and management of persons.

References

Armstrong, D. (1983) *Political Anatomy of the Body: Medical Knowledge in Britain in the Twentieth Century*, Cambridge: Cambridge University Press.

Bacchi, C. (1980) 'The nature/nurture debate in Australia 1900–1914', *Historical Studies*, **19** (October).

Berry, R.J.A. (1929) *Report of the Edward Wilson Trust on Mental Deficiency in the State of Victoria with Suggestions for the Establishment of a Child Guidance Clinic*, Melbourne: Argus.

Donald, J. (1985) 'Beacons of the future: schooling, subjection and subjectification', in Beechey, V. and Donald, J. (Eds) *Subjectivity and Social Relations*, Milton Keynes: Open University Press.

Fitzpatrick, B. (1949) *The British Empire in Australia 1834–1949* (2nd edn), Melbourne: Melbourne University Press.

Gillis, J.R. (1974) *Youth and History: Tradition and Change in European Age Relations 1770–Present*, New York: Academic Press.

Gordon, L. (1988) *Heroes of their Time: The Politics and History of Family Violence, Boston 1880–1960*, New York: Viking.

Hacking, I. (1986) 'Making up people', in Heller, T. *et al.* (Eds) *Reconstructing Individualism: Autonomy, Individuality and the Self in Western Thought*, Stanford: Stanford University Press.

HENRIQUES, J. *et al.* (Eds) (1984) *Changing the Subject: Psychology, Social Regulation and Subjectivity*, London: Methuen.

HOFSTADTER, R. (1945) *Social Darwinism in American Thought 1860–1915*, Philadelphia: University of Pennsylvania Press.

KENNEDY, R. (1988) *Charity Warfare*, Melbourne: Hyland House.

LAWRENCE, R.J. (1965) *Professional Social Work in Australia*, Canberra: ANU Press.

MARKS, R. (1980) 'Legitimating Industrial Capitalism', in ARNOVE, R.F. (Ed.) *Philanthropy and Cultural Imperialism: The Foundations at Home and Abroad*, Bloomington: Indiana University Press.

MCCALLUM, D. (1990) *The Social Production of Merit*, London: Falmer.

MINSON, J. (1985) *Genealogy of Morals: Nietzsche, Foucault, Donzelot and the Eccentricity of Ethics*, New York: St Martin's Press.

RICHMOND, M. (1917) *Social Diagnosis*, New York: Russell Sage.

ROSE, N. (1985) *The Psychological Complex: Psychology, Politics and Society in England 1869–1939*, London: Routledge and Kegan Paul.

ROSE, N. (1990) *Governing the Soul: The Shaping of the Private Self*, London: Routledge.

ROSE, N. (1996) *Inventing Ourselves: Psychology, Power and Personhood*, Cambridge: Cambridge University Press.

SEMMEL, R. (1960) *Imperialism and Social Reform: English Social-Imperial Thought 1895–1914*, London: Allen and Unwin.

TYLER, D. (1997) 'At risk of maladjustment: the problem of child mental health', in PETERSEN, A. and BUNTON, R. (Eds) *Foucault, Health and Medicine*, London: Routledge.

WEEKS, J. (1985) 'The population question in the early twentieth century', in BEECHEY, V. and DONALD, J. (Eds) *Subjectivity and Social Relations*, Milton Keynes: Open University Press.

YOUNGHUSBAND, E. (1964) *Social Work and Social Change*, London: Allen and Unwin.

Chapter 5

Project 2000 and the Nature of Nursing Knowledge

Liz Meerabeau

Introduction

In this chapter I shall discuss the reforms of pre-registration nursing education in the UK, generally known as Project 2000, and the debates that the reforms have given rise to within nursing, before going on to examine how these debates illuminate the nature of nursing knowledge. It is easy to forget how recent the move of nursing into higher education is; although there have been degrees in nursing in the UK for over 30 years, they were very much in the minority, and most of nursing education has moved only in the last five years. At the same time, higher education has changed, with an increase in the age participation rate, and the abolition of the binary divide between the universities and the polytechnics (although in many ways the divide remains, demonstrated by the differential in resources between the 'old' and 'new' universities, and the alliances formed within the Committee of Vice Chancellors and Principals, the so-called 'Russell Group' of elite universities). At the time of writing, the report of the Dearing Committee on higher education (NCIHE, 1997) has just been published. Major discussion so far has been on the recommendation that students should pay tuition fees, and the government's plan to replace means-tested maintenance grants with loans. There are concerns about the level of graduate debt this may lead to, and whether this will adversely affect recruitment to degrees in nursing, particularly for mature students. Nursing unions are pressing for the extension of bursaries (currently restricted to diploma students) to cover degree students and thereby mitigate the effect.

Clinical nursing has been squeezed by the introduction of general management in the mid-1980s, and the internal market in the 1990s; it seems likely that at least some of the features of the internal market in health care will disappear with the change in government, but the potential effects on nursing education are not clear. This chapter examines the interaction between two occupations, that of the nurse, and that of the university lecturer. It is debatable whether the latter is a distinct occupation (that of the 'don', to use rather antiquated language) or whether the primary identity of the university lecturer, particularly in vocational courses, derives from the discipline which they teach. In academic nursing there is an interaction between an occupation – nursing – which is largely female, and university teaching, which is heavily dominated by men in senior positions (Swain, 1997).

Occupational Socialization

There are several sociological studies in the UK of the process by which students become practitioners in nursing (e.g. Melia, 1987; Smith, 1992) but they predate the educational reforms. Broadly speaking, there are two analytic approaches to occupational socialization:

1 the induction approach, which derives from functionalism, focuses on the acquisition of professional roles, but takes motivation for granted and neglects the expectations which individuals bring with them. This approach also sees the training institution as a subsystem of the larger occupational system, and assumes a continuity of norms between the two;
2 the reaction approach, which analyzes how students react to their educational experiences, explores their motivation, and regards the training institution as an independent social unit.

A key theme in both the sociological and educational writing on nurse training prior to the reforms was the theory–practice gap, indicating a disjunction between what was taught in school and what was practised on the wards – in particular that care on the latter was routinized and not patient-centred. Reducing the theory–practice gap was one of the rationales behind the reforms. It is also worth noting, however, that preparatory socialization is important in general nursing (if less so in the other branches), since nursing is a highly visible occupation to which many small girls aspire. One of the themes which recurs in the ongoing debates on nursing education in the nursing press is that preparatory socialization is currently discrepant with the reality, and that students are disconcerted to find themselves in the lecture room or out 'in the community' rather than on a ward taking blood pressures.

The Process of Education Reform

Prior to 1989, when the first pilot schemes for the reforms were introduced, 98 per cent of nursing education took place within schools of nursing (Royal College of Nursing, 1985). These were usually in the grounds of a training hospital and were managed by Directors of Nursing Education who were generally accountable to the management of the District Health Authority, the health care provider, and students were employees of the District Health Authority. The different types of nurses – general nurses, mental nurses, children's nurses and mental handicap (now learning disabilities) nurses – trained separately. Intakes took place several times a year, as frequently as six times a year in some schools offering RGN training. The major part of the three-year programme took place on the wards; apart from a six-week introductory block, sessions in the school were generally confined to one week before, and one week after, a placement, and did not make great intellectual demands since in the latter, students were recuperating from about eight weeks of shift work. Summative assessment was by means of a national examination until the late 1980s, and the nursing qualification did not have any academic currency.

Enrolled nurses constituted about 85,000 of the 280,000 nurses employed by the NHS in 1987 (Humphreys, 1996). They had a two-year, largely practically-based, training period, with poor career prospects, since they could not progress beyond the status of senior enrolled nurse. The degree of autonomy they were allowed varied, largely depending on whether there were registered nurses on duty, and the UKCC (1986) concluded that they were both 'misused' and 'abused'.

Few nurse tutors had a degree; their preparation usually consisted of several years of nursing experience after registration, plus a postgraduate certificate in adult education. The UKCC (1986) summarized what it saw as the deficiencies of this approach: the constant grind of up to six intakes a year; repeated teaching with no time for research or professional development; and the need to make educational compromises to make sure the wards were staffed.

In 1985 there were also 22 degrees in nursing based in the universities and polytechnics, representing about 2 per cent of students (Royal College of Nursing, 1985). The development of degree level programmes in nursing is reviewed by Bedford *et al.* (1995). The first UK programme was validated at Edinburgh in 1960, followed by Manchester and Surrey. There were variations in the nature of the degrees offered, and in the extent to which the content of the degree was linked in to nursing (in my own, the degree was almost entirely separate from the nursing experience, which was undertaken in two large blocks). Undergraduate students were reported to feel markedly different from other student nurses (e.g. Luker,

1984) although evaluation of how they did actually differ from 'traditionally' trained nurses in their practice was sparse (Bircumshaw and Chapman, 1988), apart from follow-up studies to see in what areas they practised after qualification (e.g. Kemp, 1990).

The training system of the majority of nurses was criticized for many years. As Davies (1985) points out, the history of nursing was littered with reports on education, with little action, but considerable jockeying for power between the Ministry of Health (later Department of Health and Social Security, then Department of Health), the main professional body (the Royal College of Nursing) and the statutory body (the General Nursing Council, later the United Kingdom Central Council for Nursing, Midwifery and Health Visiting and the National Boards for Nursing, Midwifery and Health Visiting). White (1985) attributes the lack of progress in nursing education to the conflict between three main interest groups in nursing: generalists – the 'rank and file' who maintain that nursing is a practical occupation; specialists/professionalizers; and managers, including policy makers and civil servants. This has led to tensions between the Royal College of Nursing, the statutory bodies and government. For example, following mounting discontent, the RCN produced the Platt Report in 1964, drawing an angry riposte from the General Nursing Council (GNC, 1965). Platt was largely ignored by the Ministry, which was preoccupied with the Salmon enquiry on nursing management (Ministry of Health, 1966). The Briggs Report (DHSS, 1972) recommended a new statutory structure for nursing, midwifery and health visiting, and educational preparation with a single point of entry followed by specialization, but only the former was acted upon, by 1979 legislation which came into full operation in 1983. Both shadow bodies (the UKCC and the national boards) produced papers on nurse education in 1982, but they were not acted upon. Even when the elected bodies were in place, the way forward for educational reform was not easy to see. In 1984, the UKCC in agreement with the National Boards produced a five-year plan, one objective of which was to produce an education policy for preparing nurses, midwives and health visitors to meet the needs of society in the 1990s and beyond. A working group was set up which eventually became Project 2000. The Royal College of Nursing, meanwhile, impatient with gradualism, set up its own commission (Royal College of Nursing, 1985). This argued for the wholesale move of nursing education into higher education, supernumerary status for students, a broader-based common core curriculum, and a simpler pattern of qualifications. At the same time, the English Nursing Board produced a similar strategic document to the UKCC (English Nursing Board, 1985) giving some concern that it was trying to exceed its remit. As Lathlean (1989, p. 7) comments, 'it seemed to some of those involved that an enormous number of red herrings were being raised'. The UKCC Project Group for Project 2000 used the evidence amassed by both the English Nursing Board and Royal College of

Nursing, which included work produced by the Institute of Manpower Studies at Sussex and the Centre for Health Economics at York. The UKCC report was published in May 1986 for consultation; the reforms included:

- a move to one level of training (with cessation of second level enrolled nurse training);
- supernumerary status for students, who would receive a bursary rather than a grant; the workforce contribution previously made by students would be partly met by support workers;
- conjoint professional and academic validation of courses providing both eligibility to register and a recognized academic award (Diploma in Higher Education);
- a broadly-based common foundation programme for all students (including, originally, midwives) followed by 18 months' specialization;
- links with higher education;
- a curriculum which focused on health promotion as well as care of the sick, and placements which would equip diplomates to work both in hospital and in the community on qualification.

There was general agreement, but the unions were not happy about the cessation of enrolled nurse training, the RMNs did not want the gains of their 1982 syllabus to be lost, the RMHNs thought their role was narrowly conceptualized, and the midwives found much of it unacceptable. The report was eventually agreed in January 1987, the Boards signed up to it, and it was presented to the four UK Health Departments in February 1987. These then consulted with the NHS, other government departments (principally the Department of Education and Science, now the Department for Education and Employment), and the Treasury. Many doctors criticized the proposals and lobbied against them, and there were concerns as to how much the reforms would cost. The Ministerial announcement was made by the Secretary of State, John Moore, at the RCN Congress in May 1988; the broad thrust was accepted, but further work was needed on the support worker role, and the discontinuation of enrolled nurse training was delayed. The Secretary of State's response (DHSS, 1988a) and the NHS Management Board (DHSS, 1988b) were not prescriptive about the links with higher education, but envisaged links with one or two named institutions, and possibly some provision of 'theoretical instruction' in higher education.

Lathlean (1989) also examines the local policy-making machinery, both at regional and district level. What is striking retrospectively is the variability and, in some instances, the lack of machinery for implementing changes, and the varied range of advice given by the 'inspectors' from the English Nursing Board. Lathlean (1989, p. 19) questions why at that stage implementation was only partial, and concludes that 'The drive for efficiency and effectiveness in public services gave supremacy to the wishes of the Treasury over the desires of other agencies and ministries'. Increased costs included the estimated greater cost of tuition, and replacement costs for students who were no longer part of the workforce, totalling £32m at 1982/3 prices (Goodwin and Bosanquet, 1986). £580m was subsequently committed for the introduction of Project 2000 over ten years.

Humphreys (1996) argues that in the last decade there have been two distinct but interacting policy processes in non-medical education and training (the phrase used by the NHS Executive). In retrospect the adoption of Project 2000 can be seen as the high point of professional influence on nursing education. It raised the level of training to diploma level, thereby giving it academic currency, and distancing it from service priorities. The profession could now reinforce its core values, extend into new skills, and shed some of its unskilled work. Professionalization theory provides a plausible explanation for many of the Project 2000 proposals (Cox, 1992), but Project 2000 was a threat to the large numbers of 'traditionally' trained nurses, and also to enrolled nurses. As might be expected, the unions which represented enrolled nurses – COHSE and NUPE (now Unison) – had more mixed views on Project 2000 than the Royal College of Nursing.

As Humphreys (1996) states, one of the remarkable aspects of Project 2000 is the way that it was adopted by a Conservative government which generally seemed set on eroding the power of the professions. One factor was the concerns about workforce supply and retention, the so-called 'demographic time bomb', which established that there would be insufficient numbers of 18-year-olds with sufficient educational preparation to recruit into nursing to replace the high number of leavers (30,000 in 1987). Nursing shortages have remained a politically sensitive issue. One argument commonly used (although not very well supported by evidence) was that, if the educational preparation were a more enjoyable experience, more newly-qualified nurses would see themselves as standing on the threshold of their career, rather than leaving after three years' work as an apprentice. However, a (cheaper) government solution to the problem could have been reducing the entry qualifications to nursing (Salvage, 1988). Humphreys (1996) identifies the overlapping membership of the UKCC and the National Boards, and their access to the Department of Health, as important factors in achieving cohesive support for the reforms, whereas the opposition such as COHSE did not have this access. The Royal College of Nursing, although a trade union, is also a professional body, and is often an important ally for the nursing group within the Department of Health in implementing professional developments. Unlike the other nursing unions, the RCN Congress is secondary in policy formation to its Council, thus disadvantaging those outside the nursing 'establishment' who might oppose Project 2000.

Purchasing Education

After Project 2000 had been agreed, the periodic review of the UKCC and the National Boards took place, undertaken by the management consultants, Peat Marwick McLintock (1989). The report criticized the arrangement for funding Schools of Nursing, since the Boards paid the salaries of teaching staff for preregistration courses, whereas the DHAs employed them and also paid the salaries of staff on postregistration courses, plus indirect costs such as buildings. Financial and managerial lines of accountability were therefore confused. The recommendation was that the Boards should take over the management of the Schools of Nursing, which would therefore break their links with the NHS. However, as the review was being undertaken, the climate was profoundly altered by the publication in January 1989 of the White Paper, *Working for Patients* (Department of Health, 1989a), which established the internal market in the NHS. Under the provisions of the NHS and Community Care Act of 1990 which arose from the White Paper, providers of health care became independent from the District Health Authorities in four waves of NHS trusts, and the DHAs became purchasers of health care from the trusts, together with fundholding GPs. If DHAs had continued to fund nurse education, trusts would have been in the peculiar position of obtaining education from the organizations which purchased health care from them, and this would have considerably distorted the market principle. Working Paper 10: *Education and Training* (Department of Health, 1989b) appeared two months after the PMM report, with a radically different solution. Regional Health Authorities, in consultation with employers, would have the main funding role in nurse education, shifting the balance of control back to the employers. By early 1992, the PMM option of National Board ownership of schools had been rejected, continued ownership by the District Health Authorities was seen as untenable, and independent status looked unlikely, partly because the annual financial turnover was not great enough for most schools to be viable; higher education increasingly looked like the preferred setting. Over three years, the market arrangement emerged, rather than being planned *ab initio* (Humphreys, 1996). Humphreys argues that the main purpose of Working Paper 10 was not to establish overall arrangements for nursing and midwifery education, but to ensure that education costs did not corrupt the market mechanism for health care provision, an argument similar to that used later for separating out research costs (Culyer, 1994). A subsequent review of the NHS, set up in 1993, recommended the amalgamation of some Regional Health Authorities – a reduction from 14 to 8 – and their subsequent abolition and replacement by Regional Offices which would be part of the NHS Executive. Education purchasing would be undertaken by consortia of NHS trusts. This got underway in April 1996; the consortia are currently guided by Regional Education Development Groups, but the intention is that purchasing of nursing and midwifery education should devolve completely to the consortia once they have 'matured' as purchasers, it is hoped in April 1998. Their functions include collating workforce plans and estimating the need for newly trained staff, and, increasingly, individual trusts are also grappling with changes in health care provision, changing professional roles, and the implications of these for education purchasing, particularly in postregistration education.

As Humphreys (1996) states, it is arguable that there are no precedents in the field of mainstream education for the direct influence which employers now have over the universities in this area. Humphreys (1996) claims that nursing education is a hybrid, lying somewhere between conventional professional education and high-level, in-house training such as that for commercial pilots, whereas, in other countries such as Australia, when nurse education was transferred to the universities, the funding was transferred across as well. There is a quasi-market in the UK, since the purchaser is not the recipient (Le Grand and Bartlett, 1993); it is complicated by local purchasers being involved, and the extent to which they act as informed purchasers – not to mention their level of machismo – probably varies widely. Their influence is considerable, and there has been considerable debate as to whether the educational reforms have produced nurses who are appropriately skilled; the 'fitness for purpose' of Project 2000 diplomates has become a frequently-used phrase. In my own region, biannual meetings with the trusts take place, in which a detailed questionnaire designed by the regional office is completed, rating the responsiveness of the education provider. To use White's (1985) terms referred to earlier, the balance of power between professionalizers in higher education and managers shifted with the implementation of Project 2000, and is shifting back again; it is not, however, a return to the *status quo*, since the managers are themselves more likely to be graduates than at any other time in nursing.

Implementation of Project 2000

As has already been discussed, the implementation of Project 2000 involved a wide range of competing interest groups, and a tight timescale. In England implementation in the first demonstration sites took place while the links with universities and polytechnics were still somewhat tenuous. An evaluation of the implementation of Project 2000 in England was commissioned by the Department of Health (Jowett *et al.*, 1994) mainly using case studies of 6 of the 13 demonstration districts. Although the findings were generally positive, nurse teachers were put under great pressure to develop and deliver the courses at the same time as they themselves were being expected to acquire academic qualifications, and there were upheavals as clinical managers organized replacement for the students, sometimes with overreliance on bank and agency staff. The question of who would teach the students in the clinical areas remained unresolved; in practice teaching was generally undertaken by clinical staff, some of whom had not been well prepared for Project 2000 and had reservations about it. This was made more difficult by the removal of several tiers of senior nurses in the Griffiths reforms, so that in many settings there was now no intermediary between the 'ward manager' and the Nurse Executive Director. The course was over-taught and over-assessed, and the initial 18-month Common Foundation Programme was seen to be dominated by adult nursing. There were reservations about whether the trusts were taking account of the three-year lead time in forecasting numbers, and whether the needs of the private sector were being taken into account (National Audit Office, 1992). Many of those interviewed saw an unwelcome future in terms of a highly educated but dwindling cadre of registered nurses becoming the managers of care delivered by support staff.

Two-thirds of the 77 Welsh managers interviewed for a study on the service perspective (Nursing Research Unit, 1994) were uncertain of the benefits of Project 2000 and felt that they did not know enough about it (implementation in Wales occurred several years after England). A diary and questionnaire study of both 'traditional' and Project 2000 students in Northern Ireland, which also implemented it after England (O'Neill *et al.*, 1993) found that the latter students were less dismissive of the relevance of their curriculum and were socialized into nursing on the wards more slowly. They took a more optimistic view than the 'traditional' students of the capacity of their training to prepare them for a life in nursing, and were less prone to consider leaving, although assessment was causing them some anxiety.

McIntosh *et al.* (1997) evaluated the implementation of Project 2000 in Scotland, which was the only one of the four countries to implement new programmes simultaneously in all of its 12 colleges. Methods included non-participant observation in the colleges, interviews and documentary analysis, and detailed case studies of six of the colleges. As in England, there was some confusion about the level of diploma study, and some students felt inadequately prepared to deal with ill-health in their clinical placements because of the health orientation of the curriculum. There was a lack of support in the clinical environment, and the range of placements was affected by ward closures. However, McIntosh *et al.* conclude that, if the students are able to retain their sense of difference and combine it with assertiveness, they may foster a new culture. Veitch *et al.* (1997) in a paper from the same evaluation claim that the reforms to health care delivery have frustrated many of the aims of the educational reforms, such as holistic, patient-centred care.

Elkan and Robinson (1995) reviewed the findings of all the English studies to date: all were fairly small-scale and had concentrated on the 13 demonstration districts and the earlier cohorts. Common findings included the speed of implementation, problems finding clinical placements and supervision, and more reliance on the goodwill of the service (one virtue of several intakes a year was that each individual intake was considerably smaller). There was uncertainty about what constituted diploma-level work and whether some students could manage it in view of the wide range of entry qualifications, as well as struggles by students to find relevance and coherence in the Common Foundation Programme. There was felt to be an overemphasis on adult nursing, and suspicion that the course might be a precursor to a generic training, as occurs in the United States. There was confusion over the role of the nurse teacher in the practice setting. The early stages of the links with higher education were 'fraught with difficulties' and mutual misunderstandings, but more substantial links led to greater satisfaction. Several of the problems were not new – for example, the so-called theory practice gap, and other vocational courses, such as teaching and social work, face similar issues about whether the employment focus leads to employment domination of the curriculum.

Hallett (1997) discusses the implementation of the community-based aspect of the course, drawing on data from an English Nursing Board-commissioned study (Orr and Hallett, 1991; Hallett *et al.*, 1992; 1993). Community managers faced sometimes conflicting pressures, between the needs of the students, their own staff, and clients, at a time when the services were being restructured.

Maben and Macleod Clark (1996 a and b) discuss the transition from student to staff nurse, and the extent to which new diplomates were supported on the wards. They were prepared to ask when they did not know something, but this was perceived by some staff as showing a lack of confidence; it may be necessary to reconsider what is expected of a new staff nurse.

Luker *et al.* (1995) studied a random sample of 267 nurse teachers and 56 midwifery teachers, plus clinicians, using a case study of one college, a modified Delphi study and telephone interviews. It was seen as probable that other lecturers would teach the 'ologies', while nurse teachers would teach nursing theory and practice. Most did not engage in clinical practice on a regular basis. They foresaw increased travel between sites, fewer opportunities for promotion as the result of amalgamations, and the possibility of redundancies, but also access to increased expertise as the result of the move into higher education. Nearly half thought that they would not be given equal academic status to other higher education lecturers, and that research and publication might not be realistic expectations.

In the case study, site staff were given the choice of whether to stay on health service contracts, which had better pensions and redundancy terms, but less favourable holidays and working hours. Full relocation into higher education was not regarded favourably, and, where nursing education was on the main university site, it was often peripheral and the students did not mix with other students. Staff felt that the larger groups had reduced their opportunities for close contact with the students, although other research has indicated that nurse teachers were not viewed by students as the influential figures they believed themselves to be (French, 1992). A more coherent strategy for pastoral support and joint workshops on teaching larger groups were needed. Luker *et al.* (1995) suggest that the requirement that nurse teachers have a teaching qualification should be relaxed, since it might lead to a loss of clinical skills; however, this does not seem likely in view of the current pressures for all new higher education teachers to be accredited in 'professional achievement in the management of learning and teaching', a recommendation of the Dearing enquiry (NCIHE, 1997).

B. Everett, a regional assistant general secretary of the Association of University Teachers, commented in 1995 on the integration of the North Trent College of Nursing and Midwifery into Sheffield University that the new lecturers were experienced teachers, but many had no experience of research, and no requirement in their university contract that they should undertake it, drawing a riposte from the subdean that they were not as ill-prepared as he stated (Roberts-Davies, 1995). B. Banks, a professor of physiology at University College, London, claimed in 1994 that nurse teachers were deficient in their knowledge of the biological sciences, and contrasted the position of the full-time student taught by highly-qualified staff with the holder of a 'degree in nursing picked up by part-time study under traditional nurse teachers'. T. Bunnell, a biology lecturer, in 1994 highlighted the variability in the students' background knowledge.

Elkan *et al.* (1993, 1994) evaluated the implementation of Project 2000 in one district. They drew particular attention to the effects on the service of the withdrawal of student labour, which the Department of Health funding formula had not adequately replaced, leading to a more 'bottom heavy' skill-mix and a more routinized approach to care. Students' opinions varied on the relevance of the subjects they were being taught. Some found the social sciences less relevant, others the biological (and also found them anxiety-provoking). As Elkan *et al.* (1993) point out, such differences are related to the nature of nursing itself, and whether it is viewed as an art or a craft. Similarly, there were differences between the educationalists and the clinical staff as to the relative weighting of communication skills and practical skills. Elkan *et al.* (1993) comment that, although education staff tend to subscribe to holistic models of care, in practice physical care-giving has been relegated to a subordinate position. Many students, particularly the younger ones, had difficulty with self-directed learning, and said they did not know what they had to learn. While educationalists increasingly favour student-centred learning, there have been few studies of students' views, apart from Burnard and Morrison (1991) who found that students preferred a more structured, teacher-centred approach. The average level of qualifications of entrants fell slightly during the implementation of Project 2000, and as a result many students struggled with the course. Of those who entered with the DC test (for students without the minimum 'O' levels or GCSEs), 44 per cent were referred in their exam in the site studied by Elkan *et al.* (1993), compared with 27 per cent of those who had at least five 'O' levels. There was thought to be an overemphasis on the adult branch (although ironically adult branch students also complained more, perhaps because they had the clearest ideas of what they thought nursing was about). There were disparaging remarks from ward staff, who with the removal of student labour were under greater pressure.

Bedford *et al.* (1995) illustrate similar pressures in delivering nursing degrees in England (many nursing lecturers teach on both). An expansion of undergraduate programmes was recommended in 1988 by the University Grants Committee Panel on Studies Allied to Medicine (English Nursing Board, 1993). The Polytechnics and Colleges Funding Council also supported growth, but recommended a reduction in length from four to three years. An advisory group concluded that such degrees could be developed without loss of quality, provided that institutions 'responded imaginatively'. Bedford *et al.* (1995) explore the experiences of delivering preregistration degree programmes in nursing and midwifery and the pressures of the market (although degrees are funded by HEFCE, not through consortium purchasing). Pressures included the trauma of mergers, the poor showing of nursing in the 1992 Research Assessment Exercise, the pressure of 45-week academic years, and staff who were themselves undertaking degrees. There were competing demands on students and restrictions on participation in student activities; many students also had family commitments. Bedford *et al.* concluded that stress was endemic, and lecturers who were themselves overstretched had to support the students. They also refer to managers' expectations of the new graduate, and conclude that nursing and midwifery are in a position to make a major contribution to the general debate concerning professionality and the role of universities in delivering undergraduate programmes for a profession.

Jowett (1996) draws on the four-year evaluation of the Project 2000 reforms commissioned by the Department of Health, to reflect on current dilemmas in both vocational and higher education, including course content, delivery, the extent to which critical thought can be developed in a course which aims to produce 'appropriate' professional attitudes, and the difficulties of achieving widespread normative changes. The major points that she raises are:

- the disjunction between the health-promoting philosophy of Project 2000 and the vocationalism that students bring to the course, which at least for general nurses has been shaped by a lay view of what nursing is about;
- the negligible absorption of students into the HE environment;
- standard course delivery, for a heterogeneous student population;
- confusion between developing potential and vocational preparation;
- students being seen as the personification of the new course, and having to deal with their own anxieties at the same time as presenting a positive view of their course.

She refers to the 'internally condemning stance' which frequently occurs in the nursing literature, (e.g. French, 1989) which often seems unaware that the dilemmas and problems experienced are inherent in vocational education. For example, in both architecture and law (Argyris and Schon, 1977) students became competent professionals after graduation, not before, and the expectations of new nursing diplomates may not, therefore, be realistic. Roberts and Higgins' (1992) large-scale survey of HE institutions found that many students felt ill-prepared in terms of study skills, and modular courses were often seen as poorly co-ordinated. Roizen and Jepson's (1985) study of engineering referred to the 'see-saw' production from graduates who lacked theory to those who were seen as overly academic. Warren Piper (1984) referred to the trend towards 'academicization' in vocational education, whereby emphasis gets placed on high-status, abstract parts of the syllabus, often to the detriment of competent professional practice.

Changes in Higher Education

Higher education has become the centre for the production of professional knowledge (Larson, 1977). House (1993) claims that the split between theory and practice becomes more pronounced as the professional field develops, but as Bedford *et al.* (1995) point out, there is a countervailing pull away from universities as centres of advanced knowledge production, with the growth of knowledge creation in large businesses and electronic media. Barnett, Becher and Cork (1987) refer to the triangular relationship between academics, practitioners and students; Bedford *et al.* (1995) argue that it is now a polygon, as practitioners become absorbed into market structures, and the locus of knowledge creation changes.

In addition, in the last fifteen years, public sector institutions in the UK, such as universities, have undergone great pressures on their resources and have taken on some of the features of the private sector. This shift has occurred to varying degrees in different settings, depending on the extent to which professional groups are able to resist change, and how much of a unified 'production process' and 'product' there is (e.g. Tuckman and Blackburn, 1991). Pollitt (1990) concluded that there was little evidence of cultural change in the public sector, but that there was demoralization and 'pragmatic acquiescence' to the concepts of the private sector. The government cuts of 1981 heralded a new era of external regulation for the universities – for example, the Leverhulme Report (1983) and later, the Research Assessment exercise and the Teaching Quality Assessment, downward pressure on resources, greater student choice but expectation that in future more of the costs of higher education will be borne by the individual, better visibility of institutional performance, mass participation, and questioning of the single subject degree (HEQC, 1994). There have been complaints from the business community about how higher education in general meets its needs, and debates about whether the economy requires so many graduates (Baty, 1997; Harvey *et al.*, 1997). Barnett (1995), commenting on the National Council for Vocational Qualifications' consultation paper, *GNVQs at Higher Levels*, sees it as an attempt by the state to set a national curriculum for higher education. There is also an emphasis on predefined behavioural competences and occupational standards, which could be seen as an attempt to reduce indeterminacy and professional artistry.

The management structure of universities (particularly the old universities) has not been conducive to change, with its diffuse authority, weakly defined offices and heads of departments who are primarily academics and only secondarily, and often reluctantly, managers (e.g. Becher, 1987). Harrow and Willcocks (1990) state that managers are more constrained in the public sector than in the private, and the influence of stakeholders is more complex. Kouzes and Mico (1979) used the framework of domain theory to explore what they saw as inevitable conflicts in public sector organizations between the domains of policy, management and service. Raelin (1991) claims that culture clashes between professionals and their managers will be inevitable, since the former have external loyalties to their disciplinary network, whereas the latter are loyal to the organization; professional middle managers may help to bridge the gap. Mintzberg (1983) argues that many professionals used to work in professional bureaucracies, in which the influence of managers was limited, whereas they now work in what Mintzberg terms 'dominated meritocracies'. In the dominated meritocracy, the organization becomes split between the professional operators and junior managers on one hand, and the government, technostructure and senior management on the other. Mintzberg sees this model as dysfunctional and conflict-ridden, and concludes that there is a danger that professional artistry will be lost. Nursing lecturers, therefore, have moved from a situation in the schools of nursing in which they were part of a management hierarchy, to universities, which have (in theory at least) been collegial, but are becoming more managerial.

Creating an Academic Discipline

The creation of an academic community is dependent on the interrelationship between epistemological factors (the nature of the knowledge base) and social factors (the creation of academic networks and communities). Here the emphasis will be on the latter, although the two cannot be separated. There is, for example, an ongoing debate in nursing about the teaching of contributory subjects such as sociology in the nursing curriculum, in which it is likely that questions of how knowledge is used in professional practice (Eraut, 1985; Eraut *et al.*, 1995; Bedford *et al.*, 1995) are intertwined with issues about the status of nursing lecturers *vis-à-vis* other more established lecturers, and the defence of jobs.

Cooke (1993) discusses the creation of nursing as an academic subject, drawing on Bernstein's (1971) distinction between collection codes (which involve strong boundaries between subjects) and integrated codes (which imply weak boundaries), and concentrating on a survey of nursing colleges' use of sociology in the curriculum. Boundary closure stakes out a subject's territory and lays claim to the resources that go with it; claims to the label 'scientific' are particularly useful for raising status (Fisher, 1990), and reinforcing the precarious status of nursing knowledge as it tries to establish its identity distinct from biomedicine. However, the argument is a complex one. Webb (1981) argued that the introduction of the nursing process required greater synthesis in the curriculum, and that this required greater sophistication than in the traditional model, in which, much as in a junior school, a tutor covered much of the curriculum for his or her set. Cooke (1993), like Bernstein, links the development of the integrated curriculum, with its blurred boundaries, to the greater distancing of the middle class from the means of production, and argues that nurse teachers have more control over their working lives than clinicians and are, therefore, more like the 'new middle class'. However, although this is not fully developed in the paper, the integrated curriculum blurs the distinctive contribution of the disciplines, and is not high-status knowledge academically.

Parry *et al.* (1994), in a book discussing postgraduate education and training in the social sciences, also draw on Bernstein to discuss the specific cases of social anthropology, development studies, urban studies and town planning. The last three of these are termed by Parry *et al.* 'secondary disciplines', since they are multidisciplinary; however, academics in both urban studies and development studies had a strong disciplinary identity, since all came from single disciplines. Town planning did not, which Parry *et al.* attribute to its strong vocational element, and the policy-led nature of its research. Doctoral candidates who had undertaken multidisciplinary first degrees (as in nursing), or who wished to change subjects, were perceived as a problem, since in the words of one supervisor, they were 'too far from the frontier' to make a serious contribution. Hill *et al.* (1994) in the same volume compare psychology and education students; while the former were training to be future academics, education students were interested in a problem, not in an academic career, and were more likely to be part-time students.

Robinson (1991) examines the relationship between medicine and nursing in higher education, in particular the difficulty of developing the formal knowledge base for emotional labour, which is central to nursing. Orr (1997) explores her position as a nursing academic, and refers to the devaluing of practice disciplines, but also to nursing's anti-intellectualism. Wise (1997), in the same volume, reflects on academic social work and its low status, concluding that it is hard to feel that social work academics are taken seriously, because 'I do not have the option of an ivory tower existence, since my work has a grounded instrumentality' (1997, p. 124), and abstract knowledge has greater status.

There are some parallels between the position of nursing in academe, and that of business studies (although they should not be overstated). Bain (1990), the principal of London Business School, quotes a professor of English who considered that business studies was 'educationally suspect' because it was not a discipline, but 'an agglomeration of various subjects', did not have much to do with 'the disinterested pursuit of knowledge' and, because of its size and close links to industry, could be a 'Trojan horse' in the university. Bain concludes that many university subjects have similar characteristics, and that Cardinal Newman's idea of a university as a unified community of scholars is seldom realized in modern universities. Business and management may, he argues, be singled out for disparagement because they are relative newcomers:

> the history of universities is to some extent a history of the struggle of new disciplines and fields to win acceptance, with each of them, like each group of immigrants to the new world, tending to look down on those that come later. (Bain, 1990, p. 13)

In business studies there may also be an element of the genteel poor looking with disdain at the nouveaux riches, less applicable in nursing (although Banks (1994) notes somewhat testily that nurse teachers are 'much better paid' than university teachers). Bain also identifies a tension between the academic and vocational models within the business faculty, as did Simon (1969) and Schon (1988). The primary objective of those pursuing the academic model is the discovery of new knowledge through research, and their primary reference group is other academics; the primary objective of those pursuing the vocational model is the teaching of current best practice, and their primary reference group is practitioners. Currently, the latter orientation predominates in business schools. Simon and Schon had differing solutions, since the former proposed a 'rigorously scientific' approach, whereas the latter, in what has now become a very overused metaphor in nursing, advocated exploring the 'swampy lowlands' of actual practice. Like nursing, management departments performed poorly in the 1992 Research Assessment Exercise; as a result, the Economic and Social Research Council set up a commission on management research, chaired by George Bain. The report called for more funding to create time for research, and for improved communication between researchers and the user community. Best and Brook (1993) criticize the commission's failure to examine epistemological issues in management research, and its call to set an agenda of priorities for research. More generally, they present a critique of the transformation of the 'craft' of management into a scientific (quantitative) profession (Whitley, 1992), and of the tendency to pursue research problems as defined by business, and short projects which provide pragmatic solutions, with the consequence that researchers do not address fundamental issues such as the nature of management. The dominant role of business interests also limits the extent to which academic institutions control the definition and assessment of managerial skills (Whitley, 1992).

Becher (1990) compares higher education for pharmacy, education, and (pre-Project 2000) nursing. Compared to medicine, lecturers in the latter had peer networks largely confined to nursing, and were stretched between academic and professional demands. Establishment figures in academic nursing were called upon to serve on statutory bodies, thus reducing the time they had available for research, but nursing departments were also seen as aloof and elitist. They considered the majority of practising nurses to be underqualified; Becher (1990, p. 140) suggests that they could be portrayed as 'colonialists, regarding the native population with some contempt . . . and endeavouring to superimpose their own norms and values'. At that time, nursing lecturers on degree courses, unlike those on the diploma courses now, taught the learners on the wards; theoretical knowledge was heavily practice-oriented, but 'the practice of an idealized professional world'. Becher (1990) claims that, whereas pharmacy theory was middle range, nursing theory was mainly low-level generalizations (models, taxonomies and procedural rules) derived from practice. Education theory, like nursing theory, derived from reflective practice, but at a higher level.

There are several competing drivers in the development of nursing knowledge. In the 1970s and early 1980s, nursing writers in the UK (e.g.

Macleod Clark and Hockey, 1981) argued that nurses should be able to defend decisions on a scientific rather than an intuitive basis; since then intuition and professional artistry have been reclaimed and revalorized (e.g. Benner and Wrubel, 1989), drawing heavily on US and Australian work. Hagell (1989) uses sociological and feminist theory to argue that nursing has a distinct knowledge base which is not grounded in empirico-analytic science, but which stems from the lived experience of nurses as women, and their involvement in caring relationships with their clients. Her anxiety is that 'As nurses become more scientific they will lose what is essential to nursing, i.e. caring itself, because science cannot conceptualize caring nor can caring be measured, only experienced' (Hagell, 1989, p. 231). There has also been a reclamation of the bodily nature of much nursing activity, notably the work of Lawler (1991) on 'somology', and Savage (1995) on 'new nursing'. Dunlop (1986, p. 664) argues that some nursing theory, particularly the literature on caring, 'etherealizes' the body, and removes 'the mess and dirt of bodily life'. This literature may be seen as a way for nursing to reclaim a previously stigmatized subject (women's knowledge and work); for example, James (1992) compares domestic care work with hospice nursing. Since this work is not openly discussed, it becomes invisible, which poses problems for articulating the breadth of the nurse's role and its knowledge base (Reed and Procter, 1993).

The Department of Health, however, is promoting the concept of evidence-based medicine (*sic*), a somewhat linear model in which problems are identified, the literature searched and analyzed, preferably using techniques such as meta-analysis, and guidelines for practice are synthesized. The randomized controlled trial (RCT) is seen as the gold standard; it is not clear what space nursing has to develop a uniprofessional research agenda (Traynor and Rafferty, 1997). Many of the gatekeepers in health care – journal editors, ethical committees, and funding bodies – are perceived to have difficulties in judging the quality of research other than RCTs. Another example of a wider agenda in which nursing must find its space is the Research Assessment Exercise. Nursing came last in both the 1992 and 1996 Research Assessment Exercises, with a long tail of departments, particularly from the new universities, scoring a 1. Tierney (1994), Robinson (1993) and Smith (1994) all discuss why nursing should have performed so poorly and what the remedies may be: Robinson suggests alliances with cognate disciplines, and Tierney siting nursing departments in universities which generally perform better than the average, since there was a correlation between the nursing score and that of the host institution. It seems likely that, if there is an RAE in 2000, institutions will be very rigorous in deciding who will be allowed to enter, since the institution gains no financial benefit from a tail of low-scoring departments, and suffers damage to its reputation. This is particularly likely if Dearing's recommendation (NCIHE, 1997) is implemented, that research funding for high-quality departments should be differentiated from funding for research and scholarship to underpin teaching. Unless the financial climate in higher education changes greatly (and the indicators are that it will not), it is probable that, as predicted by Luker *et al.* (1995), only a minority of nursing lecturers will develop as researchers.

Conclusion

As someone who has been involved in Project 2000 for the past eight years, as a lecturer involved in course design and interviewed for the evaluation, as the research manager of that evaluation in the Department of Health, and now as an education manager, I find it difficult to see the wood for the trees. It is, after all, very early to tell whether the reforms will have their anticipated effects, and how nursing will evolve as an academic discipline. There are undoubted pressures in providing education which is purchased by local health care providers, rather than funded by the Department for Education and Employment, and it seems likely that academic nursing will remain heavily centred on teaching rather than research, albeit also developing scholarship and reflective practice. On the positive side, these pressures, and the crowded curriculum, do force nurse educators to examine the relevance of what they teach, and how that knowledge is used. The newness of the move, and the large scale of it, may also mean that the mechanisms of culture change are available for analysis and have not yet become submerged. Many nursing lecturers have gained their degrees as part-time, mature students, after forming their professional identity as a nurse teacher. They may therefore, in Schutzian terms, (1964) be 'strangers' and particularly aware of features of higher education which others take for granted. As Bedford *et al.* (1995) state, nursing is in the position to make a major contribution to the general debate concerning professionality and the role of the universities in delivering professional education.

References

Argyris, C. and Schon, D. (1977) *Theory in Practice – Increasing Professional Effectiveness*, San Francisco: Jossey Bass.

Bain, G. (1990) 'A vocational vortex', *The Times Higher Educational Supplement*, (23 February), p. 13.

BANKS, B. (1994) 'Failed cosmetic surgery', *The Times Higher Educational Supplement*, (18 March), p. 15.

BARNETT, J. (1995) 'HE's national curriculum', *The Times Higher Educational Supplement*, (17 November), p. 13.

BARNETT, R., BECHER, T. and CORK, N. (1987) 'Models of professional preparation: pharmacy, nursing and teacher education', *Studies in Higher Education*, **12**, pp. 56–63.

BATY, P. (1997) 'Graduates "too good for the job"', *The Times Higher Educational Supplement*, (28 March).

BECHER, T. (1987) 'Disciplinary discourse', *Studies in Higher Education*, **12**, pp. 261–74.

BECHER, T. (1990) 'Professional education in a comparative context', in TORSTENDAHL, R. and BURRAGE, M. (Eds) *The Formation of Professions*, London: Sage.

BEDFORD, H., LEAMON, J., PHILLIPS, T. and SCHOSTAK, J. (1995) *Evaluation of Pre-Registration Undergraduate Degrees in Nursing and Midwifery*, London: English National Board for Nursing, Midwifery and Health Visiting.

BENNER, P. and WRUBEL, J. (1989) *The Primacy of Caring: Stress and Coping in Health and Illness*, Menlo Park (CA): Addison Wesley.

BERNSTEIN, B. (1971) *Class Codes and Control Vol. 3: Towards a Theory of Educational Transmissions*, London: Routledge and Kegan Paul.

BEST, A. and BROOK, P. (1993) 'The politics of epistemology in management and business research', paper given at the British Sociological Association Annual Conference, Essex.

BIRCUMSHAW, D. and CHAPMAN, C. (1988) 'A study to compare the practice style of graduate and non-graduate nurses and midwives: the pilot study', *Journal of Advanced Nursing*, **13**, pp. 605–14.

BUNNELL, T. (1994) 'Learning the facts of life', *The Times Higher Educational Supplement*, (3 June), p. 13.

BURNARD, P. and MORRISON, P. (1991) 'Preferred teaching and learning strategies', *Nursing Times*, **87** (38), p. 52.

COOKE, H. (1993) 'Boundary work in the nursing curriculum: the case of sociology', *Journal of Advanced Nursing*, **18**, pp. 1990–8.

COX, D. (1992) *Working Paper 10 – Professional Education in Transition*, paper presented to the International Sociological Association Conference, *Professions in Transition*, April, Leicester.

CULYER, A. (1994) *Supporting Research and Development in the NHS*, London: HMSO.

DAVIES, C. (1985) *Policy in Nurse Education: Plus Ça Change?* Proceedings of the 19th Annual Study Day of the Nursing Studies Association, University of Edinburgh.

DEPARTMENT OF HEALTH AND SOCIAL SECURITY (1972) *Report of the Committee on Nursing*, London: HMSO.

DEPARTMENT OF HEALTH AND SOCIAL SECURITY (1988a) *Letter from the Secretary of State for Social Services to Chairman of UKCC, 20 May*, 1988, London.

DEPARTMENT OF HEALTH AND SOCIAL SECURITY (1988b) *Project 2000 Implementation, EL(88) MB/166*, London: DHSS.

DEPARTMENT OF HEALTH (1989a) *Working for Patients*, London: HMSO.

DEPARTMENT OF HEALTH (1989b) *Education and Training: Working Paper 10, Cmnd 555*. London: HMSO.

DUNLOP, M. (1986) 'Is a science of caring possible?', *Journal of Advanced Nursing*, **11**, pp. 661–70.

ELKAN, R. and ROBINSON, J. (1995) 'Project 2000: A review of published research', *Journal of Advanced Nursing*, **22**, pp. 386–92.

ELKAN, R., HILLMAN, R. and ROBINSON, J. (1993) *The Implementation of Project 2000 in a District Health Authority: The Effect on the Nursing Service*, Nottingham: University of Nottingham.

ELKAN, R., HILLMAN, R. and ROBINSON, J. (1994) 'Project 2000 and the replacement of the traditional student workforce', *Journal of Nursing Studies*, **31**, pp. 413–20.

ENGLISH NATIONAL BOARD FOR NURSING, MIDWIFERY AND HEALTH VISITING (1985) *Professional Education/Training Courses: A Consultation Paper*, London: ENB.

ENGLISH NATIONAL BOARD FOR NURSING, MIDWIFERY AND HEALTH VISITING (1993) *Three Year Undergraduate Nursing and Midwifery Courses Leading to Admission to the Professional Register*, London: ENB.

ERAUT, M. (1985) 'Knowledge creation and knowledge use in professional contexts', *Studies in Higher Education*, **10**, pp. 117–33.

ERAUT, M., ALDERTON, J., BOYLAN, A. and WRAIGHT, A. (1995) *Learning to Use Scientific Knowledge in Education and Practice Settings*, London: English National Board for Nursing, Midwifery and Health Visiting.

EVERETT, B. (1995) 'Innocents in the research jungle', *The Times Higher Educational Supplement*, (31 March).

FISHER, D. (1990) 'Boundary work and science', in COZZENS, S. and GIERYN, T. (Eds) *Theories of Science in Society*, Indianapolis: Indiana University Press.

FRENCH, P. (1989) *Educating the Nurse Practitioner: An Assessment of the Pre-registration Preparation of Nurses as an Educational Experience*, PhD Thesis, University of Durham.

FRENCH, P. (1992) 'The quality of nurse education in the 1980s', *Journal of Advanced Nursing*, **17**, pp. 619–31.

GENERAL NURSING COUNCIL FOR ENGLAND AND WALES (1965) *Platt Report on a Reform of Nursing Education: A Memorandum from the General Nursing Council for England and Wales*, London: GNC.

GOODWIN, L. and BOSANQUET, N. (1986) *Nurses and Higher Education: The Costs of Change*, York: University of York, Centre for Health Economics.

HAGELL, E. (1989) 'Nursing knowledge: women's knowledge. A sociological perspective', *Journal of Advanced Nursing*, **14**, pp. 226–33.

HALLETT, C. (1997) 'Managing change in nurse education: the introduction of Project 2000 in the community', *Journal of Advanced Nursing*, **25**, pp. 836–43.

Hallett, C., Williams, A., Butterworth, C.A. and Collister, B. (1992) *The Provision of Learning Experiences in the Community for Project 2000: Five Papers*, Manchester: University of Manchester.

Hallett, C., Williams, A., Butterworth, C.A. and Collister, B. (1993) *The Provision of Learning Experiences in the Community for Project 2000: Research Highlights*, London: English National Board for Nursing, Midwifery and Health Visiting.

Harrow, J. and Willcocks, L. (1990) 'Public service management: activities, initiatives and limits to learning', *Journal of Management Studies*, **27**, pp. 281–304.

Harvey, L., Moon, S. and Geall, V. (1997) *Graduates' Work: Organisational Change and Students' Attributes*, Birmingham: Centre for Research into Quality.

HEQC (1994) *Choosing to Change*, London: HEQC.

Hill, T., Acker, S. and Black, E. (1994) 'Research students and their supervisors in education and psychology', in Burgess, R. (Ed.) *Postgraduate Education and Training in the Social Sciences: Processes and Product*, London: Jessica Kingsley.

House, E. (1993) *Professional Evaluation: Social Impact and Political Consequences*, Newbury Park (CA): Sage.

Humphreys, J. (1996) 'English nurse education and the reform of the National Health Service', *Journal of Education Policy*, **11**, pp. 655–79.

James, N. (1992) 'Care = organization + physical labour + emotional labour', *Sociology of Health and Illness*, **14**, pp. 488–509.

Jowett, S. (1996) 'Challenges in vocational education: where does nurse education stand in the debate?', paper presented at the BERA conference, University of Lancaster, September.

Jowett, S. and Walton, I. with Payne, S. (1994) *Challenges and Change in Nurse Education – A Study of the Implementation of Project 2000*, Slough: NFER.

Kemp, J. (1990) 'Career patterns of graduates in nursing', *Nursing Standard*, **5** (4), pp. 36–9.

Kouzes, J. and Mico, P. (1979) 'Domain theory – an introduction to organizational behaviour in human service organizations', *Journal of Applied Behavioural Sciences*, **15**, pp. 449–69.

Larson, M. (1977) *The Rise of Professionalism: A Sociological Analysis*, Berkeley (CA): University of California Press.

Lathlean, J. (1989) *Policy Making in Nurse Education*, Oxford: Ashdale Press.

Lawler, J. (1991) *Behind the Screens*, Melbourne: Churchill Livingstone.

Le Grand, J. and Bartlett, W. (1993) *Quasi Markets and Social Policy*, London: Macmillan.

Leverhulme Report (1983) *Excellence in Diversity*, Guildford: SRHE.

Luker, K. (1984) 'Reading nursing: the burden of being different', *International Journal of Nursing Studies*, **21**, pp. 1–7.

Luker, K., Carlisle, C. and Kirk, S. (1995) *The Evolving Role of the Nurse Teacher in the Light of Educational Reforms*, Liverpool: University of Liverpool.

MABEN, J. and MACLEOD CLARK, J. (1996a) 'Making the transition from student to staff nurse', *Nursing Times*, **92** (44), pp. 28–31.

MABEN, J. and MACLEOD CLARK, J. (1996b) 'Preceptorship and support for staff: the good and the bad', *Nursing Times*, **92** (51), pp. 35–8.

MACLEOD CLARK, J. and HOCKEY, L. (1981) *Research for Nursing: A Guide for the Enquiring Nurse*, Chichester: Wiley.

MCINTOSH, J., ALEXANDER, M., VEITCH, L. and MAY, N. (1997) 'Evaluation of nurse and midwife education in Scotland', *Nursing Times*, **93** (19), pp. 46–7.

MELIA, K. (1987) *Learning and Working: The Occupational Socialization of Nurses*, London: Tavistock.

MINISTRY OF HEALTH (1966) *Report of the Committee on Senior Nursing Staff Structure*, London: HMSO.

MINTZBERG, H. (1983) *Power In and Around Organizations*, Englewood Cliffs (NJ): Prentice Hall.

NATIONAL AUDIT OFFICE (1992) *Nursing Education: Implementation of Project 2000 in England*, London: HMSO.

NATIONAL COMMITTEE OF INQUIRY INTO HIGHER EDUCATION (1997) *Higher Education in the Learning Society*, London: HMSO.

NURSING RESEARCH UNIT (1994) *Project 2000 Nurse Education: The Service Perspective*, Cardiff: Nursing Research Unit.

O'NEILL, E., MORRISON, H. and MCEWEN, A. (1993) *Professional Socialization and Nurse Education: An Evaluation*, Belfast: Queen's University.

ORR, J. (1997) 'Nursing the academy', in STANLEY, L. (Ed.) *Knowing Feminisms*, London: Sage.

ORR, J. and HALLETT, C. (1991) *Community Experience for Project 2000 Students: An Interim Report for the English National Board for Nursing, Midwifery and Health Visiting*, Manchester: University of Manchester.

PARRY, O., ATKINSON, P. and DELAMONT, S. (1994) 'Disciplinary identities and doctoral work', in BURGESS, R. (Ed.) *Postgraduate Education and Training in the Social Sciences: Processes and Product*, London: Jessica Kingsley.

PEAT MARWICK MCLINTOCK (1989) *Review of the United Kingdom Central Council and the Four National Boards for Nursing, Midwifery and Health Visiting*, London: Department of Health.

POLLITT, C. (1990) *Managerialism and the Public Services*, Oxford: Blackwell.

RAELIN, J. (1991) *The Clash of Cultures: Managers Managing Professionals*, Harvard: Harvard Business School Press.

REED, J. and PROCTER, S. (1993) *Nurse Education: A Reflective Approach*. London: Edward Arnold.

ROBERTS, D. and HIGGINS, T. (1992) *Higher Education: The Student Experience*, Leeds: HEIST/PCAS.

ROBERTS-DAVIES, M. (1995) 'No innocents in the jungle', *The Times Higher Educational Supplement* (7 April – letter).

ROBINSON, J. (1991) 'Educational conditioning', *Nursing Times*, **87** (10), pp. 28–31.

ROBINSON, J. (1993) 'Nursing and the research assessment exercise: What counts?', *Nurse Researcher*, **1**, pp. 84–93.

ROIZEN, J. and JEPSON, M. (1985) *Degrees for Jobs: Employer Expectations of Higher Education*, Guildford: SHRE/NFER.

ROYAL COLLEGE OF NURSING (1964) *A Reform of Nursing Education*, London: RCN.

ROYAL COLLEGE OF NURSING (1985) *The Education of Nurses: A New Dispensation*, London: RCN.

SALVAGE, J. (1988) 'Professionalization – or struggle for survival? A consideration of current proposals for nursing in the United Kingdom', *Journal of Advanced Nursing*, **13**, pp. 515–19.

SAVAGE, J. (1995) *Nursing and Intimacy*, London: Scutari.

SCHON, D. (1988) *Educating the Reflective Practitioner*, San Francisco: Jossey Bass.

SCHUTZ, A. (1964) *Collected Papers: Vol II Studies in Social Theory*, The Hague: Martinus Nijhoff.

SIMON, H. (1969) *Administrative Behavior*, New York: Macmillan.

SMITH, L. (1994) 'An analysis and reflections on the quality of nursing research in 1992', *Journal of Advanced Nursing*, **19**, pp. 385–93.

SMITH, P. (1992) *The Emotional Labour of Nursing*, London: Macmillan.

SWAIN, H. (1997) 'Females fail in power game', *The Times Higher Educational Supplement*, (25 April).

TIERNEY, A. (1994) 'An analysis of nursing's performance in the 1992 assessment of research in British universities', *Journal of Advanced Nursing*, **19**, pp. 593–602.

TRAYNOR, M. and RAFFERTY, A.M. (1997) *The NHS R&D Context for Nursing Research: A Working Paper*, London: Centre for Policy in Nursing Research.

TUCKMAN, A. and BLACKBURN, D. (1991) 'Fitness for purpose – TQM in the Health Service', paper given at the British Sociological Association Conference, Manchester.

UKCC (1986) *Project 2000: A New Preparation for Practice*, London: UKCC.

VEITCH, L., MAY, N. and MCINTOSH, J. (1997) 'The practice-based context of educational innovation: Nurse and midwife preparation in Scotland', *Journal of Advanced Nursing*, **25**, pp. 191–8.

WARREN PIPER, D. (1984) 'Sources and types of reform', in GOODLAD, S. (Ed.) *Education for the Professions*, Guildford, SRHE/NFER.

WEBB, C. (1981) 'Classification and framing: A sociological analysis of task-centred nursing and the nursing process', *Journal of Advanced Nursing*, **6**, pp. 369–76.

WHITE, R. (1985) 'Political regulators in British nursing', in WHITE, R. (Ed.) *Political Issues in Nursing: Past, Present and Future Vol. I*, Chichester: Wiley.

WHITLEY, R. (1992) *Formal Knowledge and Management Education*, Manchester Business School, Working Paper No. 236.

WISE, S. (1997) 'What are feminist academics for?', in STANLEY, L. (Ed.) *Knowing Feminisms*, London: Sage.

Chapter 6

Evidence-based Practice: a Dilemma for Health Visiting?

Kate Robinson

A millennialist age is inclined to adopt mantras, and one of the most popular amongst practitioners and managers within the UK health service is 'evidence-based practice' (EBP). 'Evidence', in this context, is shorthand for 'scientific evidence of effectiveness', and while practice means what it says – that is, the health care offered to patients and clients – there is less clarity about who should manage the transfer of the evidence into practice. So, while it works excellently as a slogan, the practicalities involved in implementation are the subject of debate. Unsurprisingly, in a health care system with a dominant medical voice, evidence-based *practice* began as evidence-based *medicine*, and there are now a number of different manifestations: evidence-based *health care*, evidence-based *purchasing*, evidence-based *nursing*, etc. Each of these may be used at the level of the simple slogan designed to appeal to a particular constituency, but the choice of any particular one also reveals ideas about the preferred roles of groups and organizations within the health service. Within this chapter, EBP will be the chosen term on the basis that it is the most inclusive of the options, and encompasses initiatives to include effectiveness as a core criterion in choices about health service delivery at the level of the population, the group and the individual. While the development of the EBP initiative has received substantial support within some sections of the National Health Service and is being actively promoted and funded by the National Health Service Executive (NHSE), it is not without its critics. Criticism may be based on conceptual or political grounds, and in both areas the initiative is vulnerable. However, the proponents of EBP are not as naive as they may appear. They understand that they are engaged in a marketing exercise as well as an intellectual debate, and at the end of this chapter we will return to the question of whose hearts and minds count as trophies.

What is Evidence-based Practice?

The concept of evidence-based medicine has been available to UK doctors for many years. Its origins are popularly ascribed to a paper by Archie Cochrane published in 1972 and entitled 'Effectiveness and Efficiency: Random Reflections on Health Services'. However, Walshe and Ham (1997) track the rise of EBP from 1991, and place it firmly on the foundation of the creation of the NHS research and development strategy. The purpose of this strategy was not necessarily to increase overall the amount of research going on within and around the NHS, but rather to focus on the needs of the NHS rather than on the interests of the research investigators (Department of Health, 1993). The NHS Director of R&D argued that 'The lack of information on cost-effectiveness, for example, is a real handicap to purchasers and providers of care' (Department of Health, 1993, p. 1), and the strategy can be seen as an attempt to introduce an industrial model of research and development into the NHS. The size and complexity of the NHS ensures that this is no easy task: many new initiatives, programmes and organizations have been established in pursuit of this goal. The core of the strategy involved establishing a central research and development function within the NHSE, and linked R&D directorates in each NHS Region. Together these would fund various central and regional programmes of research and assist in dissemination into practice. The importance of dissemination was particularly recognized by the creation of the NHS Centre for Dissemination and Review at York. The links between the R&D directorates were drawn tighter in the NHS reorganization of 1997 which brought the regional offices into the NHSE. At the same time, the distribution of funding became a much more serious enterprise as it incorporated the first allocation within what was known as the 'Culyer' methodology. In essence this methodology sought to identify the moneys spent within NHS Trusts on R&D which were disguised within the funding allocations from Health Authorities; to levy those moneys into an R&D budget, and to reallocate them to the service according to strict quality and utility criteria.

The degree to which the 'development' component in R&D should be the business of the R&D directorates rather than that of the service providers in the NHS has always been contentious. However, it was recognized that producing good research would not, of itself, have the large-scale impact on the service that was desired. The gap between research 'findings' and the managers and practitioners in the service was to be filled by a process of 'dissemination', which included publishing research findings in 'user-friendly' forms and producing short guidelines for practitioners to follow. The circle of dissemination included clients and patients, and there were a number of initiatives to promote evidence-based patient choice (see, for example, Hope, 1996). Access to information became a key theme, as did the potential of information technology to deliver the required knowledge to the apocryphal 'district nurse on the North Norfolk Coast'. The predicted development of the provision of evidence about therapies directly to patients via their home computers was also a driver in this debate.

The idea of evidence-based practice developed from the focus on dissemination. The possibility of receiving major funding had inspired researchers to focus on the needs of the NHS as defined through the R&D programme, and most invitations to bid for research funding were hugely oversubscribed. But it was clearly going to be very embarrassing if this substantial funding stream added to the sum total of human knowledge, but had no 'pay-off' in terms of changes in the service. Some motivating factor was needed to inspire the managers and practitioners to read the research and, better still, incorporate the findings into practice, and the idea of EBP filled that gap. The development of EBP was not a single managed programme, but consisted of a number of initiatives and great deal of rhetoric. The assessment of which of these initiatives was particularly significant could depend on your occupation, your training and your geographical base, but Walshe and Ham (1997) highlight a number of key steps, starting in 1992.

In 1992 the UK Cochrane Centre was founded, and the first Effective Health Care Bulletins were published. In 1993 the Health Technology Assessment programme was established to co-ordinate the assessment of healthcare interventions (the notion of technology was broadly conceived as any intervention, although this does not reflect the commonsense usage of the term). In the same year the Centre for Evidence Based Medicine was set up in Oxford. In 1994 the NHS Centre for Reviews and Dissemination was set up in York and the newsletter *Bandolier*, which was intended to provide information on effectiveness in an accessible way, was first published by a group in Oxford. In 1995 the *Evidence Based Medicine* journal was published; the *Evidence Based Nursing* journal followed in 1997. In 1996 the NHSE provided yet more evidence of its clear support by publishing *Promoting Clinical Effectiveness* (DH, 1996).

In addition to these accumulating contributions to a culture of clinical effectiveness, Walshe and Ham identify six supportive Executive Letters being issued between 1993 and 1996. They conclude,

> Five years ago, the ideas of evidence-based healthcare would have been unfamiliar to many clinicians, public health physicians and managers. Now there is a widespread understanding of what policy on improving clinical effectiveness is trying to achieve, and why it is important. (Walshe and Ham, 1997, p. 25)

It should be noted that they go on to question whether the practice within health authorities and trusts matched the rhetoric, but the case was well made for the importance of the initiative.

It is worth noticing the importance of the 'old' Oxford NHS Region (subsequently incorporated into the Anglia and Oxford Region) in the development of EBP, if only as an illustration that ideas may have a time but people still need to make them happen. Key players in the initiative included Muir Gray, Director of Public Health, Henry McQuay, R&D Director, and David Sackett, brought from Canada to head the Centre for Evidence Based Medicine and give the work in the UK some serious academic and practical muscle. Other important projects were also generated in Oxford. The *Getting Research into Practice* (GRIP) initiative is almost a paradigmatic illustration of some of the issues involved. The challenge of changing practice was to be met by a sustained programme involving a range of stakeholders – purchasers of health care, clinicians and the general public. Each of the four county-based health authorities in the region adopted an area of health care where there was strong research evidence about how care should be managed, and where the size and scope of the services involved offered a strong incentive for change. The therapies they chose included:

- the use of D&C for dysfunctional uterine bleeding;
- insertion of grommets for children with 'glue ear';
- management of services for stroke patients;
- the use of cortico-steroids in preterm delivery.

In the case of the first two therapies the desired outcome was reduction in the instances of use; and in the latter it was an increase or a reorganization. The idea of not doing things is an important one in EBP, and may have particularly enthused local and central managers who saw the potential to release substantial savings.

A linked project built on the lessons learned in GRIP was designed to improve the ability of health care decision-makers focusing on the needs of groups or populations to appraise research literature. The *Critical Appraisal Skills for Purchasers* (CASP) programme was set up in 1994 and promoted 'short, sharp' workshops, commonly half a day, which explain how to make a judgement about the evidence presented in a research paper. Although the original workshops were heavily biased towards the appraisal of quantitative research methods, notably the randomized controlled trial, a second version was developed in 1997 which focused on evaluating qualitative research reports. The CASP initiative has been taken up elsewhere in the country and has expanded rapidly through the methodology of 'training the trainers'. Although CASP was not originally intended for practitioners, they have inevitably become involved and by 1996 the acronym was used to stand for Critical Appraisal Skills Programme.

But is EBP Quite What it Seems?

The reasons why the slogan 'evidence-based' and the emphasis on clinical effectiveness became so important in the late 1990s await sustained analysis. However, a number of key elements can be identified, although their relative influences cannot yet be disentangled. Looking broadly at the last three decades, Gray (1997), writing as a missionary, places it as the latest in a series of methodologies for reviewing the provision of health care. In the 1970s the concern was with efficiency, in the 1980s, with quality, and in the 1990s, with effectiveness. In the language of management, the first two concerns may combine to answer the question 'Are we doing things right?' The latter moves on to answer the question 'Are we doing the right things?'. One of the specific drivers may have been the creation of the purchaser–provider structure:

> . . . some of us in the former Oxford Regional Health Authority believed the separation of purchasers and providers offered a real opportunity to use knowledge about effectiveness to improve health services and health. (Dunning *et al.*, 1994, p. 25)

Writing as a critical observer, Harrison (1997) defines the supportive context as the increasing need for rationing within health care. Specifying the effectiveness of any particular intervention has 'strong appeal as a criteria for rationing'. This appeal rests on three assumptions: first, the apparent link with 'science' which is assumed to be value-neutral; secondly, that it does not offer a direct challenge to the authority of the doctors; thirdly, that it sounds like 'common sense' and is therefore more likely to be accepted. Gray (1997) also accepts the link with rationing, putting the necessity for cost containment within the future context of an ageing population, new technologies and rising patient expectations. With reference to the latter, it is likely that some of the enthusiasm for making evidence explicit is a response to the increasing threat of litigation.

Harrison's (1997) critique of EBP rests on three arguments: first, that the complexities of changing practice have been grossly underestimated. He regards the production of clinical guidelines as central to the development of EBP, and argues that they will not be implemented unless attention is also paid to other social and economic elements of the context of practice; secondly, he focuses on the use of EBP as a means of rationing health care and suggests that this is only one among many possible methodologies. For example, as there is no public consensus that care should be effective, heroic interventions which have only a remote possibility of being successful, for example, may receive widespread support; and thirdly, he brings to the fore the epistemological base of EBP, and suggests that the explicit notion of what counts as sound evidence is, at best, a contested arena. The hierarchy of evidence with the randomized, controlled trial at the top which is accepted within EBP (see, for example, Gray, 1997) is not, he argues, supported by doctors who have been trained in the scientific tradition of the natural sciences. Interestingly, he does not refer to the other potential challenge which comes from the social science-based epistemologies espoused within nursing.

There is much in this critique which suggests that nurses might experience discomfort in a clinical effectiveness culture. However, the culture may, in practice, be less threatening than the picture Harrison paints. Gray, for example, acknowledges that effectiveness is only one element of decision-making. Therapies should be assessed according to criteria of effectiveness, safety, acceptability, cost-effectiveness and appropriateness. While the clinical effectiveness literature inevitably focuses on the development and use of measures of effectiveness, this is in part because it is proposed that this is the *missing* element of decision-making rather than the *only* element.

Harrison's focus on the use of guidelines picks up key issues in EBP, but ignores the existence of a tension about the degree to which individual practitioners may themselves search for and assess evidence and change their own clinical work. Certainly there is evidence that practitioners as well as managers and purchasers are targets for EBP initiatives. The Centre for Evidence Based Medicine focuses on clinicians, and universities in Anglia and Oxford Region have been given funding to promote EBP within the preregistration and postregistration nursing and midwifery curricula. In practice, the tension between a managerialist and a clinician-based use of effectiveness data runs through the EBP debate. On the one hand, it can be seen as an attempt to control clinicians in order to resolve the dilemma of the well-known variations in clinical medical practice (see, for example, Anderson and Mooney, 1990); on the other, it can be seen as providing the opportunity for clinicians to resolve the problem themselves and thereby retain clinical autonomy. The clinicians may be 'drinking in the last chance saloon'; self-regulation is being offered as an alternative to organizational regulation. Interestingly, Gray (1997) stresses that physicians in the US health care system are more highly regulated than those in the UK. The emphasis on the scientific basis of effectiveness appraisal can be seen in this context as the sugar coating on the pill which makes the insistence on self-regulation palatable to the medical profession. Gray puts it slightly differently:

> The most important step in facilitating change is to ensure the professionals want to change. The most effective way of encouraging professionals to change is to help them see evidence-based decision making not as a management imperative but as an intellectual challenge. (Gray, 1997, p. 219)

Research in Nursing

In 1972, the year of Cochrane's seminal EBP paper, the Briggs Report (DHSS, 1972) proposed that nursing should be a research-based profession. In the years following, an elite group of nurses struggled to make this notion real, or at least credible. Support was not universal from an occupation which valued experiential and traditional knowledge, and which deferred to medical knowledge and decision-making. However, the naive belief that the creation of an occupational research base was one of the necessary preconditions for recognition as a profession, as well as a genuine desire to improve the knowledge base, sustained the pursuit. While the generation of an independent body of nursing knowledge was one goal, an equally important one was to see research used in practice. Nursing has continually castigated itself for the low level of use of research, in part perhaps because of a belief, unsustained by the evidence, that medical practice was research-based. There is a long history of work by senior researchers, strengthened by interaction with similar work in North America, on research utilization which has continued throughout the 1990s (see, for example, Sleep, 1992; Closs and Cheater, 1994; and Kitson *et al.*, 1996). The Nursing Development Units initiative of the King's Fund added to knowledge about how practitioners might bring external evidence into a practice setting, and it would therefore be reasonable to assume that nursing would be well placed to join the EBP initiative.

However, the nursing 'utilization of research' tradition is not wholly compatible with the EBP initiative. The nursing tradition does not highlight effectiveness as a particular issue, although it is on the menu of important knowledge available from research. This may be in part because nursing values evidence of other aspects of care more highly, such as acceptability to the patient. From the viewpoint of nursing research, a problem is that nurse researchers in general subscribe to a much bigger range of definitions of validity, many coming from a social science or philosophical epistemological position. Their work is not primarily oriented to the hierarchy of knowledge which underpins the EBP initiative. Wholehearted involvement with EBP would therefore involve a considerable epistemological reorientation.

A further issue is that nursing practice may not be compatible with the implicit assumptions about clinical practice contained within EBP. Perhaps the best example of these is contained in a paper by David Sackett in which he describes the way in which he, as a clinician, practises EBM and balances the needs of his patient against the needs of society as expressed in guidelines and policies (Sackett, 1996). He takes it for granted that his role is to provide 'manoeuvres' (which he defines as diagnostic, therapeutic and other clinical actions) direct to each patient. When conflicts of interest arise, he believes that he has the right and authority to resolve them:

> . . . when I judge a clinical policy, guideline, or restriction to access to be *invalid for my patient* (due either to low-quality evidence or because individual, unique features of my patient render the guideline inapplicable to them), I ignore it. . . . (Sackett, 1996, p. 15) [original emphasis]

The account of nursing activity encapsulated in Davies' (1995) phrase 'patient care encompasses a very wide variety of activities' stands in stark contrast to the conceptual simplicity of Sackett's activity. Although some of the nursing activities, such as wound care, can fit easily into an EBP model, there is no apparent place for the housekeeping, co-ordination, monitoring, clerical and other tasks that are the daily reality of nurses. (Such work is often hidden, and its value consequently poorly understood, so the need to map and evaluate it has been identified as a research priority (Kitson *et al.*, 1997)). She concludes:

> The nurse is not engaged in the 'fleeting encounter', . . . where the work has clear conceptual and practical boundaries; instead she is in a more sustained relationship with the patient or client and her work has a much more open-ended character. (Davies, 1995, p. 91)

Nevertheless, some nurses have seen the importance of making links with the EBP initiative, and interest in it is growing. For example, Kate Seers from the National Institute for Nursing teaches on the Oxford programme on evidence-based practice, and nurses are involved in the CASP initiative (although it is interesting to note that evidence about their participation remained anecdotal up until 1997, because they were not distinguished as an occupational group in the evaluation). Perhaps more importantly, there is beginning to be some convergence in views on knowledge validity. Closs and Cheater (1994) suggest that: 'Meta-analysis is beginning to be used in nursing in an attempt to clarify the status of knowledge in relation to defined areas of practice and theory development.'

When in 1997 the Royal College of Nursing and the Centre for Policy in Nursing Research initiated a trial process to generate a nursing research agenda, it was explicitly tied to the clinical effectiveness agenda. In the descriptive account of the work (Kitson *et al.*, 1997) links are explicitly made to work by Lomas who was a leading figure in the EBP movement in North America. The account also focuses on an area where nursing could make a substantial contribution to EBP – that is, in elucidating the *process* of transforming information into changes in practice:

> . . . an explicit policy on clinical effectiveness needs to articulate very clearly how it supplements existing evidence with the interpretations of various stakeholders . . . and how it resolves legitimate conflicts over values in order to choose between priorities or courses of clinical action.

Nursing, it can be concluded, has not, to date, been a major player in the EBP initiative. From the nursing point of view this was partly because of genuine disagreement about definitions of research validity, partly because there are only a few areas of nursing practice with the necessary research base, and partly because of the profound differences that exist between the clinical practice of medicine and that of nursing. EBP was not designed to be relevant to nurses or nursing practice. However, it is clear to nurses that it is an important initiative and that some enthusiasm on their part might be politically sensible. For example, the lack of a research base to underpin decisions about effectiveness can be redefined from a weakness to an argument to increase research funding for nursing research. Does this analysis of the relationship between nursing and EBP also hold true for health visiting?

Health Visiting

Health visiting practice has elements in it which appear similar to the doctor–patient encounter. Much of the health visitor's work is done in one-to-one interaction with a single client, although this takes place in the client's home rather than in a health care setting. From this point of view the definition of practice implicit in EBP is not an obvious deterrent. Health visitors were also well placed to be at the forefront of the development of a research base for nursing. Health visiting education has always been based within higher education and the teaching teams always included academics from disciplines with a research tradition, such as sociology and psychology. However, other factors have constrained the ability of the occupation to capitalize on this potential, and health visiting research, despite some formidable work by individual researchers, remains inadequate to sustain evidence-based practice on any large scale.

One major problem is that health visiting is a relatively small occupation, whose members (about 10,000) are scattered in small groups throughout the UK. In this they share a common problem with community nursing in general. While such a group might seem large by academic standards, practitioners operate within tight management structures which rarely include research as a legitimate activity. Even those lecturers in health visiting with academic contracts may not, because of the nature of educational contracting for nursing, be given the resources to develop sustained research programmes. It is difficult within such a group to generate a serious research culture without outside support from a group with congruent research interests. Midwifery, which is also a relatively small occupational group, seems to have enjoyed such external links, notably in the field of obstetrics, and has a growing research base. Health visiting has no such natural ally, and is somewhat undecided as to where to seek alliances.

Despite the lack of a research base, health visiting has not been indifferent to the need to demonstrate its effectiveness. Both researchers (Cowley, 1995b; Barriball and Mackenzie, 1993) and commentators (Fatchett, 1990; Goodwin, 1992; Billingham, 1991) acknowledge the importance of demonstrating the outcomes of intervention in terms which make sense to policy makers and purchasers. Appleby (1991) attempted to summarize evidence of outcome, including effectiveness, but the article illustrates the paucity of significant research rather than the reverse. Interestingly, the article was reprinted by the Health Visitors' Association in a promotional booklet: *A Power of Good: Health Visiting in the 1990s* (HVA, 1994). Unsurprisingly, Kendall's research, which documents actual practice, suggests that much work is still required; she concludes:

> Much of the practice analysed in this study appeared to be based on a 'common-sense' approach to health promotion rather than a sound knowledge base. (Kendall, 1993, p. 108)

Barriball and Mackenzie (1993) review the literature on measuring the impact of nursing interventions in the community and conclude that 'little progress' has been made. They suggest there are four main difficulties: first, making a firm link between an outcome and a particular intervention; secondly, that preventive work is particularly difficult to measure in terms of outcome and input; thirdly, generating measurable and acceptable outcome criteria; fourthly, isolating the nursing contribution from that of others in the multidisciplinary team. These can be identified as methodological problems, but they can also be defined as arising from dissonance between the core beliefs of health visiting and those of the clinical effectiveness agenda.

Methodological Problems

Research on effectiveness depends on making a clear connection between an intervention and the outcome. Part of the methodological problems lie in the nature of health visiting practice which makes defining both an intervention and an outcome difficult. A core technology, or in Sackett's terms, 'manoeuvre', in health visiting is the interaction between health visitor and client. Frequently this takes place in the client's home and consists of a conversation between the health visitor and the client in which it difficult to unravel an agenda or a list of topics which have been addressed (Robinson, 1986). Olds (1996), when reviewing research on the link between home visiting and reduction in childhood injury within an EBP framework concludes:

> Home visitation is not a monolithic service but is a means of delivering a complex set of educational and socially supportive interventions in the home.

He also notes that it was difficult to decide what constituted an 'injury' and therefore to measure the outcome. However, this is not just a problem in health visiting:

> A problem with most meta-analyses, however, is that the outcomes and the interventions that are examined can vary considerably among studies, even when they appear to reflect similar constructs. (Olds, 1996)

These problems were also discussed in a review of the effectiveness of home visiting conducted in Canada (Cilisk *et al.*, 1994).

Nevertheless, unlike other technologies in nursing, home visits have been extensively researched (see Sefi, 1985; Robinson, 1986; Kendall, 1993). In the context of evidence-based practice, the research literature makes available a detailed description of the intervention which could potentially underpin more precise definitions of interventions.

Accounts of Health

However, the problems of reconciling health visiting with EBP are not all methodological; they are also ideological. Beattie (1993) proposes four ways of accounting for health. He connects the first two categories – the biopathological model and the ecological model – to a paternalist or 'top-down' approach to policy-making and to a natural science approach to validity. The second two he connects with a 'bottom-up' approach to policy-making and to a sociological approach to validity. The EBP initiative has, to date, largely been based in the biopathological model. However, it adapts easily to the ecological model which would place health visitors as applied public health practitioners aiming to prevent accidents, find and eliminate threats to disease, etc. Indeed a report in the *Observer*, prompted by a planned closure of health visiting services, suggests that this remains the popular image of health visiting. It defines the outcomes of health visiting as reduction in child neglect and abuse, finding physical impairment, improved immunization rates, reduced accident rates, detection and reduction of postnatal depression, and so on. However, there is evidence to suggest that health visiting has grown out of an ecological model, and is now espousing a biographical model. Cowley's 1995 analysis of health visitors' accounts of health places it within a humanistic, developmental perspective, linking health to personal development. Here, care has a value in itself:

> It needs a human being to give her [client] some support and show that we care, that we're going to listen, even if we haven't got a magic formula to offer . . . (Cowley, 1995b, p. 437)

There is within the data cited by Cowley an explicit rejection of the social engineering model.

> I think it's very good . . . to have them [clients] actually disagree with you over some policy. . . . Not do what I think is best, but what they think is best . . .

Here the outcome of the intervention is deemed to be the personal growth of the mother; nothing remains of the concept of child surveillance advocated in Dingwall and Robinson (1990) or the promotion of explicit strategies for health gain. This raises the issue clearly underlying much of the EBP debate. Once a specific intervention is fully described and linked to an outcome, the state may consider explicitly whether to include it within the health care or other services. While personal growth doubtless has a value to the individual, it is difficult to believe that hard-pressed purchasers would fund it in preference to, say, an oncology service. And in August 1997 Cambridge and Huntingdon Health Authority was reported as having 'killed off' the health visitor as we know her (*Observer*, 31 August 1997, p. 11) in a move away from universal home visiting and towards targeted objectives that was widely reported by the national media.

The biographical model is itself under threat as some health visitors wish to move towards the communitarian model. This has been the subject of debate throughout the 1990s, in part as a response to perceived government neglect of health visiting. In the 1980s debates about the organization and management of community nursing culminated in the Cumberlege Report, which was published in 1986. Two years later Shirley Goodwin was to ask 'Whither health visiting?' (Goodwin, 1988). In the following year she published, under the title 'Storm Clouds Ahead', a paper which explored issues about the management of the health visiting service. Her writing struck a note for the debate which was to follow: she was concerned about where health visitors would fit in the new structures which seemed to favour general practice; she was doubtful about the extent of GPs interest in health promotion; and most important of all, she was 'surprised and puzzled' by the government's lack of interest in health visiting.

Fatchett (1990) posed the debate in stark terms, asking 'Health visiting: a withering profession?' Again there is a noticeable element of surprise and bewilderment:

> It might be thought that health visitors should have been given that key role because they work with, and for, both the well and unwell in the population, often including many, e.g. travellers and prostitutes, who may not be registered with a doctor.

The political naivety of this view is contained in the suggestion that occupational groups get what they deserve, and shockingly illustrated by the assumption that the ability to work with travellers and prostitutes is likely to impress a Thatcherite government!

So, by the early 1990s we have an occupation which feels threatened by external change, but knows it has to articulate some role which is comprehensible to managers and provides space for an independent profession. The nature of that role is by no means clear. Fatchett concludes:

> . . . health visitors need to indulge in some painful decision-making, in order to prevent the withering away of their profession within the newly emerging context for primary health care.

In this context of uncertainty a lobby for a new public health role emerged. Kate Billingham, at the 1990 HVA conference, responded to the perceived confusion in health visiting by offering both an analysis and a solution. The analysis suggested that both health visitors and clients had experienced pressure from changes in government policy and this had caused the tensions inherent in the role to come to the surface. She suggests that health visitors are trying to perform three different roles:

- as health promotion specialist in family health;
- as parental support and child protection;
- as public health worker.

And she urged them to begin to choose between them.

A series of papers by people in key posts in health visiting (Goodwin, 1992; Williams, 1992; Cernik and Wearne, 1994; Naish, 1994; Jackson, 1994; Nicholas, 1996) attempted both to unravel exactly what was meant by the public health role and to enthuse health visitors about it. There is some lack of clarity about a role which contains at least two elements: on the one hand, public health visiting work can consist of generating an ethnographic account of health need in a particular locality to sit alongside the quantitative descriptions of public health medicine; on the other, it can involve intervening in the community as a community development worker in alliance with a range of other agencies. Of course, the two roles are by no means incompatible, but the second perhaps offers a more radical change of practice for most health visitors. Naish (1994) argues that the multiplicity of potential roles is unsurprising, because public health includes both a set of skills and an ideological position.

It is difficult to see in this climate of confusion and uncertainty how a sustained exploration of the effectiveness of practice could take place. If the occupation cannot decide where its future lies, it cannot predict what the research problems are, nor is it likely to attract the interest of researchers. In addition, Beattie's model suggests that both the biographical model and the communitarian model are equally antipathetic to the notions of evidence espoused within EBP. This is largely on the grounds of conflict over definitions of validity. Although it is unlikely that most health visitors would express their difficulties in those terms, it is the case that the language of EBP is uncomfortable outside of a medical sphere (and possibly also inside it, although for different reasons). Davies (1995) highlights the importance of masculine metaphors within health policy:

> It is not simply a matter, important as this is, of the predominance of men in positions of power, it is also a matter of metaphors of masculinity and how these have come at all levels of activity to shape visions of what is to be achieved.

There can be few more obvious examples of this than the title of the newsletter designed to 'sell' the concept: *Bandolier*. The logic of the title is that the newsletter would hand 'bullets' of evidence to purchasers and practitioners for them to fire. This is not an image that appeals to an occupation such as nursing, still less to that part of the occupation which works almost exclusively with women and has incorporated ideas from feminist politics. The contrast between the language of health visiting – personal, empowerment, care – and that of EBP – odds ratios, bias, randomized control trial – is profound.

More prosaically, much of the energy within a small occupation which might have gone into producing a more substantial research base, including evidence on effectiveness, was directed at debates and disagreements on the future of the profession. This has placed the occupation at a disadvantage, because there are issues surrounding EBP which are relevant to their needs. An obvious example would be finding ways of demonstrating that no-one else can do health visiting tasks effectively either better or cheaper than health visitors. Because the process of health visiting looks much like everyday social interaction (although as Robinson, 1986, and Sefi, 1985, have shown, there are important differences) there is little of the mystique of expertise surrounding the work. It may be true that a plumber could undertake a number of surgical tasks, but the public does not think so. In contrast there is clear evidence that lay members of the public, such as National Childbirth Trust teachers, perform many of the tasks undertaken by health visitors. The article in the *Observer* cited above offered unintentionally faint praise to the health visitors:

> There is strong evidence that home based social support *like that provided by health visitors*, improves the health outcome of families with children. (*Observer*, 1997) [this author's emphasis]

Note that the commentator is supporting home-based social support, and not health visiting *per se.*

Light at the end of the tunnel – or just the oncoming train? Questions about the future organizational arrangements in primary care were the subject of particular government interest in 1996, and one manifestation of this was a commitment to increasing research in and for primary care. A National Working Group on R&D in Primary Care examined a range of issues, including the purpose and definition of primary care research and the capacity to do it, and reported in 1997. They conclude that there is a considerable need for urgent action if primary care is to have the research base it requires for evidence-based practice, and make a number of proposals for 'boosting' primary care research. These proposals are intended to apply to all disciplines working in primary care but, unsurprisingly, the report assumes that the major focus of primary care research development will be general practice. The confirmation of general practice as the central delivery point of primary care is to be reflected in the organization and management of research. If health visitors wish to generate a research base and bring it into their practice, co-operation with researchers in general practice will be essential. At this point in time it is difficult to see that health visiting is either willing or able to go down that road.

References

ANDERSON, T.F. and MOONEY, G. (Eds) (1990) *The Challenges of Medical Practice Variations*, Basingstoke: Macmillan.

APPLEBY, F. (1991) 'In pursuit of excellence', *Health Visitor,* **64** (8), pp. 254–6.

BARRIBALL, K.L. and MACKENZIE, A. (1993) 'Measuring the impact of nursing interventions in the community: a selective review of the literature', *Journal of Advanced Nursing,* **18**, pp. 401–407.

BEATTIE, A. (1993) 'The changing boundaries of health', in BEATTIE, A., GOTT, M., JONES, L. and SIDELL, M. *Health and Well-being: A Reader,* Basingstoke: Macmillan.

BILLINGHAM, K. (1991) 'Public health and the community', *Health Visitor,* **64** (2), pp. 40–3.

CERNIK, K. and WEARNE, M. (1994) 'Promoting the integration of primary care and public health', *Nursing Times,* (26 October), pp. 44–5.

CILISK, D., HAYWARD, S., THOMAS, H., MITCHELL, A., DOBBINS, M., UNDERWOOD, J., RAFAEL, A. and MARTIN, E. (1994) *The Effectiveness of Home Visiting as a Delivery Strategy for Public Health Nursing Interventions – A Systematic Overview,* Hamilton, Ontario: McMaster University, Quality of Nursing Worklife Research Unit – University of Toronto Working Paper Series 94–7.

CLOSS, S.J. and CHEATER, F. (1994) 'Utilization of nursing research: culture, interest and support', *Journal of Advanced Nursing,* **19**, pp. 762–73.

COCHRANE, A.L. (1972) *Effectiveness and Efficiency: Random Reflections on Health Services,* London: Nuffield Provincial Hospitals Trust.

COMMITTEE ON NURSING (1972) *Report,* London: HMSO.

COWLEY, S. (1995a) 'In health visiting, a routine visit is one that has passed', *Journal of Advanced Nursing,* **22**, pp. 276–84.

COWLEY, S. (1995b) 'Health-as-process: a health visiting perspective', *Journal of Advanced Nursing,* **22**, pp. 433–41.

DAVIES, C. (1995) *Gender and the Professional Predicament in Nursing,* Buckingham: Open University Press.

DEPARTMENT OF HEALTH AND SOCIAL SECURITY (1972) *Report of the Committee on Nursing,* London: HMSO.

DEPARTMENT OF HEALTH (1991) *Research for Health: A Research and Development Strategy for the NHS,* London: Department of Health.

DEPARTMENT OF HEALTH (1993) *Research for Health,* London: Department of Health.

DEPARTMENT OF HEALTH (1996) *Promoting Clinical Effectiveness,* London: NMSO.

DINGWALL, R. and ROBINSON, K. (1990) 'Policing the family? Health visiting and the public surveillance of private behaviour', in GUBRIUM, J.F. and SANKAR, A. (Eds) *The Home Care Experience: Ethnography and Policy,* London: Sage.

DUNNING, M., MCQUAY, H. and MILNE, R. (1994) 'Getting a grip', *Health Service Journal,* (28 April), pp. 25–6.

FATCHETT, A.B. (1990) 'Health visiting: a withering profession?', *Journal of Advanced Nursing,* **15**, pp. 216–22.

GOODWIN, S. (1988) 'Whither health visiting?' Keynote speech, Health Visitors Association annual conference, Bournemouth.

GOODWIN, S. (1989) 'Storm clouds ahead', *Nursing Times,* (8 March), pp. 44–5.

GOODWIN, S. (1992) 'Community nursing and the new public health', *Health Visitor,* **65** (3), pp. 78–80.

GRAY, J.A.M. (1997) *Evidence-Based Healthcare*, Edinburgh: Churchill Livingstone.

HARRISON, S. (1997) 'Evidence based medicine: politics, policy and problems', *Contemporary Politics.*

HEALTH VISITORS' ASSOCIATION (1994) *A Power of Good: Health Visiting in the 1990s*, London: Health Visitors' Association.

HOPE, T. (1996) *Evidence–Based Patient Choice*, London: King's Fund.

JACKSON, C. (1994) 'Strelley: Teamworking for health', *Health Visitor*, **67** (1), pp. 28–9.

KENDALL, S. (1993) 'Do health visitors promote client participation? An analysis of the health visitor–client interaction', *Journal of Clinical Nursing*, **2**, pp. 103–9.

KITSON, A., BANA, L., HARVEY, G., SEERS, K. and THOMPSON, D. (1996) 'From research to practice: One organisational model for promoting research-based practice', *Journal of Advanced Nursing*, **23**, pp. 430–40.

KITSON, A., MCMAHON, A., RAFFERTY, A. and SCOTT, E. (1997) 'On developing an agenda to influence policy in health-care research for effective nursing: A description of a national R&D priority-setting exercise', *NT Research*, **2**, pp. 323–34.

NAISH, J. (1994) 'The growth of public health nursing', *Nursing Standard*, (10 August), pp. 32–4.

NATIONAL WORKING GROUP ON R&D IN PRIMARY CARE (1997) *Final Report*, NHS Executive South and West.

NHS MANAGEMENT EXECUTIVE (1996) *Improving Clinical Effectiveness*, London: Department of Health.

NICHOLAS, A. (1996) 'Making it happen: Community nurses' public health role', *Health Visitor*, **69** (1), pp. 28–30.

OLDS, D. (1996) 'Home visiting programmes reduce childhood injury: Commentary', *Evidence-Based Medicine*, (May/June), p. 112.

ROBINSON, K. (1986) *The Social Construction of Health Visiting*, PhD Thesis, London: Polytechnic of the South Bank.

SACKETT, D. (1996) *The Doctor's (Ethical and Economic) Dilemma: OHE Annual Lecture*, London: Office of Health Economics.

SEFI, S. (1985) *The First Visit: A Study of Health Visitor/Mother Verbal Interaction*, MA dissertation, University of Warwick.

SLEEP, J. (1992) 'Research and the practice of midwifery', *Journal of Advanced Nursing*, **17**, pp. 1465–71.

WALSHE, K. and HAM, C. (1997) 'Who's acting on the evidence?', *Health Service Journal*, (3 April), pp. 22–5.

WILLIAMS, S. (1992) 'Seizing the public health initiative', *Health Visitor*, **64** (2), pp. 48–50.

Chapter 7

Professionalization: Dilemmas for Midwifery

Mavis Kirkham

Throughout most of history, and in much of the world today, midwives have been part of the social group they served. They have therefore been with the women they cared for in the context of normal life, as well as in giving maternity care. In recent years this has ceased to be the case in this country. This process is probably inevitable and was certainly the declared aim of the great midwife reformers of the late nineteenth and early twentieth century. Here is an irony at the heart of midwifery: after a century of striving for professional status we find that very status and the structures of our profession separate us from the women we serve. Yet midwives exist to be 'with women'. We seek to overcome alienating and fragmented care by working towards continuity of care and the named midwife – fundamentals taken for granted by our pre-professional predecessors. This chapter seeks to examine this irony in midwifery's development, how it has come about and its effect on us today, and then attempts to look at how we can use our knowledge of our past to plan where we want to be in the future.

Midwives and Professionalization

Midwifery has clearly aimed to be a profession since the foundation of the Midwives Institute gave midwifery a leadership voice. The literature on what determines a profession has been examined in the Introduction and will not be repeated here. Two points from that literature are particularly relevant to midwifery.

First, Jamous and Peloille (1970) defined a profession as an occupation with a high indetermination/technicality ratio. Technicality (T) is the part of the work that can be codified in rules or procedures. Indetermination (I) is the knowledge and skill that cannot be contained in rules, such as clinical judgement or the ability to communicate well. Thus a high I quotient in the I/T ratio identifies a profession. This ratio, however, can only be viewed in its social setting. Midwives may well feel that recent developments have made midwifery more professional, but at the same time developments such as clinical audit and quality assurance place great emphasis on measurable standards and outcomes.

Secondly, amidst all the differing definitions of professions, Johnson (1972) gave a useful warning:

> What must be borne in mind is that the ideology is espoused, either whole or piecemeal, by occupational groups who have not achieved and are unlikely to achieve control over their own occupations.

Perhaps professionalism has been a will o' the wisp for midwifery.

What is a Midwife?

The word 'midwife' means 'with woman'. Legally the midwife is responsible for the safe conduct of normal childbearing and the detection of abnormalities. Normal childbearing, as distinct from medical intervention, is something done by the woman. There is evidence to suggest that helplessness is damaging (Seligman, 1975) and helplessness experienced by the childbearing woman adversely affects outcome (Green *et al.*, 1988). It cannot be an appropriate preparation for the activity of parenthood. The midwife needs considerable knowledge to ensure safety, but this knowledge needs to be experienced by the mother as a safety net rather than a ringmaster's whip. In giving support and exercising skill the midwife's role is an enabling one. This may be contrasted with the role of the obstetrician (derived from the Latin *obstare*: to stand before). In order to take an enabling role the midwife must listen to women to find what they as individuals find supportive and enabling, and then respond appropriately.

Yet, if a midwife feels her first loyalty is to the woman she seeks to be 'with', then tensions are created with her professional role. As technology demands more of midwives' attention in the presence of women, these tensions can deepen. It is therefore important to understand their nature and origins. We can do this by looking at the interlinked agendas of the different groups involved in maternity care as it has developed.

The Nineteenth Century

In the early nineteenth century

> the shift in the dominant location of medical services from private domestic to the public market arena sounded the death knell for women's medical practice. (Witz, 1992)

In this public setting women lacked access to the organizational means to control practice and to professional education. Medical men then prevented women from gaining the credentials with which to enter medicine, and the wider women's healing tradition of earlier times was denied the transition to modern medical practice.

Historical studies show that professions' higher status within the occupational structure does not rest on technical skills alone, but is supported by their members' origins in 'groups already enjoying high status and power in society' (Elliot, 1972). Such status was never held by the average midwife, who was poor, often illiterate, and working irregularly. The Midwives Institute, however, represented 'not the whole of midwifery, but the views and interests of the elite leadership' (Heagerty, 1990). Celia Davis has argued that a profession's ideology and strategy come not from a consensus amongst its members but

> The professional ideology is a leadership ideology, the strategy a leader strategy, or rather, it is the 'official' view as propounded by leaders. . . . (Davies, 1983)

When nineteenth-century midwives were struggling for higher training and status for midwifery and therefore for state registration, women did not have access to the resources necessary to achieve this. They therefore worked by proxy through sympathetic men. They did this with a skill which was highly developed in reforming Victorian ladies and not unknown in midwives today.

This struggle was fought within the hierarchical structure of Victorian society. The spheres of practice of female midwives and medical men had been hotly contested since the seventeenth century and

> medical men were intimately concerned with defining and controlling the inter-occupational boundaries between medical and midwifery practice. (Witz, 1992)

The view which was to prevail in 1902 assured both the continuance of midwifery and its control by medical men. In this situation the boundaries between midwifery and medicine had to be clearly set. 'What you want to educate midwives for is for them to know their own ignorance. That is really the one great object in educating midwives'. Midwifery education was to be 'kept necessarily and designedly limited' (HMSO, 1892). Witz (1992) described this as 'a demarcationary strategy of deskilling' by medical men who constructed the occupational boundaries between midwifery and medicine and thus defined midwifery. At the same time:

> The de-skilling strategy aimed to preserve midwifery as a distinct female occupational role in the medical division of labour, permitting the midwife independence in the daily provision of midwifery services and legitimating an independent practitioner–client relationship between a woman and her client. (Witz, 1992)

The ladies of the Midwives Institute thus preserved for midwives a degree of autonomy in the practice of midwifery by compliance with a limited, medically defined, sphere of practice. They achieved this aim with the support of sympathetic members of the upper classes and those leading doctors who would support them. Such supporters were able to defeat the opposition of the socially inferior GPs. With such support the price midwives paid for state registration was a large degree of medical control and 'the unenviable distinction of being the only profession controlled by a body on which its members must never be more than a minority' (Donnison, 1977).

The attainment of a legal system of registration was bound to have a profound effect on midwifery. Weitz and Sullivan (1985) observed a 'cooptation' of midwives into a medical model of care in Arizona after the introduction of an active licensing system for lay midwives. Such a process has been observed in several settings very different from those that put such pressures on Victorian midwives (Sullivan and Weitz, 1989). Reviewing the licensing of midwives in many settings, De Vries (1996) refutes a common assumption in the literature on professionalization:

> . . . most studies pertaining to medical licensure deal with physicians. It is exclusive emphasis on friendly licensure that leads to the conclusion that licensing always benefits an occupation.

The Midwifery Elite: Ladies and Women

At a time when

> in the context of late nineteenth-century medical care delivery, lay midwives offered at least as safe a service to parturient women as physicians, (Heagerty, 1990)

the campaigners for midwifery's future were a very different group. The Midwives Institute's early members trained in the most prestigious midwifery courses in this country, but few of them continued in clinical practice after qualification. They immediately moved to the highest positions of management in maternity and philanthropic institutions as befitted their position in society. Rosalind Paget, probably the best known of this elite, came from a philanthropic Liverpool family whose fortune came from shipbuilding. Her wealth supported the Institute for many years together with *Nursing Notes* which she founded and co-edited.

The midwife members of the Institute's Council were all trained nurses. Rosalind Paget (1901) wrote 'Being a nurse myself, I naturally in no way under rate, in fact I am inclined to over rate, the importance of a midwife being a good nurse'. Nursing training, in this era, strictly instilled deference to male medical authority. A doctrine of service and self-sacrifice was the ideal that defined relationships with patients and doctors. The leadership believed midwifery to be 'the inferior branch of the healing profession' and medicine to be midwifery's 'natural leader and superior' *(Nursing Notes,* April 1915).

At a time when even privileged women suffered from social and political inequality, the Institute offered a haven where they could gain mutual support and work for a high ideal. Beyond making mandatory the registration and training of midwives, they sought to improve the quality of midwifery attendance for the working class and at the same time to reform working-class habits and values. The midwife must aim to exert a wholesome influence over her patients

> . . . to raise and refine their feelings and make them see the benefit of cleanliness and order. . . . (*Nursing Notes*, March 1890)

They worked for this with missionary zeal.

The 1902 Midwives Act was the result of this zeal plus wider political concern over working-class health and the future of the British Empire. This was the first of a series of Acts increasing state involvement in public health, especially maternal and infant health. However, the midwifery elite's viewpoint was inevitably from above and not tempered by actual contact with childbearing women. They were less concerned with state intervention than with 'mental and moral qualities' *(Nursing Notes,* September 1903). The professional elite sought formal training for midwives partly to change the tone of midwifery by changing its social class structure (Heagerty, 1990).

From this viewpoint the 1902 Act was only a partial victory, as it allowed lay midwives to register and continue to practise as 'bona fide' midwives. The key argument against bona fide midwives – that their practice put childbearing women at increased risk of infection – was not substantiated. One Inspector of Midwives surveyed her 1907–18 statistics and found

> The figures show the lowest death rate amongst mothers attended by the very women that the Midwives Act 1902 was passed to do away with. (*Nursing Notes*, March 1931)

Nevertheless, the Central Midwives Board and Local Supervising Authorities showed little understanding of the realities of these midwives' lives. Routine supervision of midwives was carried out by a midwifery inspector who was not required to be a midwife, and many Local Supervising Authorities preferred 'a lady' who would be accustomed to supervising subordinates. This led to much misunderstanding, particularly with young ladies inspecting very experienced midwives.

> . . . the midwife herself was expected to conform to the moral and cultural standards of middle-class social reformers, rather than those of the working-class community in which most midwives had their roots. From this framework of stipulations and restrictions would emerge the ideal midwife: one who no longer placed the women she attended before her submission to the medical profession and her deference to her social betters. (Heagerty, 1990)

This was particularly tragic where a midwife's 'offence' was caused simply by her poverty or her respect for the poverty of those in her care. Such women's lives were 'unimaginable to those who are born in the more fortunate classes of society' (Llewelyn Davies, 1977). Rank and file midwives supported, and were supported by, the women of their community, as shown in the petitions in support of many midwives subject to disciplinary processes. From the other side of an unbridgeable social divide, midwifery reformers continued to place responsibility for the country's high infant and maternal mortality with 'ignorant working-class mothers and untrained midwives'. Yet bona fide midwives continued to support mothers, not just during labour, but by helping them with domestic work after the delivery. Qualified midwives were not willing to perform these menial but vital tasks. So, in Kate Isherwood's (1992) view, 'as well as being more expensive, they were of less use to women'.

By 1910 many local groups of rank and file midwives had been formed and in that year many of them joined together into the British Union of Midwives and the National Midwives Association. The British Union of Midwives aimed to organize midwives into 'a trades union, a democratic body' (*Nursing Notes*, November 1911). When *Nursing Notes* criticized the British Union for thus 'undermining the dignity of midwifery' a correspondent replied:

> Why should a midwife be expected to uphold the 'dignity of her calling' on the miserable pittance she is often obliged to take in payment for her services. . . . Let us combine and insist upon receiving good pay for good service and thus shall we 'uphold the dignity of our calling'. (*Nursing Notes*, November 1910)

The midwife's poverty sprang from the poverty of those she cared for and the President of the Union declared in its paper *The Midwives Record* 'What midwives really wanted was state aid and they must fight for it' (26 February 1910). Unlike the Midwives Institute the British Union sought to help directly rather than reform childbearing women. Like the women in their care

> Serious minded midwives, intent on the practice of a great science and on the elevation of their profession, do not need to be fussed over and patronised. They are tired of 'charity mongers'; they are sick of being 'bossed'. (*Midwives Record*, May 1910)

While the Union sought a salary for midwives, the Institute responded to the economic pressures on midwives by staying true to the *laissez-faire* economic beliefs of their class. In the Institute's view 'wholesome competition between midwives tends to keep up efficiency', 'independence is maintained' and by this example of independence 'pauperism is discouraged' (*Nursing Notes*, May 1918). While opinion was turning towards a salaried service, the Institute insisted that the mother pay for the midwife's services.

In the inter-war years maternal mortality rose although female mortality generally declined. For Janet Mary Campbell, Senior Medical Officer to the Maternity and Child Health section of the Ministry of Health, the main issues were preventing the spread of infection and preventative maternity care. Like the Midwives Institute she saw the broader factors leading to maternal morbidity as a matter of personal not social responsibility. Campbell sought maternity services that would educate women of 'the dangers they invite and the risks they run through neglect of themselves' (Campbell, 1924). This emphasis on education ignored the fact that for many women this 'neglect' was 'chosen' in the face of grinding poverty and family responsibilities.

The expanded antenatal care envisaged by Campbell put increasing demands on the midwife, and her emphasis on the prevention of infection led to the recommendation that for midwives to also be nurses would 'be good for the profession as a whole and the community at large' (Ministry of Health, 1929).

Organizations, Institutions and their Effects on Those within Them

Interprofessional Tensions

The expansion of antenatal care highlighted a dilemma. The law and their own professional interest supported midwives in claiming antenatal as well as subsequent care as their field. Antenatal examinations, especially the initial one, are concerned with differentiating between normal and abnormal and planning care accordingly. This could be seen as diagnosis or as a simpler skill. The Institute never suggested that the midwife could diagnose, but supported her in determining which cases fell within her field of practice and which should be referred to a doctor. Within the social and political setting of maternity care this debate has continued through the century.

The call for increased education of midwives in midwifery and nursing led again to the call to bring 'the right type of midwife' into the profession:

> If the midwife is to fulfil her functions and worthily uphold the traditions of medical science . . . she must be fitted for her calling, not only by training and experience, but also by her breeding and general education. (*Nursing Notes,* July 1925)

Within this discussion the call for working midwives, as distinct from midwifery's leaders, to be trained nurses was a call to bring into midwifery a professional tradition very different from that familiar to most practising midwives. While the authority and independence of the midwife was by this time difficult to maintain, it stood in stark contrast to nursing, which existed within a medical hierarchy strictly enforced by training and hospital discipline. The nurse

> . . . is used to calling her superior 'Sir', [while a midwife who was not a nurse tended to have] more difficulty in acquiring the calm professional manner of the trained nurse . . . however good a midwife might be at her work, it is a pity when she fails in the right tone and attitude towards the doctor – that of a subordinate. (*Nursing Notes,* October 1931)

The debate raged. In Heagerty's analysis:

> The established relationship between the doctor and the nurse stood in counterpoint to the tension between doctors and midwives over midwives' expanded responsibilities. Whilst nursing training

> legitimised midwifery's assumption of expanded responsibilities, it also reinforced the medical profession's dominance in maternity care. (Heagerty, 1990)

A Salaried Service or Free Enterprise

As time passed, the private practice of midwifery was increasingly marginalized by subsidized maternity care. Independent midwives without private financial means often found themselves 'shabby and in debt' (*Nursing Notes*, November 1920). Nevertheless, the Institute continued to oppose a salaried service which its leaders saw as 'charity on the part of the provident for the benefit of the improvident' and continued to support 'economic independence' (*Nursing Notes*, May 1920). One, predictable, reaction of the leadership was to blame the 'oversupply' of working-class midwives who were often mothers and only able to work part-time.

After fierce debate, the Institute leadership and its supporters came eventually to accept, and even to lobby for, a salaried domiciliary midwifery service subsidized by the government, a cause which ample evidence had long shown to benefit childbearing women. By 1936 salaried or subsidized midwives constituted half those practising. Although their patients were often 'overburdened, undernourished, living in insanitary conditions and far from specialist aid', many had maternal death rates half or less of the national average (Hansard, 1936, quoted by Donnison, 1977). This fits with the conclusions of Louden's wide study:

> Sound obstetric practice by well trained midwives could produce low levels of maternal mortality even in populations which were socially and economically deprived. (Louden, 1992)

The 1936 Midwives Act was 'a landmark in the professional development of midwives' (Donnison, 1977) in several ways. It required local authorities to provide a salaried, whole-time midwifery service, adequate to local need, free or at reduced cost. It also provided for the local authority midwife to be engaged as a maternity nurse in cases where the GP was in charge of the delivery, thus banning the unqualified handywoman from attending in any capacity. The Act facilitated the extension of the midwife's work into antenatal care and accelerated the provision of analgesia in domiciliary midwifery. In the situation thus created it was possible for the Central Midwives Board to extend midwifery training and require practising midwives to attend refresher courses.

Institutionalization: the Normal in an Abnormal Setting

The policy of institutional confinement was developed by the Ministry of Health following the 1924 Campbell Report. The proportion of women who delivered in institutions increased from 15 per cent of live births in England and Wales in 1927 to 64 per cent in 1958. In 1959 the Cranbrook Committee recommended provision for 70 per cent institutional confinement and this was achieved in 1965. In 1970 the Peel Committee, with no statistical backing (Tew, 1978), recommended 100 per cent hospital confinement, which was very nearly achieved within a decade. From 1946 there was also a move into larger hospitals with the closure of private maternity homes and GP units, again with no justification in terms of maternal or infant wellbeing.

The vast majority of women in this country today therefore experience labour as hospital inpatients. Often this is their first experience of hospitalization. It is preceded by a period of socialization into the patient role as an outpatient.

In hospital, as well as being subordinate to medicine, midwifery is organized in a hierarchical manner designed for nursing. Within the hospital the hierarchy is ever-present. The very reasons for the existence of hospitals – the centralization of medical expertise and equipment for maximum efficiency – to a large extent dictate the structure and, therefore, the problems of those within that structure. Freidson (1970) looked at the professional dominance of medical expertise:

> . . . the dominant profession stands in an entirely different structural relationship to the division of labour than does the subordinate profession. In essence, the difference reflects the existence of a hierarchy of institutional expertise . . . [which] can have the same effect upon the experience of the client as bureaucracy is said to have . . .

Doctors have the power to define the situation.

> Doctor and patient normally agree that it is the doctor who defines the situation, and defines what is said and what is not acceptable as appropriate for the patient to talk about. (Roberts, 1985)

For the 'subordinate profession', too, the dominant profession has the power to define. Under the 1902 Act the midwife was, within the limits set by the Act, an independent practitioner in normal cases. Pregnancies were seen as normal until judged otherwise, although there was latterly some dispute as to whether the GP or midwife should make that judgement. As maternity care moved into hospital – the doctors' territory – the definer and the definition changed. All pregnancies fell under medical management and were seen as 'normal only in retrospect'. This phrase, originally used by obstetricians (Percival, 1970), was soon to be used by the Central Midwives Board in their document *The Role of the Midwife* (CMB, 1983). 'Medical science' had become the 'predominant source of the social constructs of the culture of childbirth' (Oakley, 1993) as the Church had been in the Middle Ages. As part of that culture, midwives could not point out that 'Science is in this sense itself ideology; it is certainly not a matter of objective "fact"' (Oakley, 1993). By the logic of the medical scientific view, the midwife as a practitioner in her own right is defined out of existence, and the hospital midwife's work is either obstetric nursing or what medical staff delegate as 'provisionally normal' (Cox, 1982): a 'scientific redefinition' of birth (De Vries, 1996). Institutional management also brought its own pressures on midwives and doctors.

Technology, Power and Ideology

As men entered midwifery with their instruments, so the development of obstetrics saw the growth of obstetric technology which has profoundly affected power relationships. Brigitte Jordan (1987) analyzed this as an anthropologist:

> There is a hidden function of the tools of the trade that goes beyond their efficacy: it has to do with their symbolic function as indicators and enforcers of the social distribution of knowledge and power to act in childbirth. I suspect this symbolic function is partly responsible for the uncritical acceptance of the fetal monitor in high-technology settings. (Jordan, 1987)

The growth of such technology has a profound effect on the woman and her attendants because information is now available to them that the mother did not consciously provide.

> High technology, thus, draws in its wake a hierarchical distribution of knowledge and social authority that reflects the equally hierarchical social position of birth attendants in medicalised settings. (Jordan, 1987)

Thus the woman is on the professionals' territory, surrounded by equipment that only they can interpret. The midwife often appears to take the role of machine minder.

Monitoring symbolizes a fundamental change in the obstetric view of childbearing. It concerns all pregnancies and, compared with a statistical assessment of risk, normality seems a crude and possibly irrelevant concept. Arney (1982) has given us a rich analysis of obstetric knowledge and concludes:

> Monitoring and surveillance deal with the problem of residual normalcy by ignoring it. Under this new regime no distinctions between normal and abnormal exist.

Obstetrics has moved from a defined area of abnormal childbearing to a much wider view, while at the same time accommodating demands from consumers for alternatives to the traditional medical model of birth.

> The social organization of obstetrics extended outwards from the hospital over large areas, putting in place a flexible system of obstetrical alternatives as it went. Even so, every aspect of birth became more carefully controlled, a structure of control I call 'monitoring' was deployed across a greatly expanded obstetrical space. (Arney, 1982)

This ability to respond to a demand for flexibility whilst widening its area of power is a clear example of the 'chameleon-like qualities', the possession of which Saks (1992) sees as 'one of the reasons why the medical profession has been so successful to date in defending its interests'. Midwifery appears more like a well-trained domestic animal. No parallel, wide midwifery ideology exists beside the 'flexible system of obstetrical alternatives'. By Arney's analysis obstetrics has, in outgrowing its role of concern with the abnormal, threatened the adjacent role of concern with the normal. It could, therefore, be argued that the midwife has become, by default, a doctor's handmaiden, albeit a highly technological handmaiden. Perhaps this accounts for the increasing emphasis on teamwork when describing the midwife's role.

What Do Women Want of Midwives?

While women are not a homogeneous group, some themes run clearly through the research on consumers' views on the maternity services. The most frequently recurring of these themes are women's desire for information, continuity of care and to be treated with kindness (Reid and Garcia, 1989). Research clearly shows that women want intelligible, consistent information with which to orientate themselves to their situation (Cartwright, 1979; Oakley, 1980; Kirke, 1980). Surveys of the literature show appropriate information to be therapeutic (Reid and Garcia, 1989). The desire for information runs through all stages of maternity care and is a crucial determinant of women's satisfaction with that care.

Though the need is apparent across all social groups, the giving of the right information in the right way for each individual woman is a very subtle skill. In Perkins' (1991) view:

> Part of the explanation for midwives' failure to identify some women's needs lies with the difficulty they may have in expressing them. Women may lack practice in identifying their own needs, lack confidence in expressing them or have no expectations that the service will be interested in them anyway.

So midwives need well-developed skills in supporting women and listening to them before they can ascertain the needs of those many women who do not expect to be listened to. Such support can improve outcome (Oakley, 1992; Oakley *et al.*, 1996). To give continuity of care and to treat women with kindness similarly require of midwives such skills in giving support and relating to all women, not just to the articulate.

> Our 'social support' midwives gave no clinical care. When asked what they had appreciated about this type of help, the mothers put the fact that 'she listened' first: eighty per cent of them said this was important. (Oakley, 1988)

Information, similarly, is not of value only for its own sake. It enables women to orientate themselves to their situation, to weigh options and make choices. This is critically linked to the issue of control. In a large prospective study of childbearing women, Green *et al.* (1988) concluded:

> Women who feel informed about and involved in the management of labour and are able to retain some degree of 'external' as well as 'internal' control have better outcomes. The quality of staff care and how things are done are as important as what is done.

These outcomes included postnatal emotional wellbeing and relationship with the baby, significant outcomes in view of the prevalence of postnatal depression. There are, of course, major dilemmas here, as Perkins (1991) said:

> Asking women what they want used to be seen as a somewhat radical move, likely to undermine professional authority and professional judgement.

The underlying dilemma is, however, deeper than the current fashion for consumer satisfaction which professions must accommodate in a market situation. Professions keep a specialist body of knowledge and control the consumer's construction of reality. Yet midwives are most successful both in their clients' view and in measurable postnatal outcome when they give information generously, and when they empower women to feel in control of both themselves and their attendants.

A Midwifery Body of Knowledge?

Before looking further at what midwives should do with their knowledge, it is useful to see how far there is a unique midwifery body of knowledge and to examine the tensions within the working knowledge of midwives.

Knowledge of Medicine and Physiology

Midwives have a considerable amount of medical knowledge. No-one could now justify the early plans to limit this knowledge. Knowledge of physiology and of medicine is important for safe practice. There is also a body of knowledge and skill that has been delegated by medicine:

> innovations by doctors which once routinised are then delegated to nurses or other paramedical occupations. (Hughes, 1971)

In Jennifer Sleep's (1992) view:

> . . . these newly acquired skills do not represent midwifery innovations prompted and directed by the needs of normally labouring women. Many are developed as a consequence of practitioners' frustration and consumer dissatisfaction and as such provide a means of reducing the time spent waiting, for junior doctors to make and implement clinical decisions.

Dingwall *et al.* (1988) cautioned:

> . . . this downward delegation of routinised, albeit skilled, medical tasks is at the expense of the [midwives'] role as a spiritual, or in modern times, psychological support for the mother.

Not only is there less time, and less status, for the traditional support skills but the values of the delegating profession are implicit in the delegated tasks. In Schwartz's (1990) view:

> One of the tasks assigned to the midwife in her new role as sub-contractor to the (obstetric) engineering programme is to explain and to make mothers feel at ease with the new technologies.

Is this facilitating choice or ensuring acquiescence?

There is a deep dilemma in the knowledge in midwifery that comes from medicine. Medicine has taught us basic processes of normal child-bearing and a great deal about the abnormal. It has also taught us important things about what to do when things go wrong. Medicine, however, whilst deeply involved with how actively to adjust deviations from the parameters it has established, has little study of the extent of normality and how normality can be retained. Yet there must also exist a vast area of study concerned with the nature of normal childbearing, and factors that support or oppose that normality which extends far beyond the medical and pulls on many other disciplines. If midwives are concerned with normal child-bearing, surely this vast area of knowledge is one midwives must explore.

Beyond this, medical knowledge is identified with the medical profession's power to define, thus turning that knowledge into a lens through which the world is viewed. This can create a situation where

> Midwives' self-understandings were circumscribed by a medium through which they unconsciously accepted already fixed 'truths' about practice. (Moloney, 1992)

Yet there are many other sources of midwifery knowledge.

Knowledge from Midwifery Research

A body of knowledge is beginning to be built from midwifery research. This has affected practice as shown in the great reduction in routine pre-delivery shaves and enemas. More importantly, in the words of a very experienced midwife researcher, this creates an attitude:

> . . . fostering a greater sense of uncertainty in our approach to care: admitting that 'we do not know' can provide an impetus to the discovery and evaluation of ways in which practice can be improved. (Sleep, 1992)

Chalmers (1983) suggests that one of the features of scientific enquiry is its anti-authoritarian nature. Midwifery research is new. Few aspects of midwifery have yet been researched. How does the questioning that must apply to all these areas fit with our claim to professionalism, with its assumption of expert knowledge and status?

Knowledge from Other Midwives

There is, and always has been, knowledge and skill passed from midwife to midwife or student. The clinical part of midwifery education acknowledges this, although medical delegation and proceduralization have deeply affected the role models available. In the apprenticeship learning in midwifery, knowledge is transmitted in very different ways from the didactic methods of the classroom. We can all remember the hands that gently guided ours during our first deliveries.

> To master the skill means to acquire expert body behaviour. . . . In a real sense, the knowledge is in the hands and transferred by the hands. It is truly embodied knowledge . . . (Jordan, 1989)

The importance of learning through touch and learning through socialization as an apprentice are relatively little acknowledged now education has become professionalized. In Jordan's view:

> . . . the apprenticeship mode is good for learning how to do something, the didactic mode is for learning, how to talk about doing something.

Perhaps this accounts for the many occasions (Kirkham, 1989; Cutts, 1993) when midwives say they do something in caring for women which they are not observed to do in practice.

In midwifery practice knowledge is often conveyed to students and to mothers by means of stories. 'I once looked after a woman who. . . .' is an opening that always commands attention.

> These stories, then, are packages of situated knowledge, knowledge which is not available abstractly, but is called up as the characteristics of the situation require it. To acquire a store of appropriate stories and, even more importantly, to know what are appropriate occasions for telling them, is part of what it means to become a midwife. (Jordan, 1989)

It can be argued that such means of learning give more power to the learner than does didactic teaching. Here the student is not required to verbalize what she accepts into her body of operating knowledge.

Midwifery skill can be most clearly seen where midwives have most autonomy, in tiny units and amongst community midwives. There are now attempts to make such skill more widely available by research (Kirkham, 1989), by teaching students to observe and analyze role models and, more recently, by writing the stories of 'extra-ordinary, ordinary' midwives (Aspinall *et al.*, 1997). Much work is still needed to develop and reclaim this area of midwifery knowledge and to create the language and concepts needed for such development.

Knowledge from Women

Midwives also gain knowledge from women: both individuals in their care, and the women's organizations and publications concerning birth. In supporting women through childbearing, we need to know how these events are experienced subjectively. For example, the transition between the first and second stage of labour is an unexpected and often unpleasant experience for many women and their partners. This stage of labour has no physical, measurable characteristics and therefore does not appear in medical texts. 'Transition' has, however, been described for many years in lay texts because it can be a very different experience from what precedes and what follows it. Until we know that something is there, whether it is transition or the way a particular piece of technology may be perceived, we can neither prepare women for it nor help them through it. This is complex, as individuals have different experiences.

There is evidence that midwives gained knowledge through observation of women, which was only much later acknowledged by science. For instance, Leap and Hunter quote Elizabeth C (born 1905, trained as a midwife in Bradford in the 1930s, interviewed 1986):

> I think myself that the system has a certain amount of sedative that it releases at a time like that [labour] . . . I've seen people that just looked as if they were half sozzled – and they hadn't had anything! . . . I think the body does release something into the system. If it's not interfered with by giving dope, it will work. But I think when you interfere, it won't work then. (Leap and Hunter, 1993)

This old lady accurately described the release of endorphins in undisturbed labour without knowing that research had discovered endorphins (Odent, 1984).

Without the ability to look through women's eyes, both intellectually and in individual relationships, midwives are limited to seeing women through the eyes of experts or through stereotypes. The early midwifery leaders' stereotype of working-class women must not be repeated. Yet research now shows midwives stereotyping Asian women in their care (Bowler, 1993). This could be seen as more worrying than stereotyping by those far removed from the client.

Here too midwives learn from stories (Kirkham, 1997). Every mother has her childbearing story that she can tell for the rest of her life. The midwife needs to have the skill to analyze a woman's story so as to find 'treasures buried entirely and hidden by techniques which assume that all people share common constructs' (Stainton Rogers, 1991). The stories of a woman and her family's previous childbearing are crucial knowledge for a midwife, although they feature little in the standard 'previous obstetric history'. Yet the story tells much of its teller: her fears, hopes and concerns, which the midwife must know to be 'with' this individual woman. Similarly, the midwife is part of the building of the new story and her support can be of help as the new story crystallizes in its early tellings. She carries a responsibility to the mother to help her build a story that empowers her as a parent. Such skill can more professionally be described as 'debriefing'. The important thing is that here, as in so much of midwifery, the mother is the doer and the midwife the support.

Interpersonal Skills

Much of midwives' knowledge and skill in communication and interpersonal relations is learnt in normal life. Some of it is learnt from women in our care and some is learnt more formally from other disciplines such as counselling. Ironically, as most midwives and all of our clients are women, learning communication skills in our lives and from other women can enable us to fit neatly into the sexual division of labour in the obstetric hierarchy. There is progress, as shown in midwives' study days on assertiveness. More analysis is, however, needed to fuel the insights into our knowledge and practice that make it open to change and development.

Knowledge of Giving Support

Research shows that social support from midwives and others can improve outcomes in many aspects of maternity care (Oakley, 1992). From this Oakley (1993) concludes:

> Love is a scientific concept, and its effects on the health of child-bearing women can be quantified. . . . Love – caring – is as important as science – technical knowledge, monitoring and intervention – in the maternity services today.

Midwives must have held this knowledge long before the technical knowledge existed, and recent research on supportive care by social scientists and midwives (Evans, 1991) has added to the traditional knowledge. Today there are problems in midwives' use of this knowledge which arise from the effects of what has been called the 'as if rule'. 'By treating all women as if they are about to become abnormal, obstetricians are inclined to make them so' (Oakley, 1993). It is not surprising that this inclination is so often more powerful and culturally acceptable than midwives' ability to 'encourage the normal'. Oakley is sure that the 'goals of satisfying mothers and producing healthy babies, which are so often deemed by obstetricians to be at odds with one another, are in reality the same goal' (Oakley, 1993). Ironically, when this is realized, the response of the dominant profession is to define this knowledge into its own professional sphere. This was demonstrated in the 1960s by the incorporation of women's demands for less dehumanizing care into the new technical language of maternal infant bonding (Arney, 1982). This irony of professional power is clearly demonstrated in *The Active Management of Labour,* where the midwife is given status, but only within a very tightly controlled medical system and the benefits of supportive midwifery care provide further proof of the benefits of the total obstetric management package (O'Driscoll *et al.*, 1993). The *Active Management of Labour* is fascinating because, by British obstetric standards, it contains relatively active, though closely prescribed, roles for midwife and mother within a 'clear chain of command, which can be seen to function with military efficiency but with a human face'. Normal labour as the midwife's concern is seen as history, for

> Nowadays, senior registrars are cast firmly in the role of obstetric physicians, rather than surgeons, with most emphasis on the conduct of labour in normal cases. (O'Driscoll *et al.*, 1993)

This is the situation, which Arney (1982) equates with Foucault's (1977) panopticon, where all is constantly surveyed and controlled by those in authority.

There is a further irony that, as the midwife's professional role comes to constrain her role 'with woman', supportive companionship to the child-bearing woman is being developed as a separate role. Research in several countries has shown that a supportive female companion in labour can improve the outcome of labour in many measurable ways (Klaus *et al.*, 1993). 'Doula' labour supporters are now being trained in this country, but the doula role is seen as a separate role from that of the midwife, whose organizational constraints stop her from giving continuous support. All the women who benefit from a doula's care will also be in the care of another woman, the midwife (Walters and Kirkham, 1997). The need for a doula suggests to me that midwifery has lost its way, whatever it has gained in status.

We must not, therefore, assume that all is progress in midwifery knowledge. Knowledge that midwives hold may not be used in practice or may be used by others as shown above. With social change some knowledge is also lost. This is clear in breastfeeding, where midwives

> . . . know less and [are] less confident in breastfeeding than their illiterate grandmothers because their training (devoted in large part to artificial feeding) will have destroyed their unconsciously absorbed knowledge. (Palmer, 1993)

Jacono (1993) claims more generally that 'some things which ought to be intuitively obvious about caring have been lost' following professionalization and routinization of caring roles. Knowledge is socially constructed and changes as society changes. We can, however, develop our awareness of this so that we can make judgements as to what we value enough to endeavour to retain. The research skills are available if we have the political will to do this.

There appears, therefore, to be a midwifery body of knowledge, still in need of much development, which is drawn from many disciplines. The most promising areas in which it is developing scarcely fit the professional model. Indeed, this model may be responsible for important losses in knowledge. To claim this knowledge as exclusive sounds highly professional and very arrogant. Whom do we seek to exclude? If we exclude the women we serve, we also cut off a major source of knowledge. Is it possible for midwifery knowledge to be grounded in, and available to, the women we serve, or must we accept that

> Knowledge based on complex machinery and high technology is in principle not communicable. No amount of good will on caregivers' parts could possibly solve this problem. (Jordan, 1987)

If this is so, we may have attained the mystique of professionalism but can we claim to be with women or even working in women's best interests? Clearly a crucial issue is how we use our knowledge.

Midwifery Processes for Using Knowledge to Achieve Outcomes

Institutional Procedures and Routines

Midwifery is full of examples of knowledge and skill becoming fossilized into procedures. Schon (1987) described proceduralization as 'attempts to reduce professional practice to a set of absolute, precise, implementable procedures, coupled with controls'. By 'control' he meant 'how to get people to do what you think they ought to do', which leads to 'the multiplication of systems of control so that when things go wrong the response is to increase and improve procedures'. We have all worked in places where practice is hedged about by policies and procedures, many of which date from disasters in the history of that unit rather than being properly grounded in research.

Such a setting may help individuals to cope with anxiety (Menzies, 1970) but it can also

> serve to confine and limit the actions of the clinician, leaving little scope for professional judgement, skill, wisdom or creativity. (Sleep, 1992)

Sadly, research shows midwives believing they still exercise clinical judgement when thus confined (Henderson, 1984), a major delusion in the I/T ratio.

Personal Procedures and Routines

Beneath such proceduralization are deeper problems.

> In order to retain a sense of control we need sameness and predictability in our daily experience. (Campbell, 1984)

We therefore generalize and create routines for our own protection. Yet, for each childbearing woman, her experience is unique and for the midwife to offer really appropriate care she must step beyond generalization to be with this particular woman. In professional life

> the *pain* of keeping to knowledge of the particular is rarely sufficiently noticed. (Campbell, 1984)

We cannot do this where we ourselves feel threatened. Beyond the shelter of professional routine, care of individual excellence can be achieved. Support for the practitioner is crucial or the cost of leaving that shelter would soon be too great to bear.

Well-worn Habits

We also see today many strategies for using midwifery knowledge to achieve a desired outcome which are rooted in our history.

Deference and Working by Proxy

A classic example of this is 'the doctor–nurse game':

> . . . the nurse is to be bold, have initiative and be responsible for making significant recommendations, while at the same time she must appear passive. This must be done in such a manner so as to make her recommendations appear to be initiated by the physician. (Stein, 1967)

This picture rings very true to midwives, Kitzinger *et al.* (1990) observed from their research:

> Almost every midwife could immediately provide a list of tactics of 'how to get the SHO to do what you want'. It was as if they had all read the same manual on 'Gaining SHOs' Compliance' . . . the end result was that they were involved in a great deal of what we chose to call 'hierarchy maintenance work'.

Working 'by proxy' through men was essential for our unenfranchised foremothers and we still do it, although society and medicine have changed. The increasing numbers of non-nurses now entering midwifery may be less inclined to work in this way. Yet it is part of female culture, and as a student observed when studying the 'game' recently, 'every married woman does that'.

If we work by deference and proxy we ensure that at best the more powerful profession is 'right'. As we engage in 'hierarchy maintenance work', we also demonstrate to mothers our humble role in the hierarchy, which in turn implies that *they* are even more powerless.

Scapegoating

Attempts to raise our professional standing have often led to scapegoating within midwifery. This is shown above with bona fide midwives and later with part-time, working-class midwives, despite the evidence of good outcome from these groups. It is to be hoped that the advent of large numbers of non-nurse midwives and our growing self-awareness will prevent these historical patterns from being repeated. A cynic could, however, see a similar process in moves to raise the academic level of midwifery training without evaluation of the previous 'lower' academic qualifications.

In a relatively powerless position professionally it is easy for the midwife to fall back on her expert role relative to the client who has even less power.

> The more the specialised knowledge of the caregiver increases and becomes evident in interaction, the more the power of the client decreases. (De Vries, 1989)

'Problems in the midwifery profession and the maternity services are thus acted out upon women' (Isherwood, 1992). This is clearly neither 'with woman' nor therapeutic, but is a very real professional temptation. Indeed, the professional role of the midwife leaves a very fine line between managing care and leaving the woman feeling that her experience has been managed to the point of alienation. Elizabeth Davis (1981) sees this as destroying the essence of midwifery, which is being humble and paying attention. The many definitions of professionalism do not mention 'being humble'.

Past and Present

So our professional past and present are full of ironies. The traditional midwife was defined by her relationship to the childbearing woman. Modern midwifery was defined by the more powerful profession of medicine, and there is clear evidence that midwives internalized the values of medicine, thereby fitting the definition of an oppressed group as one 'which is controlled by societal forces which have determined its leadership behaviour' (Roberts, 1983). The analysis of Freire (1972) gives us insight into how, by internalizing the values of the masters, the original values of the subordinate group are denied, with damaging effects for those who thereby reject all value in their own group's identity and tradition. The resulting low self-esteem is highly self-destructive especially as, alongside the dominance by medicine of midwifery, the wider culture becomes increasingly medicalized. The tension thus produced was seen by Fanon (1963) as release in 'horizontal violence': conflict within the oppressed group, especially towards those seen as slightly deviant, thus reinforcing the *status quo*. A secondary process is fear of change.

Maintaining a position as an oppressed group does not imply fossilization; on the contrary, it has required constant adjustment as medicine and hospitals have changed. Midwifery managers have proved adept at learning the successive new vocabularies of medicine and management. This considerable change was, however, adaptive to limit change to the *status quo* in terms of the professional position of midwifery. Recent cultural change has affected midwifery practice more profoundly.

Changes have come from women which have proved a fundamental challenge to midwifery. Answering this challenge in New Zealand

> midwifery accepts its responsibilities as an emancipatory change agent . . . and identifies itself as a feminist profession. (Guilliland and Pairman, 1995)

Thus a new midwifery has been created in some countries where midwives were not previously licensed. Here, where midwifery has been contained by medicine, the transformation of existing structures and attitudes is a complex task.

Alongside this, the economic nature of society has led to consumerism and an expectation that service users are actively involved in decision-making around their care. Yet 'consumer empowerment mechanisms' (Ashton, 1992) are not without dilemmas. Consumer choice is not in itself empowering, because the provider defines the options from which choice can be made and the consumer may wish to choose something completely different. In these circumstances do we blame her or change the system to accommodate her? Surely childbearing women are engaged in the ultimate productive act rather than being mere passive consumers of health care.

Empowerment is a word much used, yet power has to be taken and cannot simply be given. We can learn from midwives who help women to achieve this.

> She was really reassuring and she made you feel competent . . . she really made you feel like you were the expert, and she just had a bit of knowledge which would help. (Aspinall *et al.*, 1997)

Cultural change has affected how professions are seen. In a recent book entitled *The End of the Professions?* Eve and Hodgkin (1997) examine professionalism and medicine and redefine the professional task:

> A professional task is one which requires the exercise of discretion or initiative on behalf of another in a situation of complexity

to add

> one person exercises discretion or initiative with another in a situation of complexity ensuring as far as possible that all necessary information, together with any financial incentives and constraints which the professional may be under, are transparent to the patient or client. (Eve and Hodgkin, 1997)

As significant as the potential for sharing power in the new definition and the revelation of external pressures to the client is the decision here to take a task-centred approach to professionalism. This would have been unthinkable earlier. Alongside the power-sharing and the centrality of relationships in care is a new type of reductionism coming from management. As the pressure to measure and cost the service becomes greater, attention is increasingly focused on separate tasks. This is particularly ironic in midwifery where, as research increasingly shows the benefits of continuity of care and supportive relationships, economic pressures lead to a focus on individual tasks. Where research reveals the long-term effects of good midwifery care, service funding is now on an annual basis.

Looking to the Future

As we look to the future we are inevitably affected by our past. The process of professionalization has created dilemmas in three key sets of relationships. It is perhaps useful to look to the future in terms of these relationships.

Relationships with Women

The recommendations of the Winterton Report (HMSO, 1992) and *Changing Childbirth* (Department of Health, 1993) reflect changes in the wider cultural view of childbirth with the emphasis on the experience of childbearing as well as on the knowledge of experts. These are the first government documents on maternity care in which women's experiences have been central and midwives have been seen as 'with women'. There is potential in the move from fragmented care to sustained relationships with women to transform midwifery practice (Flint, 1993). We can really develop the art of being with women, and small teams working as equals can transform the hierarchies in which we work.

There are many team midwifery schemes at present, but midwifery is not always being transformed. In *Mapping Team Midwifery*, Wraight *et al.* (1993) looked at many schemes and concluded:

> It appears that few team midwifery schemes are organised in such a way as to maximise those features most strongly associated with higher levels of continuity of care.

Perhaps this is not surprising if our aim in terms of mothers' experience is lost sight of in our concentration on the mechanics of providing the service. In Curell's (1990) view:

> . . . descriptions of 'continuity of care' are descriptions of the way professionals organise their work, not a description or definition of the nature or quality of any care that may be given within that particular organisational framework.

If we could change our focus 'away from the caregiver and towards the woman herself' (Curell, 1990), then clarity of aim could be followed by planning the means to achieve that aim. Many team midwifery schemes have been abandoned for organizational reasons but 'I have yet to hear client dissatisfaction quoted as a cause for abandoning team care' (Kroll, 1993).

Clearly midwives must support those they exist to be with. The issue of advocacy is, however, more complex. Women are not a homogeneous group and interests can conflict. Midwives often need to speak for those with least voice and greatest need rather than simply support the articulate. This is to do with enabling women to take the control that improves outcome rather than controlling them as professionals. Ruth Ashton, then general secretary of the Royal College of Midwives, declared:

> . . . midwives cannot be women's advocates because their professional status, their skills and their knowledge, by definition, set them apart from women in general . . . a midwife might find it difficult to support a woman who either demanded care that was unsafe or that would lead to the midwife transgressing her code of practice. (Ashton, 1992)

Perhaps we need to examine more closely what is meant by safety. There can be few midwives who have never given care for the safety of staff rather than clients in a climate of defensive medicine. As *Changing Childbirth* states, 'safety is not an absolute concept'. When we really understand her concept of safety and acknowledge that nothing is completely safe, does any mother want care that threatens herself or her baby? Can we use our expertise as firm ground from which to give women support while still being near enough to speak for those who cannot be heard?

Alliance with mothers does not mean that midwives do not have their own needs. In Gabrielle Palmer's (1993) words, 'if you are to care about mothers and babies, first care about yourselves'. Can we learn ways of looking after ourselves that do not create a barrier between us and those in our care? Can we learn to accept support from the women we serve and from whom we gain so much? This problem is fundamental for all women carers and solutions are likely also to be held in common. Exploration of this area could be immensely strengthening.

Relationships within Midwifery

Surrounded by more powerful groups, and intimately involved with life and death, midwives are in a vulnerable position. Seeking to be professional does not allow us to acknowledge that vulnerability and midwifery has therefore experienced considerable insecurity in the past 100 years. This insecurity, together with aspirations to higher status, has led to scapegoating, and a culture within midwifery that is quick to blame but slow to praise or appreciate midwives' achievements – a situation exacerbated by constant changes in health care.

Such insecurity at all levels in midwifery can cause rigidity and lead to change being seen as a threat. A report on team midwifery (Wraight *et al.*, 1993) tellingly observed:

> Many senior midwives and medical staff opposed the change since the need to devolve responsibility, for the total care of the woman, down to the team midwife caused them anxiety.

In such a situation of insecurity reflection on the shortcomings of our practice is often blocked. This is sadly clear to those outside midwifery who try to work with us. Gabrielle Palmer (1993) observed of her work on breastfeeding:

> I worry a lot about the feelings of [midwives] and go round in circles trying to be tactful when stating harsh truths. Why? Because

> I know there is no system of support for their wounded feelings and often denial is their only defence.

Oakley and Houd (1990) list the types of defence mechanisms midwives develop, all of which limit development and sensitivity in future practice. They conclude:

> One implication of the midwife's vulnerability is that midwives need their own support systems, and perhaps expert therapeutic help, to understand and work through their experiences. . . . They need to talk about fear and insecurity – for example, in connection with responsibility and the risk of being accused of having made a mistake. This is difficult in the hierarchical system of a hospital.

Available sources of support are embedded in that hierarchy, although changes are being made. Midwifery supervision has changed from the punitive system earlier this century (Kirkham, 1996), but it is significant that there is still no appeal against supervisory decisions. Yet midwives need to receive support and to plan how to improve their practice in a safe setting. There is much to be learnt here from supervision in other fields such as counselling (Hawkins and Shohet, 1989). Support of all sorts is essential if we are to achieve the confidence as midwives to outgrow the scapegoat responses of professionalism. Then we can develop the flexibility to find an appropriate balance between our need to feel in control of our work and each woman's need to feel in control of her experience.

Research can also be used to improve midwives' confidence and self-esteem. Are we familiar with the abundant evidence which shows that 'midwives manage normal pregnancy as well as, if not better than, physicians'? Yet 'the general rule appears to be that midwives do less than they are allowed' (Oakley and Houd, 1990). So often research is experienced by midwives as something used to bludgeon them to change. Used appropriately it can increase midwives' confidence and our level of analytical skill concerning our practice. We can then develop the skills to practise from secure basic principles, knowing why we act and to what end. Surely this is the only way to practise safely.

We also need much more research on midwifery practice, so that we can learn systematically from existing role models and develop theory. The resulting theory may apply such concepts as 'skilled companionship' and 'moderated love' (Campbell, 1984) to the existing knowledge on social support in maternity care. Such concepts call for great skill and caring which require the carer to be, in all senses, close to the mother. Such ideas stand in contrast to the divide between the mother and the carer that the enhanced status of professionalism implies.

With increasingly appropriate knowledge and support we can address the issue of midwifery management. There are tensions between the 'autonomous judgement' of professionals and the organizational role of management, yet good midwifery management can strengthen the position of midwives (Harrison and Pollitt, 1994). The rise of general management and the shrinking of midwifery management is widely seen as threatening midwives. Woman-focused care is likely to be less hierarchical, but vision is needed to support such processes of change.

Relations with Other Professionals

We have a traditional relationship with medicine that was enabling for doctors. We now need to develop relationships that are enabling for midwives and women.

The recent growth in midwifery-led care is very important and not without historical irony. Midwives are a relatively inexpensive commodity, especially when separated from the expenses of hospital stay. There is great potential here to develop our skills and expertise, but women's needs and experiences must be central. Perhaps alongside more home births and early transfer home we need to campaign for more home helps.

We need the strength to ensure that our skills are not subsumed within medical knowledge and then straitjacketed by medicine. This calls for strong leadership in alliance with women. We must ensure that research which shows how support improves outcome is widely implemented. We also need to ensure that our skills are available to all women. Not all women experience normal childbearing, and many who do also want to make some use of high technology services in, for example, antenatal screening. Yet what women want of midwives, and the skills in relating and communicating that midwives are developing, are relevant to all women, not just the normal. We need, therefore, to develop our skills in communication so that we can empower women in the presence of other professions and of technology. We live in a technical age. With a midwife's support during labour and a midwife's voice in equipment design surely it is possible for a monitor to be as immediately useful to a mother in labour as her microwave or video is to her at home?

If we really develop the skills of being 'with woman', we have much to offer medicine and related professions, as many studies (Cartwright, 1964) have shown communication failure to be patients' most commonly voiced criticism of health care in general. The values implicit in professionalization have led us to take on the values of the dominant profession, emphasizing technical skill. 'When this happened the "love" part of the work was lost' (Smith, 1992). We need now to develop the 'emotional labour' of care.

> Rather than being a soft option, it is a fundamental necessity. For those who wish to concern themselves with scientific proof, this can be demonstrated from published studies examining the effects of social support as distinct from clinical care. (Oakley, 1993)

It is historically ironic that there is much here that we can learn from nursing research (James, 1989; Smith, 1992).

We have come a long way by varying and often devious routes. Now we can learn from the patterns of that past. The decisions we make are political decisions because they state our priorities and determine our alliances. Professionalism, like the Victorian attitudes that achieved the 1902 Act, can only get us so far. We can and must go further. As Ehrenreich and English concluded after surveying our history:

> We must never confuse professionalism with expertise. Expertise is something to work for and to share; professionalism is – by definition – elitist and exclusive, sexist, racist and classist. (Ehrenreich and English, 1973)

Indeed professionalism can now be seen as 'positively damaging to health' (Oakley, 1984), not least the health of midwives.

We know what women want of us and how we can improve outcome for them. We need to view safety in the long-term context of the emotional wellbeing of families. This suggests that our service must be women-centred. We need to generate the strength to make knowledge and control available to women despite the pressures on us to retain knowledge and power. We need the humility to learn from social scientists, doulas and many, many others. Thus we can increase the knowledge available for women and not hoard our knowledge of women. If we thus give women our attention, we face the dilemma of caring and integrity for ourselves and for childbearing women. This is a female carers' dilemma for which a new model is needed. That model should not be static and defensive but dynamic and giving. We can create that model together.

A profession of belief as to where we stand and who we serve may be more useful to midwifery now than a claim to professional status.

References

ARNEY, W.R. (1982) *Power and the Profession of Obstetrics*, Chicago: University of Chicago Press.

ASHTON, R. (1992) 'Who can speak for women?' *Nursing Times*, **88** (29), p. 70.

ASPINALL, K., NELSON, B., PATTERSON, T. and SIMS, A. (1997) *An Extraordinary Ordinary Woman: The story of Ann Garner, a Sheffield Midwife,* Sheffield: Ann's Trust Fund.

BOURDILLON, H. (1988) *Women as Healers,* Cambridge: Cambridge University Press.

BOWLER, I.M.W. (1993) 'Stereotypes of women of Asian descent in midwifery: some evidence', *Midwifery,* **9**, pp. 7–16.

CAMPBELL, A.V. (1984) *Moderated Love: A Theology of Professional Care,* London: SPCK.

CAMPBELL, J.M. (1924) *Maternal Mortality Associated with Childbearing,* London: HMSO.

CARTWRIGHT, A. (1964) *Human Relations and Hospital Care,* London: Routledge & Kegan Paul.

CARTWRIGHT, A. (1979) *The Dignity of Labour,* London: Tavistock.

CENTRAL MIDWIVES BOARD (1983) *The Role of the Midwife,* Norwich: Hymns Ancient & Modern.

CHALMERS, I. (1983) 'Scientific enquiry and authoritarianism in prenatal care and education', *Birth,* **10**, pp. 151–6.

COX, C. (1982) 'Where are we now?', *Midwives Chronicle* (January), pp. 3–6.

CURELL, R. (1990) 'The organisation of midwifery care', in ALEXANDER, J., LEVY, V. and ROCH, S. (Eds) *Antenatal Care: A Research-Based Approach,* London: Macmillan.

CUTTS, D.E. (1993) *Counselling: Midwives Do Not Do What They Say Or Think They Do,* Paper to ICM Conference, Vancouver.

DAVIES, C. (1983) 'Professional strategies as time- and culture-bound: American and British nursing circa 1893', in LANGEMAN, E.C. (Ed.) *Nursing History: New Perspectives, New Possibilities,* New York: Teachers College Press.

DAVIS, E. (1981) *Heart and Hands: A Midwife's Guide to Pregnancy and Birth,* Berkeley (CA): Celestial Arts.

DEPARTMENT OF HEALTH (1993) *Changing Childbirth: Report of the Expert Maternity Group,* London: HMSO.

DE VRIES, R.G. (1989) 'Care givers in pregnancy and childbirth', in CHALMERS, I., ENKIN, M. and KEIRSE, M.J. (Eds) *Effective Care in Pregnancy and Childbirth,* Oxford: Oxford University Press.

DE VRIES, R.G. (1996) *Making Midwives Legal,* Columbus (OH): Ohio State University Press.

DINGWALL, R., RAFFERTY, A.M. and WEBSTER, C. (1988) *An Introduction to the Social History of Nursing,* London: Routledge, Chapman & Hall.

DONNISON, J. (1977) *Midwives and Medical Men,* London: Heinemann.

EHRENREICH, B. and ENGLISH, D. (1973) *Witches, Midwives and Nurses: A History of Women Healers,* New York: The Feminist Press.

ELLIOT, P. (1972) *The Sociology of Professions,* New York: Macmillan.

EVANS, F.B. (1991) 'The Newcastle Community Midwifery Care Project: the evaluation of the project', in ROBINSON, S. and THOMSON, A.M. (Eds) *Midwives, Research and Childbirth,* London: Chapman and Hall.

EVE, R. and HODGKIN, P. (1997) 'Professionalism and Medicine', in BROADBENT, J., DIETRICH, M. and ROBERTS, J. (Eds) *The End of the Professions?*, London: Routledge.

FANON, F. (1963) *The Wretched of the Earth*, New York: Grove Press.

FLINT, C. (1993) *Midwifery Teams and Caseloads*, Oxford: Butterworth Heinemann.

FOUCAULT, M. (1977) *Discipline and Punish*, Harmondsworth: Penguin.

FREIDSON, E. (1970) *Professional Dominance: The Social Structure of Medical Care*, Chicago: Aldine.

FREIRE, P. (1972) *The Pedagogy of the Oppressed*, Harmondsworth: Penguin.

GREEN, J.M., COUPLAND, V. and KITZINGER, J.V. (1988) *Great Expectations: A Prospective Study of Women's Expectations and Experiences of Childbirth Vol. 2*, Cambridge: Child Care and Development Group, University of Cambridge.

GUILLILAND, K. and PAIRMAN, S. (1995) *The Midwifery Partnership: A Model for Practice*, Wellington, New Zealand: Department of Nursing and Midwifery, Victoria University of Wellington.

HARRISON, S. and POLLITT, C. (1994) *Controlling Health Professionals*, Buckingham: Open University Press.

HAWKINS, P. and SHOHET, R. (1989) *Supervision and the Helping Professions*, Milton Keynes: Open University Press.

HEAGERTY, B.V. (1990) *Gender and Professionalization: The Struggle for British Midwifery, 1900–1936*, PhD Thesis, Michigan State University. (Copy in Royal College of Midwives Library, London).

HENDERSON, C. (1984) 'Influences and interactions surrounding the midwife's decision to rupture the membranes', in *Research and the Midwife Conference Proceedings*.

HMSO (1892) *Report from the Select Committee on the Registration of Midwives, House of Commons*, London: HMSO.

HMSO (1992) *Parliamentary Select Committee on Health: Second Report on the Maternity Services*, London: HMSO.

HUGHES, E.C. (1971) *The Sociological Eye*, Chicago: Aldine.

ISHERWOOD, K.M. (1992) 'Are British midwives "with women"? – the evidence', *Midwifery Matters*, **54** (Autumn), pp. 14–17.

JACONO, B.J. (1993) 'Caring is loving', *Journal of Advanced Nursing*, **18**, pp. 192–4.

JAMES, N. (1989) 'Emotional labour, skills and work in the social regulation of feeling', *Sociological Review*, **37**, pp. 15–42.

JAMOUS, H. and PELOILLE, B. (1970) 'Professions or self-perpetuating systems?', in JACKSON, J.A. (Ed.) *Professions and Professionalisation*, Cambridge: Cambridge University Press.

JOHNSON, T. (1972) *Professions and Power*, London: Macmillan.

JORDAN, B. (1983) *Birth in Four Cultures*, Montreal: Eden Press.

JORDAN, B. (1987) 'The hut and the hospital: information, power and symbolism in the artifacts of birth', *Birth*, **14** (March), pp. 36–40.

JORDAN, B. (1989) 'Cosmopolitical obstetrics: some insights from the training of traditional midwives', *Social Science and Medicine*, **28**, pp. 925–44.

KIRKE, P.N. (1980) 'Mothers' views of obstetric care', *British Journal of Obstetrics and Gynaecology*, **87**, pp. 1029–33.

KIRKHAM, M.J. (1989) 'Midwives and information-giving during labour', in ROBINSON, S. and THOMSON, A.M. (Eds) *Midwives, Research and Childbirth Vol. 1*, London: Chapman and Hall.

KIRKHAM, M.J. (Ed.) (1996) *Supervision of Midwives*, Hales, Cheshire: Books for Midwives Press.

KIRKHAM, M.J. (1997) 'Stories and childbirth', in KIRKHAM, M.J. and PERKINS, E.R. (Eds) *Reflections on Midwifery*, London: Bailliere Tindall.

KITZINGER, J., GREEN, J. and COUPLAND, V. (1990) 'Labour relations: midwives and doctors on the labour ward', in GARCIA, J., KILPATRICK, R. and RICHARDS, M. (Eds) *The Politics of Maternity Care*, Oxford: Clarendon Press.

KLAUS, M.L., KENNELL, J.H. and KLAUS, P.H. (1993) *Mothering the Mother*, Reading (MA): Addison-Wesley.

KROLL, D. (1993) 'The name of the game – team midwifery now', *Modern Midwife* (May/June), pp. 26–8.

LEAP, N. and HUNTER, B. (1993) *The Midwife's Tale*, London: Scarlet Press.

LLEWELYN DAVIES, M. (Ed.) (1977) *Life As We Have Known It: By Cooperative Working Women*, London: Virago.

LOUDEN, I. (1992) *Death in Childbirth*, Oxford: Clarendon Press.

MENZIES, L. (1970) *The Functioning of Social Systems as a Defense Against Anxiety*, London: Tavistock Institute.

MIDWIVES RECORD (1910) (can be found in the British Museum, London).

MINISTRY OF HEALTH (1929) *Report of the Departmental Committee on the Training and Employment of Midwives*, London: HMSO.

MOLONEY, J.A. (1992) *Midwifery Practice: Unfettered or Shackled?*, MA Thesis, Massey University, New Zealand.

NURSING NOTES (can be found in the Royal College of Midwives Library, London).

OAKLEY, A. (1976) 'Wisewoman and medicine man: changes in the management of childbirth', in OAKLEY, A. and MITCHELL, J. (Eds) *The Rights and Wrongs of Women*, Harmondsworth: Penguin.

OAKLEY, A. (1980) *Women Confined: Towards a Sociology of Childbirth*, Oxford: Martin Robertson.

OAKLEY, A. (1984) 'What Price Professionalism?', *Nursing Times*, **80** (50), pp. 24–7.

OAKLEY, A. (1988) *Who Cares For Women? Science and Love in Midwifery Today*, William Powell Memorial Lecture 1988, published in Oakley, A. (1993).

OAKLEY, A. (1992) *Social Support and Motherhood*, Oxford: Blackwell.

OAKLEY, A. (1993) *Essays on Women, Medicine and Health*, Edinburgh: Edinburgh University Press.

OAKLEY, A. and HOUD, S. (1990) *Helpers in Childbirth: Midwifery Today*, London: Hemisphere.

OAKLEY, A., HICKEY, D., RAJAN, L. and RIGBY, A.S. (1996) 'Social support in pregnancy: does it have long term effects?', *Journal of Reproductive and Infant Psychology*, **14**, pp. 7–22.

ODENT, M. (1984) *Birth Reborn*, London: Souvenir Press.

O'DRISCOLL, K., MEAGHER, D. and BOYLAN, P. (1993) *Active Management of Labour*, London: Mosby.

PALMER, G. (1993) 'Who helps health professionals with breast-feeding?', *Midwives Chronicle*, **106**, pp. 147–56.

PERCIVAL, P. (1970) 'Management of normal labour', *The Practitioner*, (March), p. 204.

PERKINS, E.P. (1991) 'What do women want? Asking consumers' views', *Midwives Chronicle*, **104**, pp. 347–54.

REID, M. and GARCIA, J. (1989) 'Women's views of care during pregnancy and childbirth', in CHALMERS, I., ENKIN, M. and KEIRSE, M.J.N.C. (Eds) *Effective Care in Pregnancy and Childbirth*, Oxford: Oxford University Press.

ROBERTS, H. (1985) *The Patient Patients: Women and Their Doctors*, London: Pandora.

ROBERTS, S.J. (1983) 'Oppressed group behaviour: Implications for nursing', *Advances in Nursing Science* (July), pp. 21–30.

SAKS, M. (Ed.) (1992) *Alternative Medicine in Britain*, Oxford: Clarendon.

SCHON, D.L. (1987) 'Changing patterns of inquiry in work and living', *Journal of the Royal Society Of Arts*, **135**, pp. 225–37.

SCHWARTZ, E.W. (1990) 'The engineering of childbirth: a new obstetric programme as reflected in British obstetric textbooks, 1969–1980', in GARCIA, J., KILPATRICK, R. and RICHARDS, M. (Eds) *The Politics of Maternity Care*, Oxford: Clarendon.

SELIGMAN, M.E.P. (1975) *Helplessness: On Depression, Development and Death*, San Francisco: Jossey Bass.

SLEEP, J. (1992) 'Research and the practice of midwifery', *Journal of Advanced Nursing*, **17**, pp. 1465–71.

SMITH, P. (1992) *The Emotional Labour of Nursing*, London: Macmillan.

STAINTON ROGERS, W. (1991) *Explaining Health and Illness: An Exploration of Diversity*, London: Harvester Wheatsheaf.

STEIN, L. (1967) 'The doctor–nurse game', *Archives of General Psychiatry*, **16**, pp. 698–703.

SULLIVAN, D.A. and WEITZ, R. (1989) *Labour Pains: Modern Midwives and Home Birth*, New Haven: Yale University Press.

TEW, M. (1978) 'The case against hospital deliveries: The statistical evidence', in KITZINGER, S. and DAVIS, J. (Eds) *The Place of Birth*, Oxford: Oxford University Press.

WALTERS, D. and KIRKHAM, M.J. (1997). 'Support and control in labour: Doulas and midwives', in KIRKHAM, M.J. and PERKINS, E.R. (Eds) *Reflections on Midwifery*, London, Bailliere Tindall.

WEITZ, R. and SULLIVAN, D. (1985) 'Licensed lay midwifery and the medical model of childbirth', *Sociology of Health and Illness*, **7**, pp. 36–54.

WITZ, A. (1992) *Professions and Patriarchy*, London: Routledge.

WRAIGHT, A., BALL, J., SECCOMBE, I. and STOCK, J. (1993) *Mapping Team Midwifery: A Report to the Department of Health*, Sussex: Institute of Manpower Studies, Sussex University.

Chapter 8

The De-professionalization of Probation Officers

Tim May and Jill Annison

Our aim in this chapter is to investigate the ability of an occupation group to control the purpose, process and outcome of its working activities. The group of people we focus upon are probation officers, but we believe that the issues we consider have relevance to those working in public sector, human service organizations in general. In order to fulfil this aim, the chapter itself is divided into three sections: first, there is a brief historical tour of the rise of probation in terms of the professional aspirations of its practitioners; secondly, an overview of the policy changes that have taken place in recent times considers their effects on the work of probation officers and the organization of the service as a whole; thirdly, we situate these changes within a body of literature on power, professionalism and organizations, in order to examine the consequences of these transformations for the occupational aspirations and practices of probation officers. Our purpose is not to provide an in-depth analysis of the history of probation (see Jarvis, 1972; Bochel, 1976; King, 1969; Haxby, 1978; May, 1991a; Page, 1992), but to highlight those events which we consider of importance for understanding the contemporary situation.

A Helping Hand: The Rise of Professionalism

The emergence of probation may be traced in the work of police court missionaries. Beginning with the Church of England Temperance Society, their work was informed by an evangelical spirit which placed absolute responsibility for a criminal act in doubt due to the idea of 'lapse' from a moral way of life (Garland, 1985). The personal qualities of the missionaries thus became of central importance, with 'men of character' being sought 'with experience and tact and full of the milk of human kindness' (Jarvis, 1972, p. 8).

The funding of these practices was via charitable sources, and by 1907 the Church of England Police Court Mission had established itself as the main employing body. Paralleling these developments was a growth in state intervention in the disposal of offenders in the community. This trend was encapsulated in the Probation of Offenders (No. 2) Bill 1907, whose list of the duties of probation officers included visiting and supervising offenders, reporting to the Court on their behaviour, and advising, assisting and befriending them and, when necessary, endeavouring to find them suitable employment (Jarvis, 1972, p. 16). This legislation marked a turning-point in terms of envisaging a public, rather than a voluntary service, and a 'statutory responsibility for social work with offenders outside penal institutions' (King, 1969, p. 1).

Despite these changes, the implementation of probation supervision remained subject to the vagaries of the approach of the local lay magistracy and, in turn, the individual practices of probation officers (Bochel, 1976). The developing probation system thereby remained subject to dual control – by the voluntary societies and the courts – and was staffed by a variety of full-time and part-time probation officers, some of whom were salaried, some who received payment by fees and others who were volunteers. At this stage, therefore, the role and identity of a 'probation officer' was ill-defined and depended on local circumstances and individual attributes (King, 1969).

Despite patchy implementation the National Association of Probation Officers (NAPO) was formed in 1912 whose aim was to promote 'the advancement of probation work' (Jarvis, 1972, p. 29). A subsequent move by NAPO to promote 'a bond of union amongst probation officers' (Bochel, 1976, p. 61) made an attempt towards a unified and professional organization, but this was weakened by the isolation and apathy of poorly-paid officers, with a membership in 1916 of less than 300 out of a total of 700–800 probation officers working in England and Wales (Jarvis, 1972, p. 29).

In 1922, the Report of the Departmental Committee on the Training, Appointment and Payment of Probation Officers noted that probation was not a profession in which people could expect to command high salaries (Bochel, 1976, p. 84). However, the publication of their findings did anticipate the 1925 Criminal Justice Act in terms of a recognition of the need for common standards and salaries. Furthermore, the 1925 Criminal Justice Act made it mandatory, rather than discretionary, for each area to have a probation officer attached to it and to designate each petty sessional division a probation area (May, 1991a). While administrative control remained at a local level through probation committees drawn from local magistrates, the Act also introduced financial grants from the Home Office for the provision of the service, accompanied by a central oversight of the appointment of permanent probation officers (Bochel, 1976, p. 101).

This state facilitation of a uniform service enabled professional aspirations to develop. This was apparent in the proceedings of the National Association of Probation Officers and in early editions of the publication *Probation*. Therefore, during the 1928 NAPO Annual Conference the future secretary, H.E. Norman, referred to the association not as a trade union, but a 'learned society', while the then Chair, Sidney Edridge, commented:

> At last our new Probation Act is on the Statute Book, and we may claim our rights and privileges as an integral part of the criminal justice administration of this country. (quoted in Jarvis, 1972, p. 40)

These changes were accompanied by the development of a new knowledge base upon which to rest claims to expertise. In 1930 we see the introduction of experimental, but official, training schemes in which trainees studied for a social science qualification at a university or college that incorporated an attachment to a probation office (Jarvis, 1972, p. 55). Probation thus begins its transition to a practice predicated upon an expertise based on the application of diagnostic science:

> The gradual movement from the religious, missionary ideal to the scientific, diagnostic ideal, depending in part, on notions of professionalism, required that probation work should be something for which people were trained to enter rather than called to follow. (McWilliams, 1985, p. 261)

The Departmental Committee on the Social Services in Court of Summary Jurisdiction (1936) then laid down two central principles which further facilitated this process:

> Firstly, the need for the courts for trained social workers to undertake the social work of the courts and secondly, the necessity for the Probation Service to be a wholly public service. (Jarvis, 1972, p. 55)

These principles were underpinned by a growing incorporation into the probation organization of people trained in a therapeutic and diagnostic approach, which further enhanced the calls for probation work to be viewed as a profession.

The recommendations of the 1936 Departmental Committee were, in part, implemented, but full legislative change was delayed by the outbreak of war. The Criminal Justice Act (1948) then consolidated and expanded the duties of probation officers. In terms of organizational responsibility, the legislation provided for Home Office control of local administration and an Exchequer grant to be paid at a rate not exceeding 50 per cent. This alteration in the service's political economy secured the beginnings of central government's involvement and oversight in the operation of the probation service. Furthermore, a formal expectation of the implementation of policy on behalf of the courts now existed within a more hierarchical administrative structure that provided a career ladder where none had previously existed. Encapsulated in these new roles were attempts to clarify clear lines of responsibility that charged the principal probation officer with, for example, advising the local probation committee on 'technical matters' (Home Office, 1962, p. 84).

The service grew over the period up to the publication of the influential Morrison Committee Report in 1962. The Committee enquired into 'all aspects of probation in England and Wales and Scotland'. This wide-ranging report described the probation officer as 'a professional caseworker, employing, in a specialised field, skill which he holds in common with other social workers' (Home Office, 1962, para. 54). An acknowledgement of the centrality of 'social casework' in probation practice again marked a shift from the 'saving of sinners', to the scientific assessment of offenders, seeking to 'treat' behavioural and psychological maladjustment (May, 1991a, p. 15). This reinforced the claim for professional status by probation officers but, at the same time, embodied inherent tensions between the individualism of casework and the underlying moves to implement a more uniform, nationwide probation system.

Although the Morrison Report did not uphold the requirement for a social work qualification to be a prerequisite for entry to the service, its findings accorded with wider developments in social work education. Probation training developed in the mid 1970s under the auspices of CCETSW (the Central Council for Education and Training in Social Work) through the Probation and After-Care Training Centre in London, with the Home Office relinquishing its active part in this process by the end of the 1970s. An acknowledgement of the Certificate of Qualification in Social Work (CQSW) as a prerequisite for being appointed as a probation officer was finally formalized in the 1984 Probation Rules, once again requiring a period of training as a prerequisite for professional status.

Concerns within the service regarding the expansion of community-based alternatives to custody during the late 1960s and 1970s centred upon their consequences for the erosion of social work values (Statham, 1992). That said, local implementation still provided for discretionary practices and differential emphases within schemes (Vass, 1990) which dissipated some of the criticism. Furthermore, these initiatives provided for continuing expansion of the service and a further entrenchment of its position within the criminal justice system. Thus, enhanced career opportunities developed within particular directions with justifications being invoked about the resulting opportunity for inventiveness among individual probation officers and the service as a whole (Statham, 1992, p. 32).

As suggested above, the moves to establish a professional base came up against the ambivalent responses to the growing range and nature of functions, but drew together in respect of the opportunities that facilitated an expansion of the organization. Within probation culture this strain tended to be contrasted with an idealized portrayal of the probation officer acting as an independent practitioner, supported and supervised in professional practice by the probation service hierarchy. Upon close inspection, however, it is difficult to locate these halcyon days (Finkelstein, 1996).

Punishment and Administration: the Process of De-professionalization

Under state sponsorship the rehabilitative and therapeutic ethos of probation work provided a rationale for the development of a professional base in the post-war period. This basis, however, came under increasing scrutiny from a variety of sources as the 1970s progressed. Any analysis of the success or failure of professionalization, therefore, requires a clear identification of the groups and organizations who influenced this process (Burrage, Jarausch and Siegrist, 1990, p. 207).

We have noted that the increasing implementation of administrative oversight was to clash with the legacy of what some have termed the '*laissez-faire*' culture of the Service (Statham, 1992) upon which the exercise of discretion was predicated. At team level these tensions were played out in 'the outspoken expression of opinion and genuine differences in attitude [which] has always been a feature of the service' (Fellowes, 1992, p. 89). Within the resulting scenario of cultural change, the established supervisory relationship between senior and main grade probation officers acted as a conduit for policy directives and administrative oversight, as well as professional supervision. The result was that senior probation officers increasingly acted as go-betweens: that is, they were expected both to support and to monitor work performance.

This functional transformation in the roles of senior probation officers found its resistance in the policy of 'seniorless teams' which was propounded by what some saw as 'an increasingly iconoclastic NAPO' in the early 1980s (Statham, 1992, p. 36). More generally, this represented underlying tensions coming to the fore over the perception that supervision was serving not to support, but to control, the main grade officer (May, 1991a). This may be encapsulated in the observation that

> the self-motivating probation officer, bound by rules of conduct and answerable mainly to the courts was gradually [being] replaced by the managerially controlled officer bound by a hierarchy of authority and answerable, through that hierarchy, to the executive. (McWilliams, 1992, p. 10)

Apart from these intra-organizational transformations, two other developments are of particular significance. First, there was the collection of forces that directly served to undermine aspirations towards professionalism as somehow benevolent for the society at large – what Brante (1990) terms the naive approach towards the study of professions. Broadly speaking, criticism emanated from within the profession that, as state-sponsored professionals, the practice of administering criminal justice simply replicated the inequalities which existed within society (Corrigan and Leonard, 1978; Walker and Beaumont, 1981). An emerging 'radical social work' then took claims to professionalism based upon expertise as its target:

> One important tool of professional social work has been casework – a pseudoscience – that blames individual inadequacies for poverty and so mystifies and diverts attentions from the real causes – slums, homelessness and economic exploitation. (Part of the 'Case Con Manifesto' in the Appendix to Bailey and Brake, 1975)

These critiques existed alongside a proliferation of Home Office studies that were designed to examine the 'effectiveness' of the criminal justice system in general (see Croft, 1978; Martinson, 1974), as well as academic studies of the injustices that resulted from discretionary decision-making (see Adler and Asquith, 1981; Bean, 1976), as well as the extent to which probation could have a significant impact on crime levels (Haxby, 1978; Radzinowicz and King, 1979). This all added to a growing era of uncertainty that led to the search for new methods of working that could retain the core values of probation work, while recognizing the societal changes that had taken place since its beginnings (Bottoms and McWilliams, 1979; Fullwood, 1987).

Another important factor affecting the professionalization was the change in the ideological climate that brought law and order to the centre of the political agenda. What we witnessed in 1979 was a fusion of a return to the apparent order of the market, accompanied by the rhetoric of individualism and autonomy. This 'authoritarian populism' (Hall, 1979) was translated into the penal sphere, with the result that attention was turned away from the criminal and on to the crime, with the emphasis being on punishment, not treatment and welfare (Hudson, 1987; 1993).

These changes were accompanied by a climate of 'new realism' that put in place an evaluatory framework of 'economy, efficiency and effectiveness' within the probation service itself (May, 1991a). The service responded to these conditions in a largely reactive way, but the result was to weaken its professional power base as it struggled to bridge the gap between practice and policy. All of this took place against an ideological background that refused to acknowledge any link between social problems and crime. Thus, in attempting to regain the legitimacy of the place of probation within criminal justice, divisions appeared, particularly when the Association of Chief Officers of Probation published a paper entitled 'More Demanding than Prison' (ACOP, 1988 – see *NAPO News*, July, 1988). Its very title was indicative of the change in thinking that had taken place, for the penal terrain was now a 'simple-minded sense of right and wrong; there are wicked people rather than complex issues' (Brake and Hale, 1992, p. 33).

In this climate the historical value base of humanism within the probation service rapidly became its 'Achilles heel' (Scull, 1983). Punishment in the community required schemes that monitored, punished and trained offenders, not those which offered them diagnosis and therapy. This 'administrative-technical' (May, 1991a; 1991b; 1994a) approach to thinking on crime provided for a rhetorical severance between politics, crime and social policy, leading, as noted above, to difficulties in providing for a coherent and united response across the various grades and different areas of the organization. The implications for the professional standing of probation officers were clear:

> A system which deals with deviance simply by punishment has no need of experts – except in the rather narrowly specialised field of technology and techniques of punishment. Punishment is according to desert and that is a matter of judgement requiring little technical expertise. (Wilding, 1982, p. 69)

Increased Home Office intervention in the work of local services in the pursuit of government objectives was particularly apparent in the 1984 Statement of National Objectives (SNOP). This marked a shift of probation language away from 'clients' to 'offenders', providing for a terminological exactitude that reinforced an increasingly individualized approach to the 'crime problem'. Once again, many sought to recover the traditional essence and value base of probation work in, for example, the following manner:

> Respect for the individual without discrimination, a commitment to providing choices and opportunities and a consequent belief that, with proper support, people are capable of growth, responsibility and change. (Mathieson, 1992, p. 146)

SNOP rendered objective setting an organizational strategy with the emphasis on national, as well as local, planning and evaluation (May, 1991a,

p. 41). Although its immediate impact on actual practice was questionable (Lloyd, 1986; Statham, 1992), it clearly represented a further extension of central government direction of local probation areas. This had been signalled, but not enacted, in the 1948 Criminal Justice Act, but was now an integral part of government policy. This was accompanied by the move to direct 'the role and function of the service in the context of the criminal justice system as a whole rather than in relation to the needs of individual offenders' (Raynor, 1984, p. 43). Thus, when circulated for discussion and response, implementation was held to be incontestable (Beaumont, 1995).

The rationale underpinning the implementation of supervision by the probation service was now being operated from a 'punishment-administrative', rather than 'professional-therapeutic' perspective (May, 1994a, p. 881), with a rule-based approach to probation work removing the room for discretion in individual cases. Again, this was enabled in 1988/1989 by the 'accounting "double whammy"' (Beaumont, 1995, p. 55) of evaluation of local services by the Audit Commission and of Home Office performance by the National Audit Office. These entrenched still further Home Office scrutiny of probation practice and heightened a regulatory culture of which guidelines and monitoring arrangements were core features (Nellis, 1995).

These changes not only created a framework of 'new managerialism' within the probation service, but set in place a structure for direct and ongoing intervention by the Home Office. This centre–periphery management model (May, 1991a) exposed the organization to increased scrutiny and control. Indeed, the strands of these developments were brought together with the publication of the Green Paper, *Punishment, Custody and the Community* (1988) that contained

> a thinly veiled threat that if the probation service proved recalcitrant the government would find other, more tractable agencies to do what was required. (Smith, 1996, p. 14)

Following this, the White Paper, *Crime, Justice and Protecting the Public* (Home Office, 1990a) put in place the key theme of 'just deserts' and rendered proportionality the primary aim of sentencing (Ashworth, 1994). Its implementation was, however, complicated by the government's upholding the traditional independence of the judiciary; a situation which left the probation service sandwiched between various official pronouncements. After all, 'The judiciary can be encouraged, exhorted, informed, reasoned with, but it can never be instructed' (Brake and Hale, 1992, p. 152). Yet still further options were then contained in the accompanying Green Paper, *Supervision and Punishment in the Community: A Framework for Action* (Home Office, 1990b), which spoke of area amalgamations, greater use of Home Office powers, changes in funding and contracting with the voluntary and private sectors. What actually occurred was a move towards the centre stage in the planned implementation of changes. Furthermore, only minor alterations were made to the structure of the service itself with the co-operation of both chief officers and their subordinates being considered as 'vital' to its success (Raine and Wilson, 1993, p. 103). Despite this, the 1991 Criminal Justice Act was heralded as a major landmark in penal legislation and the role of the probation service was crucial in the implementation of a twin-track approach that imposed

> tough, retributive and deterrent sentences for serious, particularly violent, criminals, and as far as possible, lighter and preferably non-custodial sentences for the mass of trivial offenders. (Stenson and Cowell, 1991, p. 24)

This placed increased demands on the probation service for the assessment of offenders within what were now termed *pre-sentence reports* (rather than social enquiry reports) and in supervising the anticipated rise in the numbers sentenced to 'community corrections' (Williams, 1995, p. 3). These changes were accompanied by the development of National Standards by the Home Office that were to provide a means of evaluating and overseeing probation work (Mair, 1996, p. 35). A procedural mentality thus found its outlet in objectives drawn up by the Home Office, measured against specified outcomes at local level and monitored and reported on by probation management, probation committees (redesignated Boards, but not legislatively enforced) and the probation inspectorate. Therefore, as with so many changes in the public sector, the emphasis centred upon method, not purpose:

> Nowadays we know much more about what is happening in the probation service, thanks largely to the development of crude performance indicators and the availability of information technology but we still know relatively little about why. (Shaw, 1992, p. 130) [Original Italics]

The sense of positive challenge that these changes signalled was short-lived (Raynor, Smith and Vanstone, 1994). The reality of the limitations on judicial discretion within the 1991 Act brought about a turnaround in the 1993 Criminal Justice Act, with serious ramifications for the service:

> The Criminal Justice Act 1993 modified the sentencing framework by allowing the court to look at all offences before it, not just the offence and one other associated with it as in the 1991 Act . . . Probation officers are having to modify yet again the way in which they work – particularly in assessing seriousness. A harsher penal

> climate generally means that probation is no longer seen as occupying centre stage, and cut-backs in expenditure are now planned. (Mair, 1996, p. 35)

The probation service had, therefore, to react to yet another about turn in the criminal justice system, but one which spelt a contraction of the service, rather than the proposed growth enshrined within the 1991 Criminal Justice Act. At the same time, the Home Secretary had always possessed explicit powers to challenge the professional standing of probation officers (Jarvis, 1980). The possession of a CQSW, while it was a part of entry into the service in the late 1970s and 1980s, was not legally enshrined. Furthermore, as noted previously, the inclusion of ancillary staff within 'alternative to custody' schemes led to uncertainties concerning areas of professional responsibility and a blurring of role boundaries (May, 1991a, p. 100). This combination of factors was to lead to one outcome: new forms of punishment in the community did not require professional training as previously conceptualized, but, instead, attention to the details of training, monitoring and general administration of schemes. Given this state of affairs, a consideration of the efficacy of social work training for probation officers appeared inevitable.

Two government-sponsored reports on probation training appeared at the end of the 1980s: first, the Coleman Review of probation training in 1989 (Home Office, 1989); and secondly, 'A Consumer Evaluation of Probation Training: The Courses Compared' (Davies, 1989). Coleman, in particular, signalled a move towards the idea of 'competence' that would 'reflect both the increasing ascendancy of employer interests in education and training institutions, and the more managerially defined forms of practice' (Nellis, 1996, p. 13). Despite this, links were strengthened between local probation areas and training institutions, and the probation service remained committed to this system of training, with the staggered introduction of the Diploma in Social Work in the early 1990s. Nevertheless, the Probation Training Unit, established in 1992,

> made an early commitment to a competence-based approach, candidly acknowledging that whatever benefits such an approach may have for individuals, its primary justification was managerial. (Nellis, 1996, p. 19)

These changes culminated in the findings of the Review of Probation Officer Recruitment and Qualifying Training (The Dews Report) which was published in September 1994. This focused not only upon competence, but also the cost-effectiveness of training (Home Office, 1994, p. 2). Proposals for future training included devolvement of funds to local areas to establish competence-based routes to obtain a Diploma in Probation Studies (Home Office, 1994). Reactions, such as the following, were typical:

> The Home Office's proposals for change are characterised by a disturbing anti-intellectualism that echoes the populism of recent criminal justice policy . . . The probation service now faces a gradual decline back into the kind of semi-amateur ethos that was found wanting several decades ago. (Ford and Sleeman, 1996, p. 20)

Although these proposals were widely contested (Nellis, 1996, p. 21), the recommendations were accepted by the Home Office and the intake of probation-sponsored students ceased from Autumn 1995, finishing in the Summer of 1997.

The pace of these changes promises to be slow, entailing the development of an NVQ framework for probation training (*NAPO News*, October 1996, p. 5). Despite their ideological and practical importance, it will be some considerable time before the effects of the Home Office withdrawal from the Diploma in Social Work qualification become apparent. Overall, however, chaotic changes, a lack of coherent policies and shifting underlying power bases, have significantly transformed the probation service in recent times.

Power, Knowledge and Occupational Control

Having provided an overview of the changes that the probation service has faced in recent times, our intention in this section is to consider the links that exist between the exercise of power, professional knowledge and occupational control. In this way we hope to shed light on the ways in which, more generally, occupational groups may, or may not, be successful in mobilizing resources in defence of their professional interests in relation to organizational change. With this in mind, Table 8.1 is intended to summarize the changes we have discussed in the previous section. As with our characterizations of the internal and external forces that related to the process of professionalization, the above elements cannot be separated in practice: for example, the Home Office's challenge to professionalism as characterized by the possession of a social work qualification, along with changes in criminal justice legislation clearly relates to the micro-level, whilst managerialism (mezzo) has a clear effect on interaction within the organization. This diagram does, however, enable us to consider the various strategies and tactics that have produced the contemporary situation within the probation service.

Overall, these changes may be linked to the forward march of modernity. What we have seen in the above history is the shifting relationships that have take place, over time, between central authorities, subject populations and 'intermediate officials' within systems of administrative power

Table 8.1 Changes to probation and their policy environment

Level of change	Environment
'Macro'	Changes in criminal justice system; dependent on political, economic and ideological climate which guides the perception and proposed solutions to the 'crime problem'.
	Alternatives to custody alter in their intent, and rationale and practice is monitored by the Home Office via Rules, Statute, Probation Inspections and Audit Commission; emphasis is upon outcomes in relation to objectives within cost-sensitive environment.
	Move towards competencies in relation to 'effectiveness' of criminal justice policies leads to questioning of social work training and, ultimately, the end of Home Office sponsorship of probation training.
Organization	
'Mezzo'	Emergence of new managerialism implementing policy and utilizing Management By Objectives with practices designed to target and monitor work of frontline personnel. As a result, conceptions of what it is to be a probation 'professional' are transformed.
Interactive	
'Micro'	Changes in the roles of personnel; formal accountability is emphasized over discretion and autonomy; types of client alter and professional status is transformed/undermined, all of which creates tensions in working practices and status confusion.

With thanks to Open University Press for permission to reproduce the above which is an updated version May 1991a, p. 51.

(Dandeker, 1994, p. 196). Increasing state intervention has taken place in the provision and nature of community corrections in relation to a target population, with the structure and practice of the probation service changing, as a result, over time. The service itself has moved from a voluntary-evangelical phase (up to 1925), through a professional-therapeutic phase (up to the 1970s) to a punishment-administrative phase (to the present day). (See Broad, 1991; May, 1991a; 1991b; 1994a; McWilliams, 1983; 1985; 1986; 1987.) This latter phase may be characterized as: a concentration upon the number of offenders processed as an alternative to custody schemes; a decrease in discretion informed by professional diagnosis via an increase in formal rules; and an increase in the monitoring of work performance through the setting of objectives.

In considering these relationships in the case of the position and status of 'intermediate officials', the history of probation has witnessed varying claims for the professional status of its workforce. Initially, these were enabled under the umbrella of legislative changes; an important landmark in this history being the 1925 Criminal Justice Act. From this point of view, we can say that the professional status of probation officers was state-sponsored, with the concept of third-party mediation being of central importance to the professionalization process. This involves a centralized state defining the needs of the client, as well as the manner in which those needs are to be met (Johnson, 1972, p. 46).

Following this initial condition, what then occurred were claims to professional expertise that arose within two domains: first, through the provision of training which, ultimately, came from institutions of higher education; and secondly, within the service itself, regarding the degree of discretion that was afforded in working with offenders and utilizing the casework method. We can say, therefore, that state licence was granted to carry out probation activities, while the growth of training, accompanied by an appropriate organizational context of work, provided for a mandate to define work tasks (Hughes, 1971). In this way professionalism flourished as a

> commitment to a particular body of knowledge and skill both for its own sake and for the use to which it is put – that is to say, commitment to preserve, refine, and elaborate that knowledge and skill, to do good work, and, where it has application to worldly problems, to perform it well for the benefit of others – to do Good Works. (Freidson, 1994, p. 210)

This was enabled and could develop as long as there was a broad alignment between macro-political aspirations over the direction of penal policy and the development of that expertise in the fulfilling of the objectives to meet those aims. This does not suggest that probation officers were (and are) simply the servants of various governments, for this would be to attribute intention to outcome in policy implementation where discretionary decision-making is part of the process. After all, it was the very exercise of that discretion, defined in terms of the ability to make choices among alternative courses of action, and its effects on government objectives, that was to become the object of increased regulative rules designed to inform working practices. Nevertheless, it is to suggest that state sponsorship was an initial condition for a process of professionalization that was to focus upon the technical aspects of working practice. Wider social and political issues then became bracketed together in the name of technical competence. This is not to say that, for example, matters of deprivation did not inform practice but, as Shaw (1987) notes of teachers and social workers, these macro-political issues are translated into micro-practical concerns which can be locally managed. In this way, professionalism acts to depoliticize practice and renders occupational groupings vulnerable to deskilling.

In this sense, the individualism of probation officers militated against a concerted challenge to changes whose implications were masked by their gradualism at an operational level (Haxby, 1978).

Mezzo, or intra-organizational transformations, prompted by changes in macro-political objectives, were also to challenge and alter these aspirations to professionalism. In the middle phase of probation practice (professional–therapeutic), the management of probation practice remained largely within the hands of individuals and teams. This practice was informed by a broad knowledge base whose appeal to esoteric/technical knowledge was, as argued, sustained as long as the conditions for its practice remained. Yet, this state of affairs was always less than secure. After all, not only were the macro-political conditions to change, but the employers of probation officers were magistrates; the officers themselves were accountable to local courts via local probation liaison committees; they acted as part of probation teams and worked within an organization whose hierarchy, while relatively flat by comparison with other public sector organizations, was to increase over time. Furthermore, the accountability ascribed to probation managers was to serve their political masters who, for the constitutional reason of the traditional independence of the executive from the judiciary, sought to bypass magistrates in the implementation of policy under conditions of increasing budgetary restraint. What were then to alter were both the *pace* and *the reasons* for organizational transformation.

Wider social and political changes, the very aspects that are bracketed within the situated pragmatics of local practice, came with the advent of Thatcherism – defined as both a social movement *and* a state project (Hay, 1996). In contemporary times, public sector managers walk in the corridors that the strategies of this project have served to build. In terms of probation this took place and was enabled by a number of factors. First, punishment has no need of experts, but, rather, administrators of community corrections (Wilding, 1982). With the changes in punishment in the community, from the early 1970s, came the recruitment of a critical mass of 'non-professional' staff. Secondly, studies questioned the exercise and the results of professional discretion, both in terms of the injustices it could create for the client and of their effectiveness on overall crime levels. Thirdly, radical probation officers were drawing attention to the political functions of their tasks and viewing professionalism as a technical, short-term fix that served to reproduce structural inequalities. Fourthly, a new managerialism in the public services evolved during the 1980s in response to the changing environmental conditions. As far as their effects on the process of professionalization go, we have considered the first three factors, but not the last in any detail.

The rise of managerialism may be linked with the perceived need for the public services to replicate the apparent successes of the private sector (Clarke, in this volume; Pollitt, 1993). The need for change in managerial practices in probation was backed up by the threat and practice of privatization of aspects of the criminal justice system (see Ryan and Ward, 1990). At the same time, we have challenged the idea that state intervention and the growth of professional autonomy are separable by noting that, although legislative change was a condition for professional development, subsequent practices did not simply reflect the needs of the state. Hence, Thatcherism's assault on probation, while clearly undermining claims to professionalism at one level, actually served to create new networks of expertise within the probation service – for example, in the concept of managerial competence, the practice of administration and the generation and collection of information, through monitoring systems, on frontline probation practices.

In the movement from the professional-therapeutic to punishment-administrative phases in probation, we witnessed frontline practice becoming re-politicized as the new managerialism became the agent of de-politicization: for example, NAPO has adopted more union- than professional association-oriented tactics during the 1980s and up to the present day. The province of de-politicization was not then frontline professionalism, but the practice of managers who were concerned to maximize performance through rule and objective setting and the monitoring of working practices. This represents a clear transformation in politicization/de-politicization from the middle to later phases in probation development. This can, in turn, be linked to macro changes:

> Both bureaucracy and professionalism were 'sold' to the public in the 1960s and 1970s as representing transcendent sets of rules and knowledges (expertise) which supposedly guaranteed the neutrality of state intervention. By comparison, in the 1980s and 1990s bureaucracy and professionalism have been identified as partisan interests which require the creation of new 'apolitical' disciplines (the market place, management and the evaluative state) to check their powers. (Clarke, Cochrane and McLaughlin, 1994, p. 231)

The result has been to reconstitute what it is to be a 'professional' within the probation service. Administrative officers, researchers and managers in general are able to lay claim to expertise that does not reside within frontline practice, a practice whose power to maintain a professional status has considerably diminished.

In considering the dynamics of this process from an intra-organizational point of view, Stuart Hall (1991) argues that these managers are imported into the public sector in order to educate public sector organizations in the mysteries of market calculation. In the probation service, however, this is rendered problematic, although this is not to say that consultants are not utilized. Instead, managers are mostly drawn from the ranks of probation officers who, over time, have moved up the hierarchy. As a result, nostalgic claims to professionalism, which act to ameliorate the excesses of bureaucracy through their idealizations of the past (Gabriel, 1993), are then reflected as outdated by those who also lived through such times, but now represent the 'future'. As Finkelstein notes of such claims to professional autonomy:

> As probation areas expanded, officers began to work in teams. They were no longer working alone but were part of larger organisations which assumed responsibilities for the work undertaken by its staff. (Finkelstein, 1996, p. 81)

It is these 'technicians of transformation' (May, 1994b), who once belonged to the ranks of frontline professionals, that now challenge that professionalism and, in the routines of their daily practice, point to a present and future that is constructed through alternative conceptions of what it is to be a professional and, in the process, pursue a different set of goals.

Internal conflicts about values have thus increased within probation thanks to these changing forms of practice in relation to the processes of politicization and de-politicization. Claims to expertise have changed as the probation service is expected, via programmes of intervention and treatment, to administer punishment in the community, not casework to individual offenders. Returning to our point regarding the importance of tracing the connection between the state and the process of professionalization, we can now link the following observation into the history we have charted here:

> Because governments depend upon the neutrality of expertise in rendering social realities governable, the established professions have been, as far as possible, distanced from spheres of political contention . . . However, because government policies and policy objectives change over time, these boundaries are in constant flux, having the effect of refashioning jurisdictions, breaking down arenas and neutrality, and constructing new ensembles of procedures, techniques, calculations and roles. (Johnson, 1993, p. 151)

Summary

Without doubt, probation has had a chequered history in the 125 years since its beginnings. Moving through stages of development, claims to professionalism have enjoyed periods of relative stability, but have changed considerably in recent times. This does not suggest, however, a simple process of de-professionalization. As we have argued, in the relationship between the state and occupational control, the idea of what it is to be a probation professional has changed. For those in the frontline of the service, feelings of de-professionalization are common. However, for managers of the service, new opportunities have been created, and these are the same people who have been drawn from the ranks of probation officers. Therefore, to invoke a simple distinction between 'them' and 'us' is problematic, as so many throughout such organizations have become persuaded of the efficacy of new working practices. However, this is clearly changing, as the concept of managerial competence becomes translated as applicable to public service sectors in general, allowing managers to move between, for example, the health, social and probation services.

In the process, value-based criticisms of new working methods can either be ignored or neutralized on the grounds that values are 'old-fashioned' and cloud rational judgement. The result is a diminution of morale among people who believe in the purpose of their work, since change is unsympathetic to this ethos. At the same time, for those who see 'the old ways' as outdated and launch themselves into the 'new ways', there is a social–psychological pay-off through a problem–solution connection: the old is the problem, the new is the solution. This may, as it has done throughout its history, transform itself into situations that were not envisaged; particularly as situated pragmatics of practice run counter to the new organizational ethos, with the result that a re-politicization of practice takes place. Whatever happens, the sands of work with offenders (May and Vass, 1996) will continue to shift and short-termism without the prop of substantive rationality will characterize the future of the service, as it increasingly seems to do for advanced capitalist societies in general.

References

ACOP (1988) *More Demanding than Prison*, Wakefield: The Association of Chief Officers of Probation.

ADLER, M. and ASQUITH, S. (Eds) (1981) *Discretion and Welfare*, London: Heinemann.

ASHWORTH, A. (1994) 'Sentencing', in MAGUIRE, M., MORGAN, R. and REINER, R. (Eds) *The Oxford Handbook of Criminology*, Oxford: Oxford University Press.

BAILEY, R. and BRAKE, M. (Eds) (1975) *Radical Social Work*, London: Edward Arnold.

BEAN, P. (1976) *Rehabilitation and Deviance*, London: Routledge and Kegan Paul.

BEAUMONT, B. (1995) 'Managerialism and the Probation Service', in WILLIAMS, B. (Ed.) *Probation Values*, Birmingham: Ventura.

BOCHEL, D. (1976) *Probation and After-Care: Its Development in England and Wales,* Edinburgh: Scottish Academic Press.

BOTTOMS, A. and MCWILLIAMS, W. (1979) 'A Non-Treatment Paradigm for Probation Practice', *British Journal of Social Work,* **9**, pp. 159–202.

BRAKE, M. and HALE, C. (1992) *Public Order and Private Lives: The Politics of Law and Order,* London: Routledge.

BRANTE, T. (1990) 'Professional types as a strategy of analysis', in BURRAGE, M. and TORSTENDAHL, R. (Eds) *Professions in Theory and History: Rethinking the Study of the Professions,* London: Sage.

BROAD, R. (1991) *Punishment under Pressure: The Probation Service in the Inner City,* London: Jessica Kingsley.

BURRAGE, M. and TORSTENDAHL, R. (Eds) (1990) *Professions in Theory and History: Rethinking the Study of the Professions,* London: Sage.

BURRAGE, M., JARAUSCH, K. and SIEGRIST, H. (1990) 'An actor-based framework for the study of the professions', in BURRAGE, M. and TORSTENDAHL, R. (Eds) *Professions in Theory and History,* London: Sage.

CLARKE, J., COCHRANE, A. and MCLAUGHLIN, E. (1994) 'Mission accomplished or unfinished business? The impact of managerialization', in CLARKE, J., COCHRANE, A. and MCLAUGHLIN, E. (Eds) *Managing Social Policy,* London: Sage.

CORRIGAN, P. and LEONARD, P. (1978) *Social Work Practice under Capitalism,* London: Macmillan.

CROFT, J. (1978) *Research in Criminal Justice, Home Office Research Study No 44,* London: HMSO.

DANDEKER, C. (1994) *Surveillance, Power and Modernity: Bureaucracy and Discipline from 1700 to the Present Day,* Cambridge: Polity.

DAVIES, M. (1989) *The Nature of Probation Practice Today: An Empirical Analysis of the Skills, Knowledge and Qualities Used by Probation Officers,* London: Home Office.

FELLOWES, B. (1992) 'Management and empowerment: The paradox of professional practice', in STATHAM, R. and WHITEHEAD, P. (Eds) *Managing the Probation Service: Issues for the 1990s,* London: Longman.

FINEMAN, S. (Ed.) (1993) *Emotion in Organizations,* London: Sage.

FINKELSTEIN, E. (1996) 'Values in context: Quality assurance, autonomy and accountability', in MAY, T. and VASS, A. (Eds) *Working with Offenders: Issues, Contexts and Outcomes,* London: Sage.

FORD, P. and SLEEMAN, S. (1996) 'Educating and training probation officers: the announcement of decline', *Vista,* **1** (3), pp. 14–22.

FREIDSON, E. (1994) *Professionalism Reborn: Theory Prophecy and Policy,* Chicago: University of Chicago Press.

FULLWOOD, C. (1987) *The Probation Service: From Moral Optimism, Through Penological Pessimism into the Future,* Manchester: Greater Manchester Probation Service.

GABRIEL, Y. (1993) 'Organizational nostalgia – reflection on the "Golden Age"', in FINEMAN, S. (Ed.) *Emotion in Organizations,* London: Sage.

GANE, M. and JOHNSON, T. (Eds) (1993) *Foucault's New Domains,* London: Routledge.

Garland, D. (1985) *Punishment and Welfare: A History of Penal Strategies*, Aldershot: Gower.

Garland, D. and Young, P. (Eds) (1983) *The Power to Punish*, London: Heinemann.

Hall, S. (1979) *Drifting into a Law and Order Society: Cobden Trust Memorial Lecture*, London: Cobden Trust.

Hall, S. (1991) 'And not a shot fired', *Marxism Today* (December), pp. 10–15.

Haxby, D. (1978) *Probation: A Changing Service*, London: Constable.

Hay, C. (1996) *Re-Stating Social and Political Change*, Buckingham: Open University Press.

Home Office (1962) *Report of the Departmental Committee on the Probation Service, Cmnd. 1650*, London: HMSO.

Home Office (1984) *Probation Service in England and Wales: Statement of National Objectives and Priorities*, London: Home Office.

Home Office (1988) *Punishment, Custody and the Community, Cmnd. 424*, London: HMSO.

Home Office (1989) *Review of Probation Training: Final Report*, London: Home Office.

Home Office (1990a) *Crime, Justice and Protecting the Public, Cmnd. 965*, London: HMSO.

Home Office (1990b) *Supervision and Punishment in the Community: A Framework for Action, Cmnd. 966*, London: HMSO.

Home Office (1994) *Review of Probation Officer Recruitment and Qualifying Training*, London: Home Office.

Hudson, B. (1987) *Justice Through Punishment: A Critique of the 'Justice' Model of Corrections*, London: Macmillan.

Hudson, B. (1993) *Penal Policy and Social Justice*, London: Macmillan.

Hughes, E. (1971) *The Sociological Eye: Selected Papers*, Chicago: Aldine-Atherton.

Jarvis, F.V. (1972) *Advise, Assist and Befriend: A History of the Probation and After-Care Service*, London: NAPO.

Jarvis, F.V. (1980) *Jarvis's Probation Officers Manual*, London: Butterworth.

Johnson, T.J. (1972) *Professions and Power*, London: Macmillan.

Johnson, T. (1993) 'Expertise and the State', in Gane, M. and Johnson, T. (Eds), *Foucault's New Domains*, London: Routledge.

King, J. (1969) *The Probation and After-Care Service* (3rd edn), London: Butterworth.

Lloyd, C. (1986) *'Response to SNOP': An Analysis of the Home Office Document, 'Probation Service in England and Wales: Statement of National Objectives and Priorities' and the Subsequent Local Responses*, Cambridge: Institute of Criminology.

Maguire, M., Morgan, R. and Reiner, R. (Eds) (1994) *The Oxford Handbook of Criminology*, Oxford: Oxford University Press.

Mair, G. (1996) 'Developments in probation in England and Wales 1984–1993', in McIvor, G. (Ed.) *Working with Offenders*, London: Jessica Kingsley.

Martinson, R. (1974) 'What works? Questions and answers about prison reform', *Public Interest*, **35**, pp. 22–54.

Mathieson, D. (1987) 'This is the heart of probation', *Justice of the Peace*, (18 July), pp. 458–60.

MATHIESON, D. (1992) 'The Probation Service', in STOCKDALE, E. and CASALE, S. (Eds) *Criminal Justice under Stress*, London: Blackstone.

MAY, T. (1991a) *Probation: Politics, Policy and Practice*, Milton Keynes: Open University Press.

MAY, T. (1991b) 'Under siege: the Probation Service in a changing environment', in REINER, R. and CROSS, M. (Eds) *Beyond Law and Order: Criminal Justice Policy and Politics into the 1990s*, London: Macmillan.

MAY, T. (1994a) 'Probation and community sentences', in MAGUIRE, M., MORGAN, R. and REINER, R. (Eds) *The Oxford Book of Criminology*, Oxford: Oxford University Press.

MAY, T. (1994b) 'Transformative power: a study in a human service organisation', *Sociological Review*, **42**, pp. 618–38.

MAY, T. and VASS, A. (1996) 'The shifting sands of working with offenders', in MAY, T. and VASS, A. (Eds), *Working with Offenders: Issues, Contexts and Outcomes*, London: Sage.

MCIVOR, G. (Ed.) (1996) *Working with Offenders*, London: Jessica Kingsley.

MCWILLIAMS, W. (1983) 'The mission to the English Police Courts 1876–1936', *Howard Journal of Criminal Justice*, **22**, pp. 129–47.

MCWILLIAMS, W. (1985) 'The mission transformed: professionalisation of probation between the wars', *Howard Journal of Criminal Justice*, **24**, pp. 257–74.

MCWILLIAMS, W. (1986) 'The English Probation System and the diagnostic ideal', *Howard Journal of Criminal Justice*, **25**, pp. 241–60.

MCWILLIAMS, W. (1987) 'Probation, pragmatism and policy', *Howard Journal of Criminal Justice*, **26**, pp. 97–121.

MCWILLIAMS, W. (1992) 'The rise and development of management thought in the English probation system', in STATHAM, R. and WHITEHEAD, P. (Eds) *Managing the Probation Service: Issues for the 1990s*, London: Longman.

NELLIS, M. (1995) 'Probation values for the 1990s', *Howard Journal of Criminal Justice*, **34**, pp. 19–43.

NELLIS, M. (1996) 'Probation training: The links with social work', in MAY, T. and VASS, A. (Eds) *Working with Offenders: Issues, Contexts and Outcomes*, London: Sage.

PAGE, M. (1992) *Crime Fighters of London: A History of the Origins and Development of the London Probation Service 1876–1965*, London: Inner London Probation Service Benevolent and Educational Trust.

POLLITT, C. (1993) *Managerialism and the Public Services: Cuts or Cultural Change in the 1990s?* (2nd edn), Oxford: Basil Blackwell.

RADZINOWICZ, L. and KING, J. (1979) *The Growth of Crime: The International Experience*, Harmondsworth: Penguin.

RAINE, J.W. and WILSON, M.J. (Eds) (1993) *Managing Criminal Justice*, London: Harvester Wheatsheaf.

RAYNOR, P. (1984) 'National purpose and objectives: a comment', *Probation Journal*, **31** (2), pp. 43–7.

RAYNOR, P., SMITH, D. and VANSTONE, M. (1994) *Effective Probation Practice*, London: Macmillan.

RYAN, M. and WARD, T. (1990) 'Restructuring, resistance and privatisation in the non-custodial sector', *Critical Social Policy*, **10**, pp. 54–67.

SCULL, A. (1983) 'Community corrections: Panacea, progress or pretence', in GARLAND, D. and YOUNG, P. (Eds), *The Power to Punish*, London: Heinemann.

SHAW, K. (1987) 'Skills, control, and the mass professions', *Sociological Review*, **35**, pp. 775–93.

SHAW, R. (1992) 'Corporate management in probation', in STATHAM, R. and WHITEHEAD, P. (Eds), *Managing the Probation Service: Issues for the 1990s*, London: Longman.

SMITH, D. (1996) 'Social work and penal policy', in McIVOR, G. (Ed.), *Working with Offenders*, London: Jessica Kingsley.

STATHAM, R. (1992) 'Towards managing the probation service', in STATHAM, R. and WHITEHEAD, P. (Eds), *Managing the Probation Service: Issues for the 1990s*, London: Longman.

STENSON, K. and COWELL, D. (1991) 'Making Sense of Crime Control', in STENSON, K. and COWELL, D. (Eds), *The Politics of Crime Control*, London: Sage.

VASS, A. (1990) *Alternatives To Prison: Punishment, Custody and the Community*, London: Sage.

WALKER, H. and BEAUMONT, B. (1981) *Probation Work: Critical Theory and Socialist Practice*, Oxford: Blackwell.

WILDING, P. (1982) *Professional Power and Social Welfare*, London: Routledge & Kegan Paul.

WILLIAMS, B. (Ed.) (1995) *Probation Values*, Birmingham: Venture Press.

Chapter 9

Social Work and De-professionalization

Richard Hugman

Social Work and Professionalization – an Introduction

Social work may be distinguished as one of the caring professions which has developed an overt concern with the process of professionalization. This is not to suggest that the issue of professionalization has not had a vital place in the analysis of, and debates about, nursing or occupational therapy (for example, Wallis, 1987a; 1987b; Jolley, 1989). Indeed, it could be said that this concern, even obsession, is a major feature common to both social work and nursing (Dingwall *et al.*, 1988; Jolley, 1989). What is peculiar to social work is the way in which concepts of professionalization have been used explicitly in the formation of occupational identity and related social structures at specific points in the twentieth century. Not only have social workers, like nurses and remedial therapists, sought to model their occupation on the more established professions of medicine and law, but they have also engaged more in explicit social science debates about the nature of professions and the implications of professionalization. Continued argument, not only about whether or not social work 'is' or 'should be' a profession, has been combined frequently with questions about the nature of professionalism as a concept, or professions as forms of social organization (Abbott and Meerabeau, Chapter 1 of this volume; Johnson, 1972; Simpkin, 1979; Wilding, 1982; Sibeon, 1990; 1991). As Johnson observed (1972, p. 25), a concern for the fate of social work in the late 1960s (especially in the UK) influenced the ways in which some analysts approached the topic at that time.

This apparently strong connection between the development of social work and theoretical approaches to professionalization can thus be explained, in part, by the close association of social work with the social sciences, comparable to that of nursing and occupational therapy with the biological sciences, and, in part, by the social circumstances of social work at key points in its history. It is for this reason that, although the issue is of crucial relevance to other caring professions, this chapter focuses primarily on social work, in order to consider recent developments in the analysis of professionalization and its relationship to the restructuring of social welfare in advanced industrial societies.

Social work is often regarded as a *new* profession, although in relation to similar occupations this may be something of a misattribution. The emergence of social work as an occupation can be seen to have begun in the second half of the nineteenth century, parallel with the development of nursing, and just prior to the emergence of occupational therapy as a single, distinct entity (Hugman, 1991; Abbott and Wallace in this volume). For example, early social workers such as Barnett, Hill and Loch in the UK, Addams and Parker Follett in the USA, and Clark and Spence in Australia, were not only working contemporaneously with each other, but also with nurses such as Nightingale, Dock and Osburn (although developments in Australia, Canada and New Zealand were heavily influenced by the UK and the USA – Castle, 1987; Dickey, 1987; Mowbray, 1992). Occupational therapy was given a major impetus by the Great War of the early 1900s and thereafter in a formal sense began to emerge as a single occupation slightly after nursing and social work (Diasio Serrett, 1985). In this way, although the specific influences were different, each occupation can be seen to have been engaged in a similar process. This was the claiming of a distinct occupational identity, based on a combination of skills and knowledge that could be systematized, taught, and then made accountable through collective organizations.

The early champions of the caring professions were certain that through the process of professionalization the work with which they were associated could be enhanced and the standards of society improved. It was, of course, a particular view of social improvement which these activists sought to promote, one which reflected their own cultural backgrounds as well as dominant class values (Abbott and Wallace in this volume; Parry and Parry, 1979; Forsythe, 1995). At the same time, an understanding of the process must be grounded in the historical circumstances of the period, within which it is possible to see such occupations as forming a vehicle for feminist intervention (Hearn, 1982; Witz, 1992). These were, for the most part, women's occupations, in which the central figures sought to emulate the social organization of the occupations pursued by the men of their time. This era of professionalization therefore contained contradictory strands, in which some discriminatory and divisive social relations were taken for granted (even reinforced), while others were challenged.

As Hearn (1982) notes, however, the continuing history of nursing and social work has been that of patriarchal dominance. This has been produced in two ways. The first is through the external control of one occupation by another, as of nursing and occupational therapy by medicine

(Hugman, 1991; Witz, 1992). The second is through the internal control of an occupation, in which the promotion of certain practices and values reflects the interests of some, but not all, members. Notably, the senior levels of social work have been disproportionately populated, since the middle of the twentieth century, by white, middle-class men. Women who have achieved this type of seniority have tended to share the same class and racial/ethnic origins as the men in comparable positions, although the presence of women at senior levels has been disproportionately small relative to their numbers in the occupation as a whole (Grimwood and Popplestone, 1993). So, although the origins of professionalization in social work, as in nursing and occupational therapy, were in many ways proto-feminist, they cannot be said to have been so unambiguously.

Social Work and Professionalism

What were the proponents of professionalization in social work trying to achieve? This question can be answered in one way by looking at the sociological literature on the professions, from which a list of 'traits' or characteristics can be discerned which demarcate 'a profession' from other types of occupation (such as 'trades'). The specific traits which are identified by different writers vary (cf. Carr-Saunders and Wilson, 1933; Greenwood, 1957; Vollmer and Mills, 1966; Parsons, 1968; Etzioni, 1969). Such characteristics include:

- possession of a distinct body of knowledge;
- esoteric skills;
- occupational control over qualification;
- a code of ethics;
- a corporate body or association;
- social prestige.

Such a list, it may be said, is difficult to distinguish from the claims made by the professions themselves as to why they should be regarded as a distinct social group. A common criticism of the 'trait' approach is that it has served to reproduce aspects of the professions' own ideologies within the findings of social science enquiry (see, for example, the critiques by Johnson, 1972; Wilding, 1982; Hugman, 1991). The body of literature which relies on this 'trait' approach is frequently grounded in functionalist analysis, in which the 'degree' of professionalism – that is, the number of traits which an occupation can be judged to possess – is seen as functional to the type of work undertaken and the social role performed by that occupation.

This connection can be illustrated by the argument of Simpson and Simpson (1969) that the control of social workers (predominantly women) either by managers or by other professions (predominantly men) is a function both of the nature of social work (focused on social/emotional problems) and of the nature of women (focused on the social/emotional aspects of life). These 'facts', they assert, lead to the functional (that is, sociologically 'most appropriate') location of social work within social relations where it is managed by others. Neither social workers (specifically) or women (generally), they conclude, want to be bothered with 'administration' or 'management'. So, from this perspective, social work is inevitably, and 'properly', accepted as a semi-profession, because it eschews claims to organizational or institutional independence. Thus, it is only ever able to replicate the classic, masculine professions in part: social work is as it is because of the 'nature' of women.

However, the critiques of the functionalist approach to traits argue that both control over qualification and prestige can be seen more plausibly as consequences than as causes of professional identity. They follow from, rather than leading to, some other aspect of the social organization of work through which particular occupations have become defined historically as distinct. This sociological approach, based on a more critical view of social relations, identified the underlying facet of professionalism as 'occupational self-government' or 'autonomy' (Freidson, 1970; 1986; Johnson, 1972; 1977; Larson, 1977; Wilding, 1982). From this perspective, professionalization is the process by which occupations achieve social power over their work (Hugman, 1991). A 'profession' is thus an occupation that, by making certain claims about the esoteric knowledge it possess, while at the same time being able to deliver a demonstrably skilled and effective service, is able to exercise a large measure of self-government and enjoy high social prestige (Freidson, 1986). From such a position, the functionalist approach to 'traits' is seen to be both circular and mechanistic.

An example of a more critical and historically grounded view is that of Jamous and Peloille (1970), who in a study of French hospital medicine had argued that the balance between esoteric knowledge and demonstrable skill could be understood as a combination of ambiguity and effectiveness (Sibeon, 1991, p. 98). Jamous and Peloille called this the ratio of indeterminacy to technical rationality. The successfully professionalized occupations (that is, those with high levels of self-government and prestige) are those which have been able to establish claims answering both criteria. Ambiguity without effectiveness is open to a lack of wider social support, while effectiveness without ambiguity can be easily prescribed and controlled from outside the profession itself (for example, by the state, by agency managers, or by other professions).

Making claims over the right to control occupational entry through qualifications, the use of ethical codes in regulating conduct in practice, the definition of practice standards, and so on, are thus seen as specific tactics within broader strategies for gaining and maintaining autonomy, rather than facts which may lead 'naturally' to occupational self-control. Historically, autonomy has not been achieved easily for any profession, and these 'traits', rather than being 'natural' have been pursued as elements of self-government. Moreover, negotiation and the forming of alliances with other groups to achieve wider social support are also part of the process. As Johnson (1972) shows, the social power of the professions, exercised in these ways, may be shared with others, such as the patrons of the service provided or the state (which may or may not also be a 'patron'). Indeed, such sharing may also be part of a strategic development. It is difficult to envisage any profession which is not buttressed at least in part by the state – for example, in the guarantee of monopoly through legislation, or through empowerment by law and administrative procedure.

Although the process approach does identify characteristics of professions, it points clearly to occupational control and autonomy as the core issue of professionalism. So, it is important to distinguish the elucidation of historical characteristics, some of which have been consciously grasped in the struggle to professionalize, from the functionalist manner in which the idea of 'traits' came to typify a sociological body of thought. This interpretation of the idea of 'traits' can be distinguished, in different ways, from that of Jolley (1989) or of Sibeon (1990; 1991). Each conflates the functionalist approach to traits (that which is usually regarded as 'trait theory') with reference to 'characteristics' embedded in other analyses, but they do so for different reasons. For Jolley (1989, p. 2) the central concern is to explore the variety of characteristics which have been identified in studies of professions, in order to establish why nursing may or may not have been able to achieve any specific facet. This is an implicit extension of the functionalist stance, albeit one which takes a more critical view of the social role of women and also some account of the process interpretation of professionalization. However, Jolley fails to distinguish between the assumptions of functionalism and the more critical implications of other approaches. By contrast, for Sibeon (1990, p. 92), it is important to recognize that other, more critical sociologies have also rested on a definition of professionalism through key characteristics. Although these have been less flattering to the professions, identifying issues such as privilege, self-interest, exclusion and monopolism, they are, Sibeon asserts, also traits. Yet what is at issue here, and which brings this present analysis much closer to that of Sibeon than Jolley, is the recognition that the major problem with the functionalist approach is that it isolates certain facets of occupations mechanically, taking them out of their historical and dynamic context, and so confuses cause and effect. Thus, to insist on bracketing mechanical functionalism with the dynamic analysis of critical characteristics as 'trait theory', as Sibeon does, seems curiously unhelpful. In particular, the former body of work leads to a concern with a 'check-list' attitude towards whether a particular occupation is or is not 'a profession'. A 'check-list' might be thought to be useful in the politics of health and social welfare (although the history of nursing, occupational therapy or social work raises doubts about even this), but it is lacking in rigour as sociology. It is the process approaches, including those that identify specific characteristics of the occupations which claim professional status, that have provided the more perceptive analysis of professionalization (and hence of de-professionalization – see below) because they are more methodologically and theoretically robust.

The answer to the question 'what were the proponents of professionalization in social work trying to achieve?' may therefore be stated as: a sufficient degree of autonomy to accomplish their occupational objectives. As with other professionalizing occupations, social work was to a large extent driven by particular views of the world, including a value framework about the desirability of particular goals. This is not to say that individuals or groups within social work were not also trying to pursue other, more material aims, such as social status, higher salaries, or whatever. However, the collective representations of social work (such as professional associations and service agencies) justified their concern with the expansion of occupational territory (cf. Beattie, 1995) through their claims to certain (value-based) goals, notably the 'relief of poverty and distress' (Forsythe, 1995).

Social Work and Anti-professionalism

Social work is also the caring profession which has the most developed strand of 'anti-professional' theorizing, although a similar line of thought exists in nursing (Salvage, 1988; Parkin, 1995). Largely drawn from neo-Marxist sociology, the 'radical social work' of the late 1960s, through to the 1980s, rejected the orthodox claims to professionalism (Bailey and Brake, 1975; Simpkin, 1979; Brake and Bailey, 1980; Mullaly, 1993). The common thread within this approach was that social work should be seen as an employed occupation much as any other non-manual work under advanced industrial capitalism. Not only did this mean that the pretensions to professional status were inaccurate, but that they actually impeded the pursuit of the core objectives of social work. A professional self-image that stressed 'impartiality' of theories and methods of practice, which for radical social work was a self-delusion, served only to obscure the way in which 'professionalizing' social workers failed to confront the underlying social structural causes of the problems with which they were dealing in their work. The 'relief' of poverty and distress was for this reason seen as the self-limitation of professionalizing social work's vision, because it left intact the origin of these social issues (Fisher and Karger, 1997).

Two sociological ideas are contained in this critique. The first is the reading of professionalism as self-interest, privilege and so on. Radical social work argues that, to the extent that social workers ally themselves with the dominant classes, it cannot be possible for them to deal with the root causes of poverty and other disadvantages. It is not the frustration of social work in failing to achieve the same form of professionalism as medicine or law that was (or still is) the problem, but the social divisions inherent in that type of occupational organization. Social work had attached itself to the wrong agenda early in its development and, insofar as it still looks to medicine or law as models in the contemporary era, it continues to do so.

The second sociological idea behind the radical critique was that the classic form of professionalism was itself under pressure from the social forces of advanced capitalism. Braverman (1974) had identified the process through which the work of the artisan had become drawn into the factories as that of 'deskilling'. In the craft mode of production the overview, and thus control, of the labour process had been exercised by artisans through home-based working. In factories the involvement of each worker in all aspects of production was replaced by task specialization. Managers and owners came to be the only people to have an overview and hence control of the labour process. For the radical social work critics, this was the fate of social work (and nursing or the remedial therapies) because it was also, in an analytic sense, the fate of other, more established professions. However, this is a prospect which, from the radical perspective, should be grasped rather than resisted, because it provides the basis for understanding social work as a form of skilled labour, and hence linking it in social class terms with the individuals and groups who use its services rather than with those who are seen as the cause of their problems (Simpkin, 1979). (I will return below to the implications of more recent changes in radical social work ideas.) Historically, insofar as this process continues, it is likely that medicine and law, far from being models for social work to emulate, will follow social work away from classic forms of professionalism (Cousins, 1987). In the meantime, social work was trapped in the contradiction between its professional ideology and the material reality of its predominant mode of employment in large-scale, managed, and often, state, organizations.

Social Work and Managerialism

Parry and Parry (1979) proposed the idea of agency or bureau-professionalism as a way of understanding the apparently mixed occupational form which social work had taken. The analytic model which they proposed was based on an shrewd grasp of the common feature of social work, nursing and comparable occupations – that the mainstream form of their organization, historically and in the present, has been within agencies. This is not to say that individual or 'private' practice does not or could not exist. Rather, it is observed that for the vast majority of members of these caring professions the predominant mode of practice is within or on behalf of an agency.

The implication of this perspective is that all practice is managed to some degree, because it is accountable within an agency relationship. This is the case whether practice is managed through a long hierarchy of paid officials (that is, a bureaucracy), or whether management is quite direct, as by committee of some kind (as it might be in a small non-government agency). In either instance the professional practitioner is accountable to persons or groups who are neither the immediate service user nor the peer group of the profession. It is in this way that social work (along with nursing, the remedial therapies, school teachers and so on) as seen in Johnson's (1972) now classic formulation of the mediated profession, as compared to patronage (control shared with users who pay for the service) or collegiality (control shared by members of the profession).

It is the question of mediated accountability which in this analysis distinguishes the so-called 'semi-professions' from the more classic types. However, as Johnson (1972) recognized, all professions are mediated to some extent, through state support for monopolies, and so on (see above). Cousins (1987), in a comparison of the UK and North America, noted that in the intervening decade and a half the more autonomous profession of medicine had become more subject to similar constraints. Large sections of medicine had for many years continued to be based on the prospect of private practice, thus mixing collegiate and patronage forms of accountability, even where doctors were employed by state health services. This is the direct opposite of the situation pertaining to social work, nursing or the remedial therapies. However, as the economic base of private practice has shifted from direct fee for service to mass insurance models, the relationship between doctors and their patients has increasingly become mediated by agencies. The private/state distinction has become that between types of agency rather than between individual and collective accountability.

In an earlier analysis, Mills (1956) had predicted the emergence of 'factory' forms of work in the classic professions. His main example was that of law, where already there was evidence of a large-scale agglomeration of practitioners, managed within relatively large hierarchies. This managerial 'demiurge' was, Mills argued (1956, p. 24), likely to subsume other practices currently organized on the more 'craft' model of the small-scale partnership or solo practitioner.

For social work and similar caring professions the developmental path of bureau-professionalization has resembled just such a 'factory' model. Yet, as with the 'law factories' of Mills' analysis, there are some conceptual difficulties in seeing this type of organization solely in dichotomous, social-class terms. The managers of this type of agency have, for a long period of time, been drawn from the profession which is managed (or, in multi-disciplinary agencies, from one or more of them). To be a senior social worker was, and still is in most cases, to achieve seniority in professional and organizational terms simultaneously (see Larson, 1977).

What has changed in the last two decades is that at the most senior levels of large bureaucratic organizations there has been the growing influence of a form of managerialism which separates professional and organizational seniority, giving precedence to the latter (see the chapter by Clarke in this volume). Managerialism goes beyond the grasp of good management, to become an ideological movement in which management has come to be seen as a separate type of expertise (even a distinct 'profession') which 'naturally' has the capacity to direct, in broad terms, the work of others, including professions of all kinds. Nowhere has this been seen to have greater influence than in the National Health Service in the UK (Pollitt, 1993). Medical practitioners, along with nurses and other health professionals, have increasingly become subject to managers who do not have a background in any health practice, and may even have been recruited from manufacturing industry or the commercial and financial sector.

For social work the advent of managerialism has been no less profound, although it may have had a lower public profile. A superficial analysis might suggest that there is little change, because the managers of social work may continue to be drawn from the body of practitioners. However, two factors serve to challenge this supposition. First, the theories and practices of management on which these recruits to seniority base their actions have increasingly as their reference point the ideology of managerialism. A reflection of this can be seen in a comparison of the writings of Harbert (1988) and Bamford (1990). Both were directors (chief executive officers) of large local government departments in the UK at the time when they wrote their analyses, and both had originally trained and practised as social workers. However, their orientations to the boundaries of professionalism and management are quite distinct. Harbert (1988) stresses the 'otherness' of professionals from a management perspective. There is no sense of the role of the senior manager as a senior professional. Harbert's point of reference is that of management in general and other managers in particular. For Bamford (1990), however, there are two points of reference. The first is the set of ideas about management, while the second is the professional set of objectives in the services being managed. Bamford's distinction between good management and managerialism is that, in the former, the theory and practice of management is harnessed to the effective and efficient achievement of professional goals, while managerialism directs professional activity towards ends which are defined organizationally.

The view which reflects the perspective that became increasingly dominant in the 1980s and early 1990s is that of Harbert. Yet organizational goals are not constructed in a vacuum. If their reference point is not professional values, then it will lie elsewhere. There is no evidence in his analysis to suggest that Harbert (1988) wished to diminish social welfare as such, but an important factor in the social environment of such developments, including the growth of managerialism in health and social services, has been the New Right agenda in which economic concerns have been given priority over social issues. This phenomenon is in many ways global, and particularly affects the advanced industrial parts of the world, such as Western Europe, North America, Australia and New Zealand. One of the consequences is that professional concerns with the social dimension of health and welfare have become subordinated to a particular type of economic thought. The language of 'value-for-money' (VFM), 'economic rationalism' and 'economy, efficiency and effectiveness' (the three Es) has become commonplace, reflecting this shift in orientation.

That this language patently avoids the difficult socio-political questions of how the objectives of health and social welfare might be defined cannot fully obscure the extent to which these are not taken for granted, nor could they be, but are representative of a specific ideological position. The complexities of how 'needs' are defined, with which social work and other caring professions (as well as the discipline of social policy) has been grappling for over a century, are glossed over in assumptions that they can be equated with the 'wants' of individuals. It is then seen as plausible that the individuals themselves should be responsible for meeting these needs (Gray, 1996). Issues of access and social power are negated by this position which, having constructed health and social welfare as a commodity, leaves the resolution of need and the definition of VFM to quasi-market forces as if it were purely a technical matter, free of social values (Bartlett and Le Grand, 1993). However, as Balogh *et al.* have observed (1989), there are other 'Es', namely 'ethics' and 'equity', related to the social construction and use of power, which the (quasi-) market ideology ignores, but which is still a core aspect of the language of professionalism. The present analysis will return to this point below.

Managerialism, then, may be said to have fulfilled the radical social work prophesy. Social work, along with nursing, the remedial therapies and other comparable occupations, has struggled towards professional status, only to see such status losing its autonomy and subordinated to a separate and freestanding class of management. It is now regarded, at least by those in powerful social positions, as a 'product' generated by an 'industry', to be organized and managed as such. Social workers are, indeed, defined as skilled workers. De-professionalization would seem to be the inevitable outcome. Yet there have been other changes which require elucidation, in which different forces are having an impact, namely signs of the break-up of the large-scale organization of industry and the dispersal of work. It is to this phenomenon that the discussion must now turn.

Social Work and Post-Fordism

Changes in social welfare structures and practices are part of the social and historical circumstances within which they are located. Ford's factory organization of the labour process, with automated control over highly-skilled, specialized work has now, in many instances, been superseded by dispersed work patterns. This phenomenon has thus come to be known as 'post-Fordism' (Williams, 1994). The impact of new (computer-based) technologies on the organization of work in manufacturing and commerce has been profound. Most specifically, the large-scale organization of work is being rethought as a consequence of the possibility for more dispersed organization. This is not happening because of a loss of interest in controlling the labour process on the part of those who own businesses or the managers of such businesses. Rather, it reflects the availability of alternative means to ensure that such control remains, or is even refined, while at the same time achieving greater 'flexibility'. A dispersed workforce may carry lower infrastructural costs, for example. This can be seen physically in a reduced need for office space, when employees work from home, or work is contracted. 'Contracting-out' is also an important aspect of 'flexibility', because some of the non-physical costs of employment (health insurance, holidays, training) may be passed to the contracted worker along with the costs of equipment, offices, and so on. In this sense it could be said that the miniaturization of electronics has led to the miniaturization of the workplace and even of the workforce. Reflected in systematically high unemployment levels, this is then dispersed through sections of society as the miniaturization of work as a whole. One may be left with the sense that it is employees, above all, who are required to bear the implications of flexibility (Hutton, 1995; Thurrow, 1996).

There has been a related effect in the caring professions and similar areas of social life. Hospitals, schools, universities, and social care institutions in the modern era of the twentieth century can all, in some ways, be seen as factories (Scull, 1984). The internet, modems, lap-top computers, mobile telephones and so on are all as much a part of the means towards the 'decarceration' of social workers and other caring professionals into the community as they are of 'flexibility' in the manufacturing, commercial and financial, or consumer service sectors. There has been a parallel move towards the 'contracting-out' of health and welfare services, including social work. Contracts, as much as modems, provide a means by which the practices of professionals can be held accountable, while no longer being located, socially or physically, in the main agency. The more specific the contracting agency, usually the state, can be in a contract, the more easily it can disperse responsibility for practice in social welfare provision, while retaining strong overall control. Thus, social work, in the 'Western' countries and increasingly elsewhere, is modelled on the 'tight centre/loose periphery' advocated by management theorists (Peters, 1987).

What of professionals and professionalism in the 'post-Fordist' analysis? Does the 'tight centre/loose periphery' model imply that all semblance of autonomy is finally lost in governance by contract? Indeed, has the balance of ambiguity to effectiveness been tipped so far as to preclude any sense of the esoteric in skills and knowledge claimed by the caring professions? A key issue in answering these questions is that of the definition of competence (and, by corollary, incompetence) and what has come to be known as the 'competencies' movement. This has been of crucial concern for social work in the UK, perhaps more than in any other country, from the 1980s and through the 1990s.

Sibeon (1990, pp. 97–105) identifies the debate around the social work qualification in the UK as a prime example of the way in which unintended as much as intended consequences of action by individuals or groups can shape the power exerted by an occupation in the professionalizing process. In particular, he links the type of knowledge to which social work makes claims, judged by some to be normative rather than scientific, with the relatively weak form of professional autonomy social work has ever achieved (1990, p. 104). In other words, powerful groups outside professional social work, including senior managers recruited from within the profession, were able to promote the view that there was too much indeterminacy and not enough demonstrated effectiveness in social work. The frequent criticisms of social work ideas and practices voiced as a result of high profile enquiries into the deaths of children (such as East Sussex, Brent or Lambeth), or the removal of children from allegedly abusive parents later judged to have been inappropriate (Orkney, Rochdale) might serve as indicators of the phenomenon to which Sibeon referred, and which have continued through the 1990s (Aldridge, 1994). Social workers may feel they are 'damned if we do and damned if we don't', but other powerful social sectors (barristers, solicitors, journalists) are sure they can be determinate about social work's technical competence (or its lack).

As Sibeon (1991) shows, a concern with questions of 'competence' was harnessed to managerialist goals through an emphasis on the technicality of social work practice in debates in the UK in the late 1980s. The review of social work qualifications, initiated by the Central Council for Education and Training in Social Work (CCETSW), and the subsequent proposals for a single qualification, were widely supported by senior managers (at least in their collective identity), precisely because they were based on an approach to the definition of tasks and skills that would be readily defined, monitored and appraised (in Sibeon, 1990, p. 101). As a corollary, the recognition of professional training would be based on the demonstrated skills of graduates (outcomes) rather than the prescription of the knowledge-based subject matter covered in courses (inputs).

Such a situation encapsulates the argument of de-professionalization, in that, within the constant flux of the professionalizing process, the gains towards occupational self-control were reversed through the interaction of different groups, within which the power of social work can be seen to have waned. However, the sociological perspective of Derber (1983) provides a somewhat different explanation. For Derber, the key issue is not simply the subordination of professionals to managerialism, but the way in which this is achieved. He argues that the high levels of technical competence required in the complex social and physical systems of advanced industrial (or 'post-industrial') capitalism lead to a situation in which it is necessary for a trade-off to ensure that such systems can be maintained. Professionalism is maintained in relation to the means of task performance, while the ends of such work come increasingly to be defined externally (by managers, by the state, and so on). From this perspective, the contemporary form of professionalism, is one in which 'ideological autonomy' has been abandoned as a strategy to ensure that 'technical autonomy' is maintained.

Evidence for this process can be seen in the way in which managed health care subordinates medicine as well as nursing in the definition of broad clinical priorities, while continuing to be dependent on very high levels of skill on the part of medical practitioners. In this respect, the apparent weakness of social work may be seen in its 'failure' historically to claim distinctive practices, those which are not to some extent shared with other occupations. However, there are two ways in which Derber's arguments can be seen to have been demonstrated only partly through recent developments.

The first of these is the practical difficulty of separating 'ideological' and 'technical' realms of autonomy. Managed health and social welfare systems have sought increasingly to specify the scope of services so precisely that areas for judgement are confined to 'diagnosis' or 'assessment'. Once this decision has been made, the freedom for decision by professionals is severely reduced, largely through budgets that are set according to criteria established externally to the professions in question. For example, the definitions of need used in the UK National Health Service have led to wards and operating theatres being unused for parts of each year, and medical views of urgency becoming constrained within financial constraints that are imposed according to non-medical criteria (Hutton, 1995). Similarly, for UK social workers the implementation of 'community care' has created a situation in which responsibility and accountability have increased, but within the financial context of very restricted room for manoeuvre (Means and Smith, 1994). In this sense, technical autonomy can be seen as compromised by ideological subordination. The image used by Simpkin (1979, p. 115) as a critique of an earlier phase of managerialist developments, 'put a lion in a safari-park and he'll [*sic*] think he's free', can be reapplied to the potential for post-Fordist contractual arrangements to restrict professionals' freedom of action, even in the technical performance of their work, while creating a semblance of independence. The concern of social work senior managers with a technical definition of 'competence' thus appears to be a logical conclusion (Dominelli, 1996).

Secondly, at the time and place in which Derber (1983) developed his analysis it was not possible to see how further contradictions would open up from the interplay of competing interest groups. For social work this is reflected in the very high level of indeterminacy which has pertained throughout its development. That is, the goals of social work have from its infancy been based as much on social *values* as on social *facts*. It is this which explains, not only the relative weakness of social work professionalization, but also, paradoxically, the ferocity with which more powerful groups appear to have seen social work as a major target in attacks on the professions generally (Aldridge, 1994; 1996). It is not just a matter of reformulating a profession which encapsulates the high point of social democratic consensus on welfare into the producers of the post-consensus welfare industry (although this is the case) (Parton, 1994). Conscious efforts to de-professionalize social work, through the replacement of theoretically-based education by competency-based training, are to be seen as part of the post-Fordist strategy to ensure that the loose-periphery of practitioners in social welfare services can be relied on to work within the values of the emergent tight-centre. Yet it is in this very sphere that the recent history of social work illustrates the way in which such developments cannot be determined totally, even by very powerful groups. In the final section of this chapter, therefore, the important place of values in debates about the contemporary professionalization of social work will be explored.

Social Work and 'New Social Movements': Ethics and Equity, the Other 'Es'

Sociological accounts of the last decade of the twentieth century have rapidly become focused around the question of whether the developments in social structures, including globalization, post-Fordism, changes in the family, and rapid demographic shifts (such as ageing populations) constitute a late phase of modernity (and hence of capitalism), or should be seen as post-modernity and the emergence of a new social order (Giddens, 1990; Bauman, 1992; Lyon, 1994). Part of this analysis is the identification of a diverse set of social groups which, following Touraine (1981), have come to be known as 'new social movements'. These are groups based around traditional class divisions, but also women's groups, the interests of various racial and ethnic minorities, gays and lesbians, people with disabilities, older people, youth and student groups, and environmentalism. The attention to this increased complexity of the structures and relations in contemporary society evident in the social sciences, especially sociology, has influenced the theoretical development of social work. Given the historically-close intellectual proximity of social work and social science this should, perhaps, be unsurprising. However, the implication for social work is that, at the very time in which it was subject to an apparent process of ideological proletarianization, it was simultaneously developing a theoretical awareness of the 'new social movements' and the implications these might have for practice. Precisely because the values which have emerged emphasize equity, alongside ethics (Balogh *et al.*, 1989), professionalism may confront the '3 Es' (economy, efficiency and effectiveness) of contemporary managerialism.

It is in this way that the placing of 'anti-discrimination and anti-oppression' (UK) or 'social justice' (Australia, Canada) at the core of the professional agenda for social work should be seen, not just as a superficial political gesture by an occupation based on social democratic ideals which are under threat, but as a reformulation of the ideological component of professionalism. Indeed, connections between the ideological and the technical aspects of anti-discriminatory and anti-oppressive practice have been articulated by social work theorists who approach the issue from different positions, suggesting that a new paradigm is emerging (Fook, 1993; Mullaly, 1993; Thompson, 1993; Dominelli, 1996).

Given the relationship between the origins of social work professionalism and early feminism, and a broader concern with structural economic inequality and its effects, the contemporary orientation to diverse social divisions could be seen as a 'return to previous traditions' (Forsythe, 1995). Indeed, it seems curiously to parallel, in the form of a critique, the rhetoric of the political New Right regarding so-called 'Victorian values' (Young, 1992). Yet the attention of late-twentieth-century social work to such concerns differs significantly from that of the late nineteenth century. Just as the rhetoric of the New Right draws highly selectively on the ideas and values of the late nineteenth century and places them in the current context, so too the re-emergence of a concern for social work to address social divisions and questions of 'equity' may have some formal echoes of its occupational history, but the process has a distinctively late-twentieth-century substance.

First, in the introduction to this chapter it was noted that feminist agendas in nineteenth-century social work were disconnected from the approach taken to socio-economic issues. This was reflected in both the social class composition of social work and the groups who formed its leadership at that time (as well as through much of the century). Moreover, other social divisions with which contemporary feminism interacts were simply non-existent or, at best, could be described as nascent. Recognition of the diversity and the interconnectedness of social divisions, to which anti-discriminatory and anti-oppressive practice and the values of 'social justice' are a response, is very much a late-twentieth-century phenomenon. The very notion of 'equity' which is encapsulated here was not a part of the ideology of early social work.

Secondly, although the contentious nature of concerns with social divisions has created strong debates within social work now as much as it did for the former generation (see, for example, Parry and Parry (1979) on the struggle between the charity organization and settlement movements), the shape of these debates has changed. There is not the same polarization of focus between individualistic and community responses linked to notions of conservative and critical social analysis respectively. In particular, the idea of 'community' can be said to have been incorporated within a conservative 'relief' understanding of the social work task (Means and Smith, 1994; Hugman, 1997). Likewise, counselling and casework may be infused with radical values and used to promote social justice or equity based models of practice (Fook, 1993).

Thirdly, whereas the early stages of social work professionalization were manifestly focused on the harnessing of techniques to broad socio-political values, there is today a more ambiguous relationship. In other words, there are elements of a prescriptive technocratic development in the way in which social work has grasped these issues in recent times. The incorporation of anti-racist and anti-discriminatory practice as terms within the statement of 'competencies' by the Central Council for Education and Training in Social Work in the UK (CCETSW, 1991) and a comparable, although broader, claim to 'promotion of social justice' as a social work skill by the Australian Association of Social Workers (AASW, 1994) are examples of this blurring of the line between values and techniques.

As a strategy for defending the connection between knowledge, skills and values this assertion of a particular value-orientation within social work has carried a high level of risk (Patel, 1995; Dominelli, 1996). It has received criticism from within the profession that it is in conflict with the liberal strand of ethics on which social work has also historically drawn, but, perhaps more threateningly, from external sources there have been attacks on the legitimacy of a profession engaging with 'politics' in this way (Pinker, 1993: see Patel, 1995, p. 40). Yet, in this respect, it may be argued that there are connections between contemporary social work and its historical roots, because social work in the late nineteenth century, whether of the individualistic 'relief', or the community settlement mode, was self-consciously engaged in forms of political activity. Faced by challenges not only to its autonomy but to its existence, the professionalizing and radical strands of social work appear to have moved closer together. It is possible, although by no means certain, that such a shift will be the basis for a different trajectory for the forces of de-professionalization to that envisaged only a decade ago.

Social Work and De-professionalization – a Conclusion?

This analysis could be seen as an attempt to cling to modernist constructions, of the idea of a profession as well as of social values such as equity and social justice (Rojek *et al.*, 1988; Parton, 1994). However, social work, like other disciplines which are closely linked to social science, cannot avoid the difficult choices to be made in response to the debates about modernity and post-modernity. Even here the paradoxes and contradictions are quite stark. Most important for this discussion, the very intellectual foundations of the 'new social movements', deriving from lines of thought developed in the classic modernist period (for example, in the work of Marx, Simmel, Weber and others), are built upon, while at the same time being seen as the refutation of modernism. Feminism, anti-racism, gay and lesbian rights, disabled people's rights, older people's groups such as Grey Power, and so on, are all in this sense modernist in their assumptions of social relations, social structures and social divisions.

Social work, in responding to these social divisions, has, at the same time, engaged in an implicit struggle against de-professionalization. There is an irony here which is quite profound when the earlier radical critiques of professionalism are considered. (For instance, even by the mid-1980s some 'radical social work' theorists were arguing for an autonomy in the formation of social work knowledge that paralleled the claims of orthodox professionalism, although maintaining a different view of the goals towards which the use of such theory would be directed – see, for example, Bailey, 1984). Nevertheless, the resulting pattern of the counter-assertion of the ideological autonomy of professions is one which could, potentially, open up a line of development that would at a later date be understood as a reformulation of professionalism, rather than de-professionalization as such. Indeed, there is, for some commentators on the late-modern/postmodern situation, a risk that without a commitment of this kind to social values the individualistic, market-oriented, neo-liberal future is bleak indeed (Bauman, 1994; Hutton, 1995).

The (re-)emergence of anti-discriminatory and anti-oppressive practice, and a concern with social justice and equity-based values, have some connections with the origins of social work, insofar as it is currently less secure than at the high point of the social democratic consensus. At the same time it may also be a means for mainstream social work to (re)discover its socio-political dimension, and with that a more critical drive for a professionalization which itself is based on ideas of social justice and equity. However, to paraphrase the epigram attributed to various late Chinese leaders when asked to comment on the impact of the French revolution on human history – it is, as yet, too soon to tell.

References

AASW (1994) *Australian Social Work Competency Standards for Entry Level Social Workers*, Hawker (ACT): AASW.

Aldridge, M. (1994) *Making Social Work News*, London: Routledge.

Aldridge, M. (1996) 'Dragged to market: being a profession in the postmodern world', *British Journal of Social Work*, **26**, pp. 177–94.

Bailey, R. (1984) 'A question of priorities', *Issues in Social Work Education*, **4**, pp. 58–60.

Bailey, R. and Brake, M. (Eds) (1975) *Radical Social Work*, London: Edward Arnold.

Balogh, R., Beattie, A. and Beckaleg, S. (1989) *Figuring Out Performance*, Sheffield: English National Board.

Bamford, T. (1990) *The Future of Social Work*, Basingstoke: Macmillan.

Bartlett, W. and Le Grand, J. (1993) 'The concept of the quasi-market', in Le Grand, J. and Bartlett, W. (Eds) *Quasi-Markets and Social Policy*, Basingstoke: Macmillan.

Bauman, Z. (1992) *Intimations of Post-Modernity*, London: Routledge.

Bauman, Z. (1994) *Alone Again: Ethics after Certainty*, London: Demos.

Beattie, A. (1995) 'War and peace among the health tribes', in Soothill, K., Mackay, L. and Webb, C. (Eds) *Interprofessional Relations in Health Care*, London: Edward Arnold.

Brake, M. and Bailey, R. (Eds) (1980) *Radical Social Work and Practice*, London: Edward Arnold.

Braverman, H. (1974) *Labor and Monopoly Capital*, New York: Monthly Review Press.

Carr-Saunders, A.M. and Wilson, P.M. (1933) *The Professions*, London: Oxford University Press.

Castle, J. (1987) 'The development of professional nursing in New South Wales, Australia', in Maggs, C. (Ed.) *Nursing History: The State of the Art*, London: Croom Helm.

CCETSW (1991) *Rules and Requirements for the Diploma in Social Work* (2nd edn), London: CCETSW.

Cousins, C. (1987) *Controlling Social Welfare*, Brighton: Harvester Wheatsheaf.

Derber, C. (1983) 'Managing professionals: ideological proletarianization and post-industrial labour', *Theory & Society*, **12**, pp. 309–41.

Diasio Serrett, K. (1985) 'Another look at occupational therapy's history', in Diasio Serrett, K. (Ed.) *Philosophical and Historical Roots of Occupational Therapy*, New York: Haworth Press.

Dickey, B. (1987) *No Charity There: A Short History of Social Welfare in Australia*, Sydney: Allen & Unwin.

Dingwall, R., Rafferty, A.M. and Webster, C. (1988) *An Introduction to the Social History of Nursing*, London: Routledge.

Dominelli, L. (1996) 'Deprofessionalizing social work: anti-oppressive practices, competencies and post-modernism', *British Journal of Social Work*, **26**, pp. 153–76.

Etzioni, A. (Ed.) (1969) *The Semi-Professions and Their Organization*, New York: Free Press.

Fisher, R. and Karger, H.J. (1997) *Social Work and Community in a Private World*, White Plains (NY): Longman.

Fook, J. (1993) *Radical Casework: A Theory of Practice*, St Leonards (NSW): Allen & Unwin.

Forsythe, B. (1995) 'Discrimination in social work – an historical note', *British Journal of Social Work*, **25**, pp. 1–16.

Freidson, E. (1970) *The Profession of Medicine*, New York: Dodd Mead.

Freidson, E. (1986) *Professional Powers: A Study of the Institutionalization of Formal Knowledge*, Chicago: University of Chicago Press.

Giddens, A. (1990) *The Consequences of Modernity*, Cambridge: Polity Press.

Gray, J. (1996) *After Social Democracy*, London: Demos.

Greenwood, E. (1957) 'Attributes of a profession', *Social Work*, **2**(3), pp. 44–55.

Grimwood, C. and Popplestone, R. (1993) *Women, Management and Care*, Basingstoke: Macmillan.

Harbert, W. (1988) *The Welfare Industry*, Hadleigh.

Hearn, J. (1982) 'Notes on patriarchy, professionalization and the semi-professions', *Sociology*, **16**, pp. 184–202.

Hugman, R. (1991) *Power in Caring Professions*, Basingstoke: Macmillan.

Hugman, R. (1997) 'Community and care', in Hugman, R., Peelo, M. and Soothill, K. (Eds) *Concepts of Care*, London: Edward Arnold.

Hutton, W. (1995) *The State We're In*, London: Jonathan Cape.

Jamous, H. and Peloille, B. (1970) 'Changes in the French university-hospital system', in Jackson, J.A. (Ed.) *Professions and Professionalization*, Cambridge: Cambridge University Press.

Johnson, T.J. (1972) *Professions and Power*, London: Macmillan.

Johnson, T.J. (1977) 'The professions in the class structure', in Scase, R. (Ed.) *Industrial Society: Class, Cleavage and Control*, London: Allen & Unwin.

JOLLEY, M. (1989) 'The professionalisation of nursing: the uncertain path', in ALLAN, P. and JOLLEY, M. (Eds) *Current Issues in Nursing*, London: Chapman & Hall.

LANGAN, M. and LEE, P. (Eds) (1989) *Radical Social Work Today*, London: Unwin Hyman.

LARSON, M.S. (1977) *The Rise of Professionalism: A Sociological Analysis*, Berkeley (CA): University of California Press.

LYON, D. (1994) *Postmodernity*. Buckingham: Open University Press.

MEANS, R. and SMITH, R. (1994) *Community Care: Policy and Practice*, Basingstoke: Macmillan.

MILLS, C.W. (1956) *The Power Elite*, London: Oxford University Press.

MOWBRAY, M. (1992) 'The medicinal properties of localism: a historical perspective', in THORPE, R. and PETRUCHENIA, J. (Eds) *Community Work or Social Change? An Australian Perspective*, Sydney: Hale & Iremonger.

MULLALY, R. (1993) *Structural Social Work*, Toronto: McClelland & Stewart.

PARKIN, P.A.C. (1995) 'Nursing the future: a re-examination of the professionalization thesis in the light of some recent developments', *Journal of Advanced Nursing*, **21**, pp. 561–67.

PARRY, N. and PARRY, J. (1979) 'Social work, professionalism and the state', in PARRY, N., RUSTIN, M. and SATYAMURTI, C. (Eds) *Social Work, Welfare and the State*, London: Edward Arnold.

PARSONS, T. (1968) 'Professions', in SILLS, D. (Ed.) *The International Encyclopaedia of the Social Sciences*, London: Macmillan.

PARTON, N. (1994) 'Problematics of government, (post) modernity and social work', *British Journal of Social Work*, **24**, pp. 9–32.

PATEL, N. (1995) 'In search of the holy grail', in HUGMAN, R. and SMITH, D. (Eds) *Ethical Issues in Social Work*, London: Routledge.

PETERS, T. (1987) *Thriving on Chaos*, London: Pan.

PINKER, R. (1993) 'A lethal kind of looniness', *Times Higher Education Supplement*, (10 September), p. 19.

POLLITT, C. (1993) *Managerialism and the Public Services* (2nd edn), Oxford: Blackwell.

ROJEK, C., PEACOCK, G. and COLLINS, S. (1988) *Social Work and Received Ideas*, London: Routledge.

SALVAGE, J. (1988) 'Professionalization – or struggle for survival? A consideration of current proposals for the reform of nursing in the United Kingdom', *Journal of Advanced Nursing*, **13**, pp. 515–19.

SCULL, A. (1984) *Decarceration* (2nd edn), Cambridge: Polity Press.

SIBEON, R. (1990) 'Social work knowledge, social actors and deprofessionalization', in ABBOTT, P. and WALLACE, C. (Eds) *The Sociology of the Caring Professions* (1st edn), Basingstoke: Falmer.

SIBEON, R. (1991) 'The construction of a contemporary sociology of social work', in DAVIES, M. (Ed.) *The Sociology of Social Work*, London: Routledge.

SIMPKIN, M. (1979) *Trapped within Welfare*, London: Macmillan.

SIMPSON, R.L. and SIMPSON, I.H. (1969) 'Women and bureaucracy in the semi-professions', in ETZIONI, A. (Ed.) *The Semi-Professions and Their Organization*, New York: Free Press.

THOMPSON, N. (1993) *Anti-Discrimination*, Basingstoke: Macmillan.

THURROW, L. (1996) *The Future of Capitalism*, St Leonards (NSW): Allen & Unwin.

TOURAINE, A. (1981) *The Voice and the Eye: An Analysis of Social Movements*, Cambridge: Cambridge University Press.

VALENTINE, P.E.B. (1996) 'Nursing: a ghettoized profession relegated to the women's sphere', *International Journal of Nursing Studies*, **33**, pp. 98–106.

VOLLMER, H. and MILLS, D. (1966) *Professionalization*, New York: Prentice Hall.

WALLIS, M.A. (1987a) '"Profession" and "professionalism" and the emerging profession of occupational therapy (part 1)', *British Journal of Occupational Therapy*, **50**, pp. 259–62.

WALLIS, M.A. (1987b) '"Profession" and "professionalism" and the emerging profession of occupational therapy (part 2)', *British Journal of Occupational Therapy*, **50**, pp. 300–2.

WILDING, P. (1982) *Professional Power and Social Welfare*, London: Routledge & Kegan Paul.

WILLIAMS, F. (1994) 'Social relations, welfare and the post-Fordism debate', in BURROWS, R. and LOADER, B. (Eds) *Towards a Post-Fordist Welfare State?*, London: Routledge.

WITZ, A. (1992) *Professions and Patriarchy*, London: Routledge.

YOUNG, G. (1992) 'Enterprise regained', in HEELAS, P. and MORRIS, P. (Eds) *The Values of the Enterprise Culture*, London: Routledge.

Chapter 10

Conflict over the Grey Areas: District Nurses and Home Helps Providing Community Care

Pamela Abbott

Introduction

Feminist critiques of community care have concentrated on the ways in which policies of community care exploit unpaid female carers. Indeed, Janet Finch and Dulcie Groves (1987) have suggested that it is not possible to have community care that does not exploit women. While recent studies (e.g. Arber *et al.*, 1991) have demonstrated that although more men than was previously thought provide community care, women as daughters and wives provide the bulk of informal care (Arber and Ginn, 1991). Hilary Graham (1985) argues that part of the domestic economy for women is the provision of health care and that they play a major role in providing for others in the family who are sick, disabled, elderly or in other ways dependent. Much domestic work is about health care, Graham argues: providing for health, health education and mediating professional help in time of crisis. It is women in the home who determine whether professional help is required, and in the case of children it is generally women who transport them to the doctor for examination.

The welfare state is built on the assumption that the traditional family is the norm, and that women care and provide for the members of this family. As well as caring for children, women are expected to take on the care of other relations who cannot look after themselves: community care generally means informal, unpaid care by women. It is assumed, in popular supposition and implicitly in the legislation and welfare rules, that caring is women's natural role and that they take on the burden of care relatively willingly. The extent of the burden should not be underestimated, however. I have argued previously (Abbott and Sapsford, 1987a) that the cost of normalizing life for children with learning disabilities is to denormalize it for their mothers. Nissel and Bonnerjea (1982) found that wives caring for elderly relatives spent an average of two to three hours a day carrying out essential tasks for the relative, whether or not they were in paid employment; husbands spent on average eight minutes. The burden is particularly heavy where the dependent is an adult, because the woman has no realistic expectation that the burden will be eased in some finite period of time, so that she can develop her own life and perhaps return to paid employment and some measure of economic freedom.

The emphasis on community care and, specifically, on policies aimed at keeping people in their own homes is a matter of ongoing concern for women, as is the emphasis on care being provided by relatives, friends and volunteers – especially in the light of the projected growth in the number of older people and the continuing political emphasis on familial responsibility for caring. The expectation that family members (mainly women) will provide the bulk of care for dependent relatives has not changed with the implementation of the National Health Service and Community Care legislation in April, 1993. The promised support for informal carers has not become a reality, as the available services are targeted at those most in need and withdrawn from, or denied to, others who are seen as less vulnerable. Research shows that home helps are allocated mainly to older people living alone or to elderly couples when both are very frail. Indeed, home help services are often withdrawn if a relative moves in with an elderly person who had previously received them (Abbott, 1992 b, c; 1997).

All this is common ground in the feminist community care literature. What has been less readily acknowledged is that the workers who are paid to provide community care in people's own homes – home helps/home carers – are themselves predominantly women, low-paid and often employed on a semi-casual basis (see, e.g., Abbott, 1992b; 1997). Indeed, as I shall argue in this chapter, attempts to enhance the role of these workers (and their status in their own eyes) result in their coming into conflict with another group of community care workers – the district nurses. The reasons for the conflict, I shall argue, relate not so much to professional skills and needs for nursing care as to the labour-market position of women in general and of nurses and home helps in particular. Indeed, it is possible to argue that district nurses are attempting to operate occupational closure against home helps in just the same way as doctors did against female health care workers in the nineteenth century (Witz, 1992). The chapter provides an example of the way in which the female caring professionals operate in protecting their own status against other groups of workers who threaten to challenge their claim to an esoteric knowledge base and professional expertise. In other words, in protecting their claims to professional status, district nurses operate in the same way as the medical profession used to operate.

Community Care: the Division of Labour

The main formal providers of community care are home helps, provided by Local Authority social services, and district nurses, provided by the health services. The main help required by elderly frail people can be divided into domestic care, social care, personal care and nursing care (Abbott, 1992b; 1997). Traditionally, home helps have provided domestic and social care, and district nurses personal and nursing care. Since the 1980s, however, enhanced home help/home carer services have increasingly been provided, with home helps supplying personal care as well. This change has been accompanied by arguments that the home help service and other elements of community care should be targeted on vulnerable elderly people who are otherwise at risk of having to enter residential care. At the same time, demonstration projects aimed at maintaining frail elderly people in their own homes have suggested that an adequate provision of services can be managed at a cost lower than that of residential care, given proper care/case management (but service innovations that lacked care management have not utilized home care services effectively – see Davies *et al.*, 1990). The most successful 'experiments' have been those where health and social services' inputs have been integrated under one management, and they have demonstrated that home care assistants can perform tasks successfully and efficiently that are commonly undertaken by nurses as well as home helps.

Griffiths (1988) suggested that the main employed providers of community care should be care workers, and that district nurses should be used only for those tasks that require their specific skills. However, there are problems in defining what is social and what is health care, in terms both of which agency *does* carry tasks out and which agency *should* carry them out. NAHAT (undated) tried to identify clearly those tasks which were the responsibility of the health services and those which should fall on the local authority. While they tried to minimize the overlap, a large class of personal care tasks and some which involved advising clients or their relatives on health and diet remained unallocatable. Melanie Henwood (1992), in a review of research, suggested that

> the realities of interaction between health and social care (both at strategic and operational levels) remain a formidable barrier to co-ordinated care. (Henwood, 1992, p. 5)

The Community Nursing Service operates at the point of interaction between assistance with personal tasks which are often performed by home helps and informal carers, and the more technical forms of medical intervention. This is a grey area, often exemplified by the 'social' as opposed to the 'medical' bath: personal care tasks are clearly nursing tasks, but they are not *skilled* nursing tasks and can be (and often are) performed by an auxiliary, a home help or an informal carer.

At the operational level there is often little attempt to sort out which of the two services shall provide which kinds of care:

> Research continues to demonstrate the lack of co-ordination and liaison in day-to-day practice, with resulting service duplication and overlap. (Davies *et al.*, 1990, pp. 26–7)

Thus care planning, at the level of individuals, has to take place between agencies rather than just within them (Charnley and Bebbington, 1988). While some nurses (e.g. Clark *et al.*, 1990) have stressed the danger of district nurses being excluded from the assessment of patients with nursing needs, others (e.g. Hamer, 1989) have pointed to a need for district nursing to change, handing over more tasks to care assistants and thereby freeing more time for specialized nursing tasks.

Undoubtedly it is the case that home helps/home carers can and do take on personal care tasks and to that extent substitute for district nurses. However, three problematic issues arise when they do so. First there is the extent to which personal care is seen by clients as an aspect of nursing and as something they would prefer to receive from a nurse. Secondly, the move towards personal care means the virtual disappearance of the conventional home help service, for which there is still a need. As Melanie Henwood points out,

> The withdrawal of service from clients with lesser needs may reduce the capacity of home care to operate in a preventive or rehabilitative mode. (Henwood, 1992, p. 43)

Thirdly, Local Authority Social Service Departments charge (albeit on a means-tested basis) for services provided, while Community Health Care Trusts do not charge clients for district nursing services.

Research that I carried out into the skill-mix in community care in Cornwall (Abbott, 1992 a, b; 1997; Abbott and Campbell, 1992) demonstrated a substantial overlap in the work of home helps and district nursing teams in the area of personal care. This was especially marked in those parts of the county where auxiliaries were employed as part of district nursing teams. However, what was evident was not only that both home helps and members of the district nursing team were carrying out personal care tasks for clients, but that this was an area of conflict. While home helps were keen to take on personal care, which they found rewarding, the district nurses were concerned that home helps were caring for vulnerable elderly people who needed to be cared for by the district nurse. In practice, much of this personal care work, when taken on by district nursing teams, is actually performed by auxiliaries who have no formal nursing training.

Nevertheless, the clients are patients of the district nursing team, and the district nursing team leader is responsible for supervising their care and 'treatment'. Especial concern was expressed that home helps were caring for people who needed nursing care, and that they encouraged dependency by doing things for clients, while the district nurses encouraged clients to do things for themselves. There appeared to be little co-operation or co-ordination between home helps and district nurses even with 'shared care' clients (Abbott, 1992a; 1997). While this is partly explained by the fact that home helps are employed by local authority social services and district nurses by health authorities, with different management hierarchies, I would argue it also relates to the district nurses' perception of themselves as professionals. Home helps are seen by them as being untrained domestics – precisely the image from which nursing has successfully escaped. Jane Salvage (1985) has argued that professionalizing strategies in the nursing profession militate against nurses working with relatives and other carers to meet the needs of patients/clients, and this certainly appears to apply to their relationships with home helps.

In our research district nurses often argued that clients preferred nurses to perform personal care tasks. However, we found no evidence for this, and, indeed, as I have argued elsewhere (Abbott *et al.*, 1992; Abbott, 1997), clients expressed greater satisfaction with the home help service, if anything, and few made any reference to the charges made for the service. This was partly because home helps were seen as friendly and approachable, whereas the district nurses were seen to keep a professional distance, and partly because of the working practices of the nurses. The home helps were all employed to work in their own locality, were allocated to particular clients, and the days and times of day of visits were negotiated with the clients. The district nursing teams worked large patches which they divided up geographically, working different geographical areas in rotation; this meant that clients were not visited regularly by the same member of the team. This practice was justified by the need for more than one member of the team to know a patient, and so that difficult clients could be shared among the team. The timing of visits was determined by nursing and operational considerations – a logical order for a week's/day's visits, minimizing mileage and time spent travelling. Patients were unable to specify the day or time of day when the team member would visit. Consequently, the clients were unable to build up the same friendly relationships that they had with the home helps. Home helps were seen by users as much more approachable than district nurses, and as more prepared to 'do extras' to help clients. Indeed, it could be argued that the non-remunerated extra work that home helps perform is an essential element of community care

(Warren, 1990; Abbott, 1992b; 1997; Abbott *et al.*, 1992). To use the distinction made by Gremmen (1995) in care-giving between the formal professional ethic and the ethic of care, home helps appeared, when they felt it necessary, to move more easily away from the formal rules in responding to needs in individual circumstances than did district nurses.

Professionals and Carers – the Female Division of Labour

In order to understand the conflict between female workers employed to provide community care for older people, we need to examine the female labour market. As Catherine Hakim (1979) has argued, the labour market is segmented vertically and horizontally by gender; women are concentrated in a narrow range of occupations, and in lower-status jobs within occupations. Over 60 per cent of women are in jobs which are done only by women, and over 80 per cent of men in jobs which are done only by men (Martin and Roberts, 1984). Using the occupational classifications of the New Earnings Survey, over 70 per cent of full-time female workers are in clerical work (mostly typists), 'professional and similar occupations in education, welfare and health' (where by far the largest grouping is the nurses) and 'personal services' (where the largest groupings are domestic staff, school helpers, kitchen assistants and caretakers). Within categories women are likely to hold the lower positions: more women than men are in non-manual jobs, but few are in professional or managerial positions. Within the professional group women are likely to occupy the lower-status positions as schoolteacher, librarian, nurse or social worker, while men dominate in the higher-status professions of law, accounting, architecture and medicine. Occupational segmentation is even more pronounced in part-time than in full-time work. (See, e.g., Abbott and Sapsford, 1987b; Abbott and Payne, 1990; Abbott and Tyler, 1995.)

In addition to labour-market segmentation, with women employed in certain occupational sectors and men in others, it has sometimes been argued that Britain has a dual labour market (Barron and Norris, 1976). Women are said to be part of a secondary-sector workforce – workers who are easily dispensed with in times of recession, are poorly remunerated and have poor conditions of employment. Dex (1985), however, has pointed out that some women are employed in the male primary sector, and that there is a female primary sector and a female secondary sector. Qualified nurses, especially those who are employed full-time, are clearly part of a female primary sector, while unqualified auxiliaries are part of a female secondary labour market. Home helps are also part of this secondary sector. Indeed, auxiliaries and home helps are drawn from the same pool of female labour – women with few, if any, educational credentials, seeking part-time work that is satisfying and which uses the skills they have acquired over the years.

However, at least in the area where I carried out my research, the employment conditions of auxiliaries and home helps were very different. Auxiliaries were employed on part-time contracts with guaranteed hours of work, and were on an incremental salary scale. Home helps were employed by the hour, the hourly rate of pay being lower than that paid to the auxiliaries. Although they did have holiday and sick-leave entitlement, they had no guaranteed hours of work. Furthermore, they found the personal care work satisfying to carry out, and felt it enhanced the status of the job of home help. They also suggested that their job would more appropriately be titled 'community carer' or 'home carer' (Abbott, 1997). The auxiliaries and home helps certainly saw themselves as fighting to protect their jobs. The home helps wanted to retain personal care, and do more of it, because they wanted to maintain or increase the number of hours they were employed. The auxiliaries felt that if home helps took on more personal care their own jobs would be endangered: they felt either that their jobs would disappear altogether, or that they would be forced to take on domestic and social care work. They felt that the latter was demeaning and would lower their status; they did not want to become home helps. The district nursing sisters certainly justified their taking on clients who required only personal care, in part, as protecting the jobs of their auxiliaries, and I myself was certainly seen as a threat – a researcher who might recommend that auxiliaries were no longer required.

This concern about the future of auxiliaries was exacerbated, at the time when I carried out the research, by the uncertainty surrounding what would happen when the National Health Service and Community Care Act was implemented in April, 1993. The district nurses I interviewed were concerned that, when Care Management was introduced, social services staff would make nursing diagnoses. The view was expressed that home helps would be assigned to carry out personal care for elderly frail people who needed to be cared for by nurses, and indeed it was suggested that this was already happening. They were not suggesting that such users had medical needs, but that they had nursing care needs. While the fears of these nurses that care management would fail to refer clients who need nursing care, the concern expresses another factor that underpins the conflict between district nursing teams and health visitors, on the one hand, and other professionals and care workers on the other – the felt need for nurses to be able to define an area of professional expertise that is distinct from medicine.

Nursing is a predominantly female occupation that is subordinated to a predominantly male profession – medicine. It is a highly stratified occupation, and this is reflected in the hierarchical structure of the district nursing team. The teams in the area where I carried out research typically consisted of one or more full-time district nursing sisters, one of whom was the team leader, and a number of full- or part-time state enrolled nurses and auxiliaries. All patients were under the care of the district nursing team leader, who was ultimately responsible for their nursing care, although day-to-day care might be carried out by other members of the team. However, the autonomy of district nurses in supervising direct nursing care is circumscribed by medical control. While the professionalizing strategy of nurses is to claim professional expertise and autonomy in the area of nursing care, the medical profession continues to see nurses as subordinates who should work under medical direction. Nurses' professionalizing strategy has been to claim a unique contribution to healing. In doing so, they have moved away from a biomedical model to a holistic approach, stressing the enablement of active patient-participation in care. In this model of nursing the patient is seen as a whole person for whom all aspects of healing work are crucial, including basic personal care. However, in developing this model, nurses are in danger of claiming a monopoly on caring (James, 1992).

To the extent that they do claim a monopoly of caring work and stress their role in assessing the needs of frail elderly people, nurses are emphasizing expertise over experience. This claim to specialist knowledge and skills is based on their claim to a unique training with certification and credentials. By claiming to have unique skills, nurses are able to maintain a distance between themselves and other carers – paid and unpaid – and increase their autonomy and status. Nurses' professionalizing strategies have typically been deployed in opposition to medicine and the professionalizing strategies of doctors in the nineteenth century. Doctors claimed a monopoly over healing (medical) knowledge and operated occupational closure against others who claimed to have healing skills. In the process, nursing was created as a female occupation subordinate to medicine (Abbott and Wallace, this volume; Witz, 1992). Since the late nineteenth century at least some segments within nursing have argued for its professionalization. Debate has ensued between vocationalists and professionalizers (Melia, 1987; Abbott and Wallace, this volume). In developing professionalizing strategies, nursing itself operates occupational closure against other occupational groups involved in caring work.

In arguing that district nurses should assess the care needs of frail elderly people and should manage personal care, nurses are defining an area of expertise over which they claim a monopoly. They are defining it in relationship to that of social work, the occupational group which mainly provides care managers. They are also, however, operating occupational closure against unqualified carers. They are defining themselves as a nursing elite and consolidating a professional identity. The attempt to exclude home helps from providing personal care is not based just on their lack of knowledge and skills (which would in any case be debatable, given that many of them have extensive experience of caring for frail elderly people – their own dependents), but also on the fact that home helps are not managed by the district nurses and their clients' care is not supervised by them. The district nurses' claim to a professional monopoly in defining who needs which form of nursing care is challenged by the increased scope of the home help role. When the district nursing team takes on a client whose main need is personal care or who needs personal care as well as specialized nursing care, this work is mainly undertaken by auxiliaries. In the highly stratified nursing hierarchy, auxiliaries work under the supervision of the district nurses, and the district nurses' claim to professional expertise and status is further enhanced by having unqualified, 'unskilled' staff working under their direction.

Conclusion

What I have argued in this chapter is that the jurisdictional conflict between Social Services and Community Health Care Trust staff, and especially home helps and district nurses, which I found in the research I undertook, can be understood by examining the labour-market positions of these predominantly female occupational groups. The conflict arises partly because a pool of unqualified female workers are seeking satisfying part-time employment. Home helps and nursing auxiliaries are both drawn from the same sector of the female labour pool. Home helps are seeking to gain more hours of employment and greater job satisfaction by being allowed to take on personal care work. Auxiliaries see these moves as endangering their jobs: they see their work as being taken over by social services and face either job loss or having to take on low-status domestic and social care. At the same time, district nurses are seeking to protect and enhance their occupational position by claiming a monopoly and certain expert knowledge, and consequently are trying to define a client group whose care they should supervise. While this strategy protects the employment of nursing auxiliaries, it also serves to mark the boundary between social work and nursing. It acts as a mechanism of operational closure against other groups of carers, both paid and unpaid, and increases the status of district nurses *vis-à-vis* other carers. It devalues the skills that other carers have learnt over the years as they have performed caring work, and arguably mitigates against meeting the needs of the patient/client (Salvage, 1992). However, a major factor underlying this conflict is the undervaluing of caring work in general in our society. Caring work is seen as female work, and this results in low status and low pay. In attempting to have their caring work seen as being based on professional knowledge and, consequently, to enhance their professional knowledge and occupational rewards, nurses operate a stratagem of occupational closure against other carers. Patriarchal ideologies of what counts as important work and what is to be accorded a high status underlie the conflict between nurses and other carers and result in the devaluation of both paid and unpaid female caring work.

References

ABBOTT, P. (1992a) *Stage I Report on the Skills Mix Project*, Plymouth: University of Plymouth Community Research Centre.

ABBOTT, P. (1992b) *Rationalising the Skills Mix in Community Care for Disabled and Older People: A Report of Research in Cornwall*, Plymouth: University of Plymouth Community Research Centre.

ABBOTT, P. (1992c) *Care Needs of Older People in Devon: A Research Report to Devon Social Services*, Plymouth: University of Plymouth Community Research Centre.

ABBOTT, P. (1997) 'Home helps and district nurses; community care in the far South West', in ABBOTT, P. and SAPSFORD, R.J. (Eds) *Research into Practice: A Reader for Nurses and the Caring Professions* (2nd edn), Buckingham: Open University Press.

ABBOTT, P. and CAMPBELL, S. (1992) *Stage II Report on the Skills Mix Project*, Plymouth: University of Plymouth Community Research Centre.

ABBOTT, P. and PAYNE, G. (Eds) (1990) *The Social Mobility of Women*, Basingstoke: Falmer.

ABBOTT, P. and SAPSFORD, R.J. (1987a) *Mental Handicap and Motherhood: The Origins and Consequences of a Social Policy*, Milton Keynes: Open University.

ABBOTT, P. and SAPSFORD, R.J. (1987b) *Women and Social Class*, London: Tavistock.

ABBOTT, P. and TYLER, M. (1995) 'Ethnic variation in the female labour force: a research note', *British Journal of Sociology*, **46**, pp. 339–53.

ABBOTT, P., LANKSHEAR, G. and GIARCHI, G. (1992) 'Community care: who cares?', paper presented to a conference on The Marginalisation of Elderly People, Liverpool, May.

ARBER, S. and GINN, J. (1991) *Gender and Later Life: A Sociological Analysis of Resources and Constraints*, London: Sage.

ARBER, S., GILBERT, N. and EVANDROW, M. (1991) 'Gender, household composition and receipt of domiciliary services by disabled people', *Journal of Social Policy*, **7**, pp. 153–75.

BARRON, R.D. and NORRIS, E.M. (1976) 'Sexual division and the dual labour market', in BARKER, D. and ALLEN, S. (Eds) *Dependence and Exploitation in Work and Marriage*, London: Longman.

CHARNLEY, H. and BEBBINGTON, A. (1988) *Who Gets What? An Analysis of the Patterns of Service Provision to Elderly People*, Canterbury: University of Kent (PSSRU, Living in the Community Discussion Paper 560).

CLARK, B., FEATHERSTONE, A., WALTERS, M. and WEALE, A. (1990) 'Sorting out skill mix', *Journal of District Nursing* (April), pp. 19–20.

DAVIES, B., BEBBINGTON, A. and CHARNLEY, H. (1990) *Resources, Needs and Outcomes in Community-Based Care*, Aldershot: Gower.

DEX, S. (1985) *The Sexual Division of Work*, Brighton: Wheatsheaf.

FINCH, J. and GROVES, D. (1987) 'Community care and the family: a case for equal opportunities?', *Journal of Social Policy*, **9**, pp. 437–51.

GRAHAM, H. (1985) 'Providers, negotiators and mediators: women as hidden carers', in LEWIN, E. and OLSEN, V. (Eds) *Women, Health and Healing: Towards a New Perspective*, London: Tavistock.

GREMMEN, L. (1995) *Ethiek in der Gezinsverzorging: Gender en macht van zorg*, Utrecht: Jan van Arkel.

GRIFFITHS, R. (1988) *Community Care: Agenda for Action*, London: HMSO.

HAKIM, C. (1979) *Occupational Segregation: A Comparative Study of the Degree and Patterns of Differentiation Between Men's and Women's Work in Britain, the United States and other Countries*, London: Department of Employment, Research Paper 9.

HAMER, S. (1989) 'Fresh thoughts', *Journal of District Nursing*, (July), p. 17.

HENWOOD, M. (1992) *Through a Glass Darkly*, London: King's Fund Institute.

JAMES, N. (1992) 'Care work and casework: a synthesis?', in ROBINSON, J., GRAY, A. and ELKAN, R. (Eds) *Policy Issues in Nursing*, Buckingham: Open University Press.

MARTIN, J. and ROBERTS, C. (1984) *Women and Employment: A Lifetime Perspective*, London: HMSO.

NATIONAL ASSOCIATION OF HEALTH AUTHORITY TRUSTS (undated) *Care in the Community: Definitions of Health and Social Care – Developing an Approach (a West Midlands Study)*, Birmingham: NAHAT Occasional Papers.

MELIA, K. (1987) *Learning and Working: The Occupational Socialisation of Nurses*, London: Tavistock.

NISSEL, M. and BONNERJEA, L. (1982) *Family Care of the Handicapped Elderly: Who Pays?*, London: Policy Studies Institute.

SALVAGE, J. (1985) *The Politics of Nursing*, London: Heinemann.

SALVAGE, J. (1992) 'The New Nursing: Empowering patients or empowering nurses?', in ROBINSON, J., GRAY, A. and ELKAN, R. (Eds) *Policy Issues in Nursing*, Buckingham: Open University Press.

WARREN, L. (1990) 'We're home because we care: the experience of home helps caring for elderly people', in ABBOTT, P. and PAYNE, G. (Eds) *New Directions in the Sociology of Health*, Basingstoke: Falmer.

WITZ, A. (1992) *Professions and Patriarchy*, London: Routledge.

Chapter 11

Doctor–Nurse Relationships: Accomplishing the Skill Mix in Health Care[1]

Davina Allen

Introduction

In this chapter I examine the changing boundary between nursing and medical work in the acute general hospital setting. It is set against the backdrop of developments in UK health policy (DH, 1989) and nursing and medical education (DHSS, 1987; GMC, 1993; UKCC, 1987) which created the impetus for shifts in the division of labour within the caring community, and initiated widespread professional and policy discussion as to the appropriate allocation of work. Drawing on interactionist theories of the division of labour at work (Hughes, 1984; Abbott, 1988; Strauss *et al.*, 1963; 1964; 1985; Strauss, 1978) my aim is to move on from the policy debates to examine the ways in which staff at the point of service delivery manage their occupational boundaries. I shall be using ethnographic data from doctoral research into nurses' routine management of their jurisdiction. The professional and sociological literature suggested that, owing to recent policy developments, there would be an increased need for negotiation of the work boundary between nurses and doctors and that this was likely to be subject to some tension. However, field observations revealed that although the boundary between nursing and medicine was certainly changing, ward staff accomplished these shifts in the division of labour with minimal inter-occupational negotiation and little associated conflict. The question to be addressed in this chapter is why the debates in the literature were so little in evidence on the wards. I shall begin with an exploration of the policy context. I will then outline the theoretical framework guiding the research, before going on to analyze the study's substantive findings.

Policy Background

The starting-point for the study were the professional and policy discussions about the significance of recent developments in nursing and medical education and in health policy for shaping the boundaries of nurses' work. The sort of questions that had been raised in this context include: 'In what ways should nurses be expanding their scope of practice?' 'Should they be undertaking doctor-devolved work?' One way of understanding these debates in the context of nursing is in terms of the long-standing tensions between professionalism and managerialism. The interaction of these two forces has had a major historical influence on nursing as an occupation and on the definition of its jurisdiction (see, for example, Dingwall *et al.*, 1988), but may be seen as having entered a new phase with the introduction of Project 2000 (UKCC, 1987) and its underpinning ideology, 'New Nursing' (Beardshaw and Robinson, 1990), and the advent of the NHS 'management revolution' (Klein, 1995).

Managerialism

The management 'problem' in the NHS has been a persistent feature of its evolution. The search for improved management has been the basis for successive reforms of the Service by both Labour and Conservative governments, and has resulted in the importation into the NHS of managerial concepts borrowed from industry, which reflect changing management ideologies in relation to the whole of the public sector (Clarke, in this volume; Flynn, 1990). Previously, service organizations had been seen to be unique, but this belief was replaced by the conviction that they were equally amenable to the principles of economic rationality associated with business organizations (Allsop, 1984). The direction of health policy took a crucial turn with the introduction of general management following the Griffiths Report, and at the time of the research was being further consolidated as a result of the 1990 National Health Service and Community Care Act. The 1990 NHS reforms were wide-ranging. They attempted to dismantle the old NHS bureaucracy and pave the way for competition between hospitals that were effectively self-governing units. An important aspect of this broader policy context was the introduction of a range of management initiatives which, although they did not depend on 'market' conditions, would clearly be affected by this wider policy agenda (Paton, 1993). Underpinning the NHS reforms was a particular view of 'management' (Clarke, in this volume; Flynn, 1990). Many of the changes had been introduced by people from the private sector, and the managerialist ethic that developed was grounded in the belief that managers should 'manage', that they should be in control of their organizations and be proactive. 'Active' management would replace 'passive' administration. Recurring themes included: action, decisiveness, effectiveness, thrust, urgency and vitality, consumer satisfaction, quality, and efficiency.

Changes in management arrangements involved combining tighter accountability and monitoring with an increase in devolved freedoms. Units of management became smaller and under tighter local control. One area where there was considerable devolution of responsibility was in the management of human resources. It was argued that devolution of pay bargaining and devolved responsibility to provider units for the management of human resources would lead to greater flexibility of the workforce. There was much talk of 'performance-related pay', and guidelines for Trusts on the assessment of nursing staff were drawn up (Nursing Standard, 1994). Nurses were quick to point out the difficulties of applying such principles to their work. 'Any definition of productivity is linked to speed and outcomes, a crude measure of performance. By that yard stick good nursing will almost certainly lose out' (Casey, 1993). In addition to pay, issues of demarcation of work responsibilities between different staff groups were brought centre stage (Paton, 1993). As Shaw (1993) points out, *Working for Patients* (DH, 1989) questioned the traditional parameters of registered nurse activity:

> As part of this initiative, local managers, in consultation with their professional colleagues, will be expected to reexamine all areas of work to identify the most cost effective use of professional skills. This may involve a reappraisal of traditional patterns and practices. (DH, 1989)

'Skill mix' and 'reprofiling' became vogue phrases (Paton, 1993). This could refer to senior staff extending 'downwards', or junior staff extending 'upwards'. An important parallel development in this respect was the White Paper *Opening New Markets: New policies on Restrictive Trade Practices* (DTI, 1989), as a result of which employers can now legally employ staff on the basis of competencies (Shaw, 1993). In the future non-professional staff may be employed to carry out those tasks traditionally reserved for those with the professional qualification, providing competence can be shown (Brown, 1990). Of crucial importance for nurses in this context were changes in medical education (DHSS, 1987; GMC, 1993) and the initiative to reduce the hours worked by junior hospital doctors (NHSME, 1991). The *New Deal* (1991) set firm limits on junior doctors' contracted hours (72 per week, or less in most hospital posts) and working hours (56 hours per week) which had to be achieved in all hospitals. As a means to this end the *'New Deal'* called for an increase in the number of career grade posts and encouraged new ways of organizing junior doctors' work such as shifts, partial shifts and cross-cover between specialities. Crucially, it also suggested the 'sharing' of key clinical tasks by nurses and midwives. In order to realize the objectives of the *New Deal*, task forces or local implementation groups were established throughout the UK and given the power to recommend the removal of education approval from a training post, if an acceptable standard was not achieved.

Professionalism

Project 2000 and its ideological underpinning, 'New Nursing' (Beardshaw and Robinson, 1990), is the UKCC's strategy for reform of nursing education, structure and practice. It is a clear bid for a separation of education from service – dismantling a historical bargain that was unsatisfactory from the perspectives of both learners and teachers – and also an ambitious plan to create a practitioner-based division of labour (see Meerabeau in this volume; Davies, 1995). Proponents of Project 2000 argue that it has the potential to overcome some of the occupation's most persistent problems: low status, poor retention, and a lack of a clearly defined area of expertise with a scientific basis for practice. At the heart of Project 2000 is the ideology of 'New Nursing', which attempts to address the increasing fragmentation and technical orientation of late-twentieth-century nursing through the development of a distinctive, patient-centred approach to care. It advocates a shift from the old system of hierarchical task allocation, stressing that nursing practice should be the jurisdiction of trained staff. The 'New Nursing' ideals are associated with centres of nursing excellence such as the Burford and Oxford Nursing Development Units, which, although not typical of nursing today, are held up as an example of 'the contemporary ideology of nursing in action' (Pearson, 1988, quoted by Salvage, 1985).

Managerialism and Professionalism – Sources of Strain?

Although both management and professional versions of nursing support the development of nurses' scope for practice, they approach the issue of role expansion from rather different perspectives. Part of the problem is reflected in the distinction drawn by MacGuire (1980) between 'extended' and 'expanded' nursing roles. MacGuire suggests that 'expanded' should be reserved to refer to roles in which nursing skills are drawn upon, while 'extended' should be used to refer to those roles where nursing is not a prerequisite and where the tasks are essentially medical. This is more than a quibble over terminology. The distinction between expanded and extended nursing roles underlines the different perspectives from which professionalizers and managers approach the role of nurses in the division of labour. 'New Nursing' emphasizes the distinct contribution of nursing to health care and aims to develop a knowledge base which is independent from medicine. Professionalizers advocate role development driven by patient need. For example, a great number of nurses have integrated complementary therapies into their practice (Wright, 1995). Much of the recent impetus behind nursing role developments, however, has been driven by cost considerations and the desire to improve the hours and working conditions of the medical profession (cf. Allen *et al.*, 1993; Allen and Hughes, 1993; Hughes and Allen, 1993). Furthermore, in the absence of additional resources, the expansion of nursing's jurisdiction to include activities which were formerly the remit of doctors has implications also for the dilution of the nursing workforce, therefore threatening to undermine the professionalizers' aspirations for a practitioner-based division of labour in which hands-on nursing care activities are performed by qualified staff.

Discussion

Although it is useful to consider the debates precipitated by recent policy developments in terms of the tensions between managerialism and professionalism, it would be misguided to slip into over-simplistic, dichotomous thinking. Indeed, there are a number of issues over which nurses' professional aspirations and management interests converge. For example, the nursing process has become an important tool for quality assurance programmes, and primary nursing fits with a decentralized approach to management in which ward sisters become budget holders and primary nurses are held responsible for the care they give (Bowers, 1989, cited by Savage, 1995). Moreover, nursing is an extremely heterogeneous occupation (Melia, 1987): professional status is not supported by all groups within nursing (Salvage, 1985; Porter, 1992a), and a business culture may attenuate the clinical values of nurse managers (White, 1986). Professional and service versions of nursing can thus be found within nursing, indeed in nurses' everyday talk professional and service versions of nursing are often intertwined (cf. Robinson *et al.*, 1989). As we approach the twenty-first century, the work of nurses is likely to be shaped by a complex configuration of social forces which, despite the shift from a Conservative to a Labour government following the 1997 General Election, seem likely to continue to be mediated at the level of service delivery by the interactive effects of professionalism and managerialism. At root, however, these are only ideas (albeit influential ones) about the appropriate work for nurses. The actual work of hospital nurses is likely to be the product of nurses' practical management of their work boundaries in the course of their everyday activities. Thus, while it is useful to use macro-sociological terms in order to conceptualize the research problem, such an approach ultimately fails to capture the complexity of nursing work in the hospital division of labour. This is where the sociology of work and occupations can augment understanding.

Accomplishing Nursing Jurisdiction – a Theoretical Framework

In focusing on nurses and doctors' day-to-day accomplishment of their occupational boundaries, I have drawn on a large body of sociological theory:

(i) Hughes' (1984) writings on the world of work and occupations.
(ii) Strauss and colleagues: negotiated order perspective (Strauss *et al.*, 1963, 1964, 1985; Strauss, 1978).
(iii) Abbott's (1988) work on professional jurisdiction.

Taken together, these theories suggest an approach that conceptualizes the division of labour in dynamic terms. Occupational roles, in this view, are not self-evident but have to be actively negotiated within a system of work or, to put it in Abbott's terms, jurisdiction has to be claimed and sustained in the work arena. From this perspective, then, the establishment of a bounded occupation is a practical accomplishment.

To provide a perspective that can fruitfully be employed in the analysis of nursing, however, I suggest that attention also needs to be given to issues of gender. Historically gender has been both a liability and a resource for nurses. It has been utilized by nurses as a justification for jurisdictional claims, but, because historically the division of labour between nursing and medicine was based on a sexual division of labour, gender has overdetermined interoccupational inequalities (Gamarnikow, 1978). Increasingly the insights of feminist sociologists are being brought to bear on nursing. A gender lens has been applied to the analysis of the content of nursing work (James, 1992 a, b; Smith, 1992), nursing and the trade unions (Carpenter,

1988) and patterns of nurse–doctor interaction (Porter, 1991, 1992b; Campbell-Heider and Pollock, 1987). Most recently Davies (1995) has employed a gender perspective in order to understand why nurses have been so marginal to the debates that have shaped health policy since 1948, despite the fact that they constitute over half the NHS workforce and that their services consume about a quarter of total NHS expenditure. According to Davies, the discontents of nurses have to be seen in terms of a broader societal devaluation of women and the work that they do.

To recap: in the first part of this chapter I have outlined the policy background to contemporary changes in the nursing role. I have argued that the debates precipitated by recent policy developments can be understood in terms of the deep-rooted historical tensions within nursing between managerialism and professionalism. Drawing on interactionist theories of the division of labour, I have suggested that, although this framework helps us to understand the ideas driving the policy context, it ultimately fails to get to the complexity of everyday nursing practice. It is to nurses' practical management of their occupational boundaries in the course of their everyday work activities that I wish to turn in the next section.

Method

Data were generated on a medical ward and a surgical ward within a single NHS Trust hospital situated in the middle of England. The hospital had almost 900 beds and provided general, acute, obstetric and elderly services to a local population of 254,000. At the time of the study the hospital had an annual budget of £60m and employed about 2,800 staff.

Fieldwork was carried out over a 10-month period during which time I observed and participated in the working worlds of doctors, nurses, health care assistants, auxiliaries and clinical managers. Although I am myself a nurse, I did not work in this capacity during the fieldwork. Nevertheless, I was overt about my nursing background. In addition to the observational data, 57 tape-recorded, semi-focused interviews were carried out with ward nurses (n: 29), doctors (n: 8), auxiliaries (n: 5), health care assistants (n: 3) and clinical managers (n: 11).[2] Most interviews lasted between an hour and an hour and a half. Informal interviews were also undertaken. These took the form of spontaneous extended conversations that were not tape-recorded but which had a different flavour from the briefer discussions held with staff while they worked. Much of the data on the medical perspective were from informal interviews of this kind. Data were also generated through the analysis of organizational documents and attendance at nursing and management meetings and in-service study days.

My approach to data analysis may be best described as holistic: data from different sources were compared in order to make judgements as to how each piece should be interpreted. The slices of data were then related to the larger picture in order to evaluate their meaning and, in turn, on the basis of the analysis of these different snippets the meaning of the whole would itself be modified. '*FolioViews Infobase Production Kit version 3.1*' was employed to facilitate data management. A more extensive description of the research methodology and the fieldwork process can be found in Allen (1996).

Summary of Main Findings

Guiding Assumptions

I began the research with what I considered to be well-founded reasons for anticipating an increased need for negotiation and associated inter-occupational tension at the nursing–medical boundary. The changing boundary between medicine and nursing was certainly a hot topic in the professions and professional media. For example, on 5 October 1994 *The Guardian* examined 'The Sacking of Sister Pat' (Cook, 1994), the case of the neurology sister dismissed by the Plymouth Hospitals NHS Trust for making out a prescription for medication that was not signed by a doctor. The 'Pat Cooksley affair' was closely followed by the case of 'the appendix nurse', Valerie Tomlinson, a theatre sister who, under medical instruction, removed a patient's appendix. The *Nursing Standard* on 18 January 1995, in an editorial expressing surprise at the public outcry and media furore over the Tomlinson story, announced that 'Huge numbers of nurses are now undertaking duties which doctors used to perform' (Casey, 1995a). Only six months later (19 July 1995) however, the title of the editorial conceded that 'Often "doctor jobs" [*sic*] have been thrust upon nursing and have added little to the enhancement of nursing practice' (Casey, 1995b).

That disagreements existed about the appropriate allocation of work in health care appeared to be confirmed by the literature. For example, a survey of nurses, junior doctors, and support workers had revealed rank and file staff to be deeply ambivalent about the bracketing of nursing role developments with the junior doctors' hours initiative (Allen and Hughes, 1993; Allen *et al.*, 1993). Furthermore, Walby and Greenwell *et al.* (1994), in an extensive interview study of nursing and medical personnel in the changing health service, devote a whole chapter to exploring boundary conflicts between nursing and medicine.

Proponents of the negotiated order perspective make it clear that negotiations tend to be encouraged by ambiguous and uncertain situations (see for example, Strauss, 1978; Hall and Spencer-Hall, 1982; Maines and Charlton, 1985).

> Negotiations occur when rules and policies are not inclusive, when there are disagreements, when there is uncertainty, and when changes are introduced. (Maines and Charlton, 1985, p. 278)

This was the premise on which the research was based. I felt that the policy changes that were taking place and the debates they had precipitated would throw the processes through which occupational boundaries were constituted into sharp relief.

The Boundary between Nursing and Medicine: Views from the Wards

The nurses in this study were being encouraged by hospital mangers to develop the scope of their practice in order to relieve the burden of work on medical staff. The principal areas in which ward nurses were extending their skills were: administration of intravenous antibiotics, venepuncture, ECGs, male catheterization, and intravenous infusion. In both my informal conversations and interviews with ward staff it became clear that there was uncertainty and disagreement about changing work boundaries.

Most of the ward nurses regarded doctor-devolved work as a double-edged sword. They saw advantages for patient care, but were also concerned that, if they further expanded their jurisdiction, it would be even more difficult to undertake sustained, hands-on care work. In keeping with the ideals of 'New Nursing', the nurses in this study saw patient contact work as a central reward of the job.

> Part of me wants to do it and part of me feels that if I do that then it's taking me away from the patients again. (Interview Data – Staff Nurse)

> I think that sometimes it takes us away from the simple idea of what a nurse is for and what the patient thinks we're for. I think it's a good idea when you haven't got the doctor and there's an IV to be given and you can't get one and the nurse can give it on time. (Interview Data – Staff Nurse)

The doctors in this study were more than happy for nurses to take over what they regarded as low-status menial activities: intravenous antibiotic administration, venepuncture, ECGs and cannulation. Nevertheless, many were clear that certain of these were essential medical skills that they themselves did not want to lose.

> Taking blood and putting in cannulas. Especially putting in cannulas. I think that's very important. I think it is a vital skill that doctors should have really. (Interview Data – PRHO)

However, doctors were equivocal about activities that came closer to the focal tasks of medicine – such as patient clerking and diagnostic investigations. Some thought that nurses had the skills to undertake this work in a limited sense, providing they worked within clearly defined protocols. Others felt this was moving too far towards nurses making diagnoses and this was a responsibility that most doctors (and also nurses) believed should remain with the doctor.

> I think diagnosis is likely always to remain the domain of the doctor. (Interview Data – Consultant)

Doctors were divided as to whether expanded role activities should be shared with nursing staff or permanently devolved. Most of the nurses however believed tasks should be shared with medical staff and undertaken according to the exigencies of the work.

As the above extracts make clear, there were divergent perspectives concerning changing interoccupational boundaries. Furthermore, in my conversations and interviews with staff many recounted instances of contested boundaries. Nevertheless, my field observations revealed that ward staff managed changes in their interoccupational boundaries with minimal negotiation and little explicit conflict. These findings clearly raise important sociological questions as to why the uncertainty and disagreement in both the literature and in actors' accounts were so little in evidence on the wards.

Accomplishing the Medical–Nursing Boundary

In a paper presented at the British Sociological Association Medical Sociology Conference in 1995 I began to explore the reasons for the minimal negotiation of occupational boundaries and lack of explicit conflict on the wards (Allen, 1995). One of the factors I identified was the hospital's bureaucratic approach to the UKCC guidelines on nurses' scope of professional practice. The UKCC, in issuing its guidance on nurses' scope of practice, opted to move from a bureaucratic to a professional model. *The Scope of Professional Practice* places the onus for decisions about the boundaries of nursing firmly in the hands of individual practitioners. This strategy presented difficulties for the senior nurses in this study who were responsible for nursing standards, policies and procedures in a climate which was increasingly characterized by concern with litigation and risk-management (see, for example, Annandale, 1996). They responded by developing a system of self-directed learning packages, coupled with supervised clinical practice, which nurses wishing to practise in an expanded role had to complete and sign to certify that they were competent. Hospital policy restricted role development to nurses who had been qualified for longer than a year. Furthermore, ward sisters determined which nurses should develop their scope of practice and in what areas. This meant that for a number of nurses in this study their occupational boundaries were not negotiable. It seemed then that the potential for interoccupational negotiation had been reduced by the hospital's bureaucratic approach to the UKCC's guidelines.

On reflection, however, I believe that the impact of hospital bureaucracy should not be overstated. UKCC guidance on nurses' scope of practice supports role expansion, providing it does not result in the unnecessary fragmentation of patient care or lead to inappropriate delegation of work. This still allowed those nurses who had completed training to make decisions as to whether it was appropriate for them to use their skills or not. In their accounts of their work the nurses insisted that their priority was nursing care, and that if they were busy they expected to be able to negotiate the allocation of extended role tasks with doctors. In practice, however, this appeared to be more a case of a shift in the nurse–medical boundary than a negotiated domain of work. Despite their reservations about role expansion and their commitment to nursing care activities, those nurses who had the skills to undertake doctor-devolved work did so regardless of their other work pressures.

I suggest that, in order to understand why nurses undertook doctor-devolved work with minimal negotiation and little explicit conflict, we need to focus our sights on the interactive effects of three features of nursing and medical work on hospital wards: the different priorities and perspectives of nurses and doctors arising from the fragmented temporal-spatial ordering of their work; formal organizational hierarchies; and workplace turbulence coupled with gender ideologies.

Nurses and Doctors: Perspectives and Priorities

The nurses and doctors in this study had very different priorities and perspectives which arose from the fragmented temporal-spatial organization of their work. Nursing care was provided by nursing and support staff via a three-shift system. The hospital employed a permanent night staff and a day staff who worked a combination of morning and afternoon shifts. Nurses and support workers had timed meal and coffee breaks. By contrast, junior doctors routinely worked office hours, Monday to Friday. As a result of the junior doctors' hours initiative, doctors were supposed to have a bleep-free period over lunch to allow them an opportunity to dine with their peers. Nevertheless, it often happened that meal and coffee breaks were fitted around the demands of the work – particularly during on-call hours. Outside normal hours medical cover was provided by the on-call team. Junior doctors were on-call one day in six.

Medical and nursing work also differed in terms of their spatial organization. Nurses left the ward for periods of time in order to accompany patients to different departments and, on occasion, personnel might be moved to another ward in response to staff shortages. For the most part, however, the nurses were ward-based. Although junior doctors were formally attached to a ward, their work frequently took them to other wards within the hospital and to different departments – for example, outpatient clinics and theatres.

> Ian and I, neither of us are [. . .] ward-based. We pop up to the wards in our free minutes. (Interview Data – SHO)

The difference in the temporal-spatial organization of medical and nursing work was most marked outside normal hours when doctors were on-call. The on-call period was from 9 pm until 9 am the following morning. The on-call team were responsible for all admissions in their particular directorate as well as providing emergency cover for the wards. On weekdays ward cover did not commence until 9 pm, but at the weekend and on public holidays the on-call team were responsible for ward work for the full 24-hour period. The introduction of an Admissions Unit[3] meant that doctors spent little sustained time on the wards during the on-call period.

The different temporal-spatial organization of medical and nursing work created different perspectives and priorities which were a source of strain. Nurses were mainly concerned with the needs of the patients on their wards, whereas doctors' remit included patients' requirements for the whole directorate – including new admissions. During the on-call period, doctors tried to organize their work so that they were not wasting time and energy moving backwards and forwards between the different wards. At the same time, however, they had to balance their efficiency concerns with the need to attend to patients in order of clinical priority. Compared to the doctors, nurses were much more conscious of the need to adhere to organizational timetables: considerable nursing effort went into co-ordinating patient care activities and ensuring that treatments were carried out to schedule.

The differing work priorities of nursing and medical staff are revealed in the tensions I observed over death declaration. As far as medical staff were concerned, death declaration was of low importance – their priorities lay with the living.

> PRHO: [D]ead patients they're not a priority. I think 'Well they're dead – I'll deal with the live ones'. (Fieldnotes)

The death of a patient disturbed the wards' 'sentimental order' (Glaser and Strauss, 1965) and nurses were therefore typically eager to perform last offices in order that the body could be removed to the mortuary, and the ward returned to 'normal'. Nurses were unable to begin any of their work until the doctor had declared a patient to be dead. The different agendas of nursing and medical staff are nicely illustrated in the following two extracts. The first is a recorded conversation from a day I spent with the on-call PRHO.

> PRHO: Are you writing down what the nurses do to me too? That Boxtree ward keep bleeping me and bleeping me to certify that lady.
> DA: Is that what all the bleeps have been for?
> PRHO: Yes, and the last one was not very nice. 'You've got to come and certify her now!' 'I'm busy'. 'You must come now'. (Fieldnotes)

The second extract is from notes made when I was observing the wards at night. I had answered the ward phone because the nurses were busy. It was a staff nurse from another ward trying to locate the on-call doctor. The time is about 11 pm.

> The phone rings and I answer it.
> Staff Nurse: Hello it's staff nurse on Elm ward. Is doctor Green there?
> DA: I think so. I'll just go and check. [(I checked with SN)]
> DA: Yes.
> Staff Nurse: [(There is a tone or irritation in her voice)] Well can you ask him to phone me? There's a patient he needs to certify. He's supposed to have been coming since seven and I'm on my own and I really do need to get this sorted out. So can you ask him to phone me. (Fieldnotes)

Doctors and nurses also held divergent definitions of what constituted emergency cover. Doctors perceived their on-call role in fairly narrow terms, and complained that much of the work they were expected to do fell outside their understanding of 'emergency service'.

> On-call basically means to me to provide emergency services within the hospital but to quite a large extent this is just to do things like prescribing drugs, writing ECGs, give IV drugs, this sort of thing. It's not an emergency service at all. (Interview Data – PRHO)

> PRHO: I'm really annoyed about this. I'm not supposed to be bleeped to re-catheterize patients. I'm on call for emergencies. (Fieldnotes)

Nurses also recognized that on-call doctors could only provide a restricted service and left what they considered to be non-essential requests for normal working hours. Nevertheless, unlike doctoring, nursing is not temporally limited, and, in adhering to hospital policies, nurses were dependent on the on-call doctor to carry out tasks that arose which they were unable to undertake themselves. As a consequence, the nursing definition of emergency cover incorporated a broader range of work than over-burdened doctors considered legitimate.

> The on-call PRHO came to the ward.
> Doctor: Have you got any jobs?
> Staff Nurse: I've got some jobs.
> Doctor: As long as it's only prescribing!
> Staff Nurse: Oh! [(Passing the doctor a drug kardex)] She needs that written up and a new drug kardex.
> Doctor: She needs an additional drug kardex.
> Staff Nurse: But it needs re-writing.
> Doctor: I'm not re-writing kardexes.
> Staff Nurse: But it will need doing tomorrow. Are you on? I suppose not. What should I say? You refused to do it?
> Doctor: No, that the locum on-call doesn't re-write kardexes.
> Staff Nurse 2: Well this is something you should take up with your medical colleagues then. Make sure they re-write kardexes on Friday.
> PRHO does re-write the drugs kardex. (Fieldnotes)

Much of the strain relating to the bleep system stemmed from the distinct perspectives and priorities arising from the different temporal-spatial organization of medical and nursing work. Nurses frequently complained that they could not get doctors to come to the wards. I saw that considerable nursing effort was expended in co-ordinating patient care activities and the unavailability of medical staff placed additional burdens on nurses. Equally, however, I witnessed the work pressures of on-call doctors and observed how quickly they became irritated when their work was continuously interrupted by nurses bleeping them to come and attend to work on the wards. Doctors' annoyance was heightened when nurses' requests seemed trivial in relation to their other work priorities. The PRHOs felt that other members of the health care team did not really appreciate the on-call experience.

> [S]ometimes you would get bleeped from the gerry wards 'Come and see this patient', medical wards 'Come and see this patient' – I can't because I'm seeing one ill patient and I get bleeped to see another ill patient. I can't be in four places or nine places at once and some of the nurses don't understand that and it's quite frustrating because although I don't get a chance to see an ill patient, like they might bleep me in the morning but I won't get down to see him until six or seven in the evening and then they get annoyed and I try to say 'I've been to see quite a few ill patients throughout the day'. (Interview Data – PRHO)

Interestingly, however, a dominant theme in nurses' accounts is that their clear frustration with the fragmented temporal-spatial ordering of work is intermingled with the sympathetic acknowledgement of doctors' pressures of work.

> [I]t's hard with the on-call doctors at night time because you're trying to get them to please come onto the ward and do this and they're obviously busy elsewhere and everybody needs them so they can't come on. So sometimes we have been known to get a bit angry. You know 'You've got to come now if you don't come I'll fast bleep you and you will come'. It's an effort to try and get them onto the ward sometimes. (Interview Data – Staff Nurse)

> Some of them are not very willing to do things for you. I think they're busy, which is fair enough I know they've got a lot on, but when its say, something like tablets, and the ambulance has come to pick a patient up and the tablets are not there a patient can't go and the ambulance has to go. (Interview Data – Staff Nurse)

At one level, then, nurses' willingness to undertake doctor-devolved activities despite their reservations about the changing medical–nursing boundary, can be understood as a reflection of the difficulties they had in getting medical staff to come to the ward, coupled with their sympathy for junior doctors' burdens of work. Another feature of medical and nursing work which helps to account for the ways in which nurses accomplished occupational jurisdiction is the formal organizational hierarchy in which they worked.

Organizational Hierarchies

Although nurses were prepared to negotiate with individual doctors in a direct way about certain aspects of patient treatment, within the hospital's formal organizational structures it was doctors who had higher status. This created strains because, owing to the temporal-spatial organization of medical and nursing work, nurses initiated much of the doctors' work. One of the ways in which nurses managed this potentially difficult relationship was by leaving doctors lists of jobs. At one level this reflected the fact that often doctors were absent from the ward. At another it also had the advantage of disguising the identity of the nurse as the originator of the work and allowed the doctor to set his own work priorities. I suggest that nurses' preparedness to undertake doctor-devolved tasks can also be understood in terms of the tensions arising from this disjuncture between formal organizational hierarchies and the flow of work (Allen, 1997). Quite simply, it was easier for nurses to undertake the work itself than it was to try and negotiate from a subordinate position with over-burdened doctors who had different priorities and perspectives. There are some clear parallels here with the domestic division of labour as a comparison of the following extracts indicates. The first is taken from Hochschild's (1990) study of working parents' management of the division of labour in the household.

> I do think women – should I say men as well, but actually I mean women – start nagging about little things like picking up clothes. I realise that things can really build up. Peter's father poured out to me things that go back for years. His wife would continually nag him about things, like not hanging his suit up at night. I harp at Peter about helping the kids. He'll let me ask him before he does it, and I don't like to have to ask him to help. If I'm continually harping, maybe I should make some adjustments.
>
> Given the threat of what could happen if their marriage were to flounder, Nina decided not to push Peter on the issue of housework [. . .] She could cut back her hours. She could keep on doing the second shift. (Hochschild, 1990, pp. 87–8)

The second extract is from my fieldnotes:

> Most of the time it's easier for you to go and do it yourself as long as you've got your certificates and what have you to prove it [. . .] you know what they [doctors] are willing to do and the hassle it is to get them to do the menial jobs. It's just not worth the hassle sometimes. It's just easier to get it done and get on with it and say 'Right this is the result. Do something with it'. (Staff Nurse – Interview Data)

Workplace Turbulence and Gender Ideologies

The final feature of nursing and medical work that can help us to understand why nurses routinely undertook doctor-devolved work with minimal interoccupational negotiation or conflict, is the turbulence of the workplace coupled with the gender ideologies which underpinned the hospital organization.

The modern hospital constitutes a 'turbulent' work environment (Melia, 1979). Hospitals are complex, heterogeneous, internally-segmented organizations, and patient care has to be co-ordinated 24 hours a day, 365 days a year, with numerous timetables which are often in conflict. Staff at the point of service delivery have to manage the daily tensions between the unpredictability of individual patient needs and the complex temporal structures of the hospital (Allen, 1997). Flexible working is essential in such an environment (Allen and Lyne, 1997). Indeed, there is a sense in which a 'usefulness' culture underpins hospital life. Nevertheless, in the hospital in this study the expectation of flexible working was not uniformly applied to all categories of staff. Rather, it was nurses who were expected to be the malleable workers in the system: flexibility was an institutionalized expectation of the nursing role.

> Consultant: On the last point I was going to suggest that rather than put money into ward clerks, you put money into the nursing side in some form or another, because those personnel are actually more multiskilled than just pure ward clerks [. . .] They can do clerical, they can do nursing, they can be doing fetching and carrying. (Meeting – Tape)

During the course of the fieldwork I learnt of explicit examples of resistance to shifts in the division of labour and of boundary-creating measures undertaken by ward staff. For example, when the ENB (English National Board) placed limits on the amount of night duty students could work during their training, the hospital responded by developing the skills of auxiliary nurses. A number of the auxiliary nurses had worked towards NVQs which enabled them to undertake patient observations. The auxiliaries felt that they should be remunerated for this additional responsibility, however, and protested by collectively refusing to undertake observations even though they had the requisite skills to do so. Nevertheless, the boundary-defining stance of the auxiliaries did not result in disputes with qualified staff.

Similarly, on the surgical ward the locum consultant insisted that the SHO clerked his patients even though a nurse practitioner had been employed to fulfil this function. The precise reasons for this boundary-defining stance were far from clear. The nurse practitioner maintained that this was a political gesture, the locum consultant's protest against his failure to be given a permanent post at the hospital. In practice, the nurse practitioner and SHO managed the overlap in their work without tension. The nurse practitioner undertook a 'pre-operative assessment' and the SHO used this information to inform his 'clerking' of the patient.

In both the above cases resistance to shifts in the division of labour was accommodated by nursing staff. When nurses themselves took a boundary-defining stance however, tensions ensued. For example, one of the ward managers at the hospital had refused to succumb to the pressures of the junior doctors' hours initiative and had not allowed her staff to train in the administration of intravenous antibiotics. The ward manager did not believe that it was easy in practice for nurses to pass expanded role activities back to medical staff if they were busy. Furthermore, committed to the belief that nursing role developments should be led by patient need, the ward manager elected to concentrate on training nurses in the application of plaster casts, as she felt this would bring significant improvements in patient care. Her unorthodox actions had, however, allegedly resulted in enormous difficulties between nursing and medical staff. Because nurses were routinely administering intravenous antibiotics on most of the other wards in the hospital, doctors had come to assume this was a nursing role. The difficulties were further exacerbated by the fact that the ward was situated at the far end of the hospital and created additional 'leg work' for medical staff. As the nurses on the ward had not undertaken the requisite training, their roles were non-negotiable. However, in what had become a war of attrition, the nursing staff were regularly abused by medical staff and accused of being second-class nurses. At the close of the fieldwork the ward manager was on the brink of succumbing to the pressures that were being exerted by the doctors and supporting the ward nursing staff in undertaking intravenous antibiotic administration. The stance taken by this ward sister was unorthodox, but the response of medical staff raises important questions as to the power of nursing staff in negotiating the division of labour at work.

Arguably, the expectation that nurses will be flexible workers in part reflects the legacy of nursing's occupational history, and underlines the point made by Davies (1995) that gender is embedded in the design and functioning of organizations. Nineteenth-century nurse reformers were heavily influenced by the feminist theory of Jameson, that there were natural spheres of activity for men and women. This natural division of work was believed to be rooted in the family, and thus work for women outside the home ought to resemble the domestic sphere, and complement the 'male principle' with the 'female principle' (Gamarnikow, 1978; see also Abbott and Wallace, in this volume). Hence, the occupational space nursing came to occupy in the hospital was rooted in the domestic division of labour. As Stacey (1981) points out, however, in the ever-increasing division of labour and the associated increasing specialization, it is the woman in the house who has remained the generalist. Similarly, in the hospital division of labour it is the nurse who is expected to act as the generalist when circumstances demand, notwithstanding her/his specialist skills.

There are striking similarities between nurses' patterns of work and new post-Fordist management ideologies of flexible working patterns, as James *et al.* (1993) have shown. For example, in Britain considerable attention has been given to the notion of a flexible firm developed at the Institute of Manpower Studies principally by Atkinson (Wood, 1989). Atkinson identifies four main types of flexibility of which the two most important are numerical flexibility and functional flexibility. In numerical flexibility employers are able to vary the amount of labour they employ at short notice in order to respond to different circumstances. Functionally-flexible workers are able to take on a wider range of tasks, which is considered to increase efficiency by, for example, enabling them to perform the work of absent colleagues (Walby, 1989).

Given that flexible specialists are so sought after by post-Fordist managers, it is ironic that, instead of being seen as highly skilled and worthy of investment, nurses' adaptability has left them vulnerable to being mocked as 'unskilled' (James *et al.*, 1993). As Jenson (1989) has suggested, this is a feature of 'women's work'. Secretaries, Jenson argues, are the ultimate flexible specialists, yet this is not recompensed but instead interpreted as something unexceptional, especially since the multiplication of tasks bears a resemblance to domestic labour.

Conclusion

In this chapter I have examined the changing division of labour between nursing and medicine. I began by outlining recent policy developments and suggested that the debates they have precipitated could be understood in terms of the deep-rooted historical tensions within nursing between ideologies of professionalism and managerialism. I argued that, whilst the concepts of professionalism and managerialism are useful in understanding the policy context, ultimately they fail to get to the complexity of nursing work. I have suggested that this is where sociological theories of the world of work and occupations can augment understanding. In focusing on nurses' practical management of their occupational boundaries, I have drawn on several – broadly interactionist – theories of the division of labour (Hughes, 1984; Abbott, 1988; Strauss *et al.*, 1963; 1964; 1985; Strauss, 1978) which, taken together, offer a potentially fruitful theoretical framework which can be employed in the analysis of nursing work. However, I have suggested that to be entirely satisfactory greater attention needs also to be given to issues of gender.

I have argued that, as a result of my reading of the professional and sociological literature, I began this study by anticipating that recent policy developments had generated the need for negotiation of the boundaries between nursing and medical work, and that these negotiations were likely to be subject to some dispute. Field observations revealed, however, that nurses and doctors on the wards managed shifts in the division of labour with minimal negotiation and little explicit conflict. Despite their commitment to patient care activities, and contrary to UKCC guidelines, those nurses who could undertake doctor-devolved work did so irrespective of their other work pressures. In my analysis of these unexpected findings I have suggested that nurses' management of their occupational boundaries has to be understood in terms of the context of nursing and medical work in the acute hospital.

I have argued that the difference in temporal-spatial organization between medical and nursing work generated diverse priorities and perspectives which were a source of strain. Nurses frequently complained that they could not get the doctors to come to the ward. Nurses' difficulty in negotiating with medical staff was compounded by their subordinate status within the hospital organization, and the institutionalized assumption that nurses would be flexible workers. As we have seen, however, nurses' frustration with the unavailability of medical staff was offset by their genuine sympathy for the burdens of on-call doctors. Moreover, it was nurses who had to cope with the frustrations of patients and relatives which arose when doctors were unavailable. I suggest that when we understand the ways in which nurses' work was circumscribed by the organizational context, we can begin to understand why those nurses who could function in an expanded role undertook doctor-devolved work irrespective of their other work priorities. Quite simply, it was easier for nurses to do the work themselves than it was to attempt to negotiate from a subordinate position with over-burdened doctors who held different priorities and perspectives. Indeed, in addition to the work that had formally been devolved to them, nurses routinely and informally undertook a wide range of work that officially remained the jurisdiction of medicine, such as: prescribing intravenous fluids and drugs; and making requests for investigations and blood tests.

> I am guilty of doing things I shouldn't do. I mean I do blood forms and things like that even though I know I shouldn't. Because it's an easier life and I know things are going to get done. (Interview Data – Senior Nurse)

Undertaking doctor-devolved work clearly made sense in the work context, which suggests that there may be good reasons for arguing for the incorporation of certain tasks – such as intravenous drug administration and venepuncture – into the basic nursing curriculum. Indeed failure to do so is likely to further fragment patient care.

As I have argued at the beginning of this chapter, it is only relatively recently that the nurse–patient relationship has assumed a central place in contemporary nursing ideologies, reflecting the efforts of the nursing leadership to develop an essentialist version of nursing work as part of the occupation's professionalizing project. Clearly the nurse–patient relationship provides an important peg on which to hang the diverse activities that constitute nursing work and around which to anchor nursing's occupational identity. However, attempts to fix the nursing role too rigidly must be doomed to failure. Nursing work has always been characterized by flexible work boundaries both in terms of its day-to-day practice and also historically in response to the impact of wider technological, social and economic factors. The challenge for nursing in the twenty-first century is to reconcile the new essentialism of its professionalizers with its traditional flexibility within the hospital division of labour.

Notes

1 The research on which this chapter is based was supported by a Department of Health Nursing and Therapists Research Training Studentship. The views expressed here are the author's own and do not represent those of the Department of Health. The PhD thesis was supervised by Professor Robert Dingwall (Social Studies) and Professor Veronica James (Nursing Studies), University of Nottingham.

2 These figures do not add up because one person was interviewed more than once and two auxiliaries were interviewed together.

3 The Admissions Unit was created primarily with the needs of junior doctors in mind. The unit acted as a 'buffer' for medical emergencies admitted to the hospital. Patients could stay on the unit for up to 48 hours where their condition could be assessed, and, if deemed necessary, an appropriate bed found on one of the wards. The Admissions Unit concentrated on the processing and disposal of patients; it increased the efficiency of on-call doctors by concentrating all acute medical admissions in one area rather than placing them in different wards around the hospital.

References

ABBOTT, A. (1988) *The System of Professions: An Essay on the Division of Expert Labor*, Chicago: University of Chicago Press.

ALLEN, D. (1995) 'The shape of adult nursing: the division of labour at work', paper presented at the BSA Annual Medical Sociology Conference, University of York.

ALLEN, D. (1996) *The Shape of General Hospital Nursing: The Division of Labour at Work*, PhD Thesis, University of Nottingham.

ALLEN, D. (1997) 'The doctor-nurse boundary: a negotiated order', *Sociology of Health and Illness*, **19** (4).

ALLEN, D. and HUGHES, D. (1993) 'Going for growth', *The Health Service Journal*, **103** (5372), pp. 33–4.

ALLEN, D. and LYNE, P. (1997) 'Nurses' flexible working practices: some ethnographic insights into clinical effectiveness', *Clinical Effectiveness in Nursing*.

ALLEN, D., HUGHES, D. and PICKERSGILL, F. (1993) 'Receptivity to expanded nursing roles: the views of junior doctors, nurses and health care assistants', paper presented at Nurse Practitioners: The UK/USA Experience Conference, The Cafe Royal, London.

ALLSOP, J. (1984) *Health Policy and the National Health Service*, London: Longman.

ANNANDALE, E. (1996) 'Working on the front-line: risk culture and nursing in the new NHS', *Sociological Review*, **44**, pp. 416–51.

BEARDSHAW, V. and ROBINSON, R. (1990) *New for Old? Prospects for Nursing in the 1990s*, London: King's Fund Institute.

BOWERS, L. (1989) 'The significance of primary nursing', *The Journal of Advanced Nursing*, **14**, pp. 13–19.

BROWN, J. (1990) 'Creating opportunities from challenges', paper presented to the annual conference of the Royal College of Nursing, London.

CAMPBELL-HEIDER, N. and POLLOCK, D. (1987) 'Barriers to physician-nurse collegiality: an anthropological perspective', *Social Science and Medicine*, **25**, pp. 421–25.

CARPENTER, M. (1977) 'The new managerialism and professionalism in nursing', in STACEY, M. (Ed.) *Health and the Division of Labour*, London: Croom Helm.

CARPENTER, M. (1988) *Working for Health: The History of the Confederation of Health Service Employees*, London: Lawrence & Wishart.

CASEY, N. (1993) Editorial, *Nursing Standard*, **8** (12), p. 3.

CASEY, N. (1995a) Editorial, *Nursing Standard*, **9** (19), p. 3.

CASEY, N. (1995b) Editorial, *Nursing Standard*, **9** (43), p. 3.

COOK, J. (1994) 'The sacking of Sister Pat', *The Guardian*, (15 October), p. 18.

DAVIES, C. (1995) *Gender and the Professional Predicament in Nursing*, Buckingham: Open University Press.

DH (1989) *Working for Patients: The Health Service Caring for the 1990s*, London: HMSO.

DHSS (1987) *Hospital Medical Staffing (Achieving a Balance) – Plan for Action, Health Circular 87 (25)*, London: DHSS.

DINGWALL, R., RAFFERTY, A.M. and WEBSTER, C. (1988) *An Introduction to the Social History of Nursing*, London: Routledge.

DTI (1989) *Opening New Markets: New Policies on Restrictive Trade Practices, Cmnd. 727*, London: HMSO.

FLYNN, N. (1990) *Public Sector Management*, Hemel Hempstead: Harvester Wheatsheaf.

GAMARNIKOW, E. (1978) 'Sexual division of labour: the case of nursing', in KUHN, A. and WOLPE, A.M. (Eds) *Feminism and Materialism: Women and Modes of Production*, London: Routledge and Kegan Paul.

GLASER, B. and STRAUSS, A.L. (1965) *Awareness of Dying*, Chicago: Aldine.

GMC (1993) *Tomorrow's Doctors*, London: GMC.

HALL, P.M. and SPENCER-HALL, D.A. (1982) 'The social conditions of the negotiated order', *Urban Life*, **11** (3), pp. 328–49.

HOCHSCHILD, A. (1990) *The Second Shift: Working Parents and the Revolution at Home*, London: Judy Piatkus.

HUGHES, D. and ALLEN, D. (1993) *Expanded Nursing Roles, Junior Doctors' Hours and the Hospital Division of Labour: A Pilot Study*, London: SETRHA.

HUGHES, E.C. (1984) *The Sociological Eye*, New Brunswick: Transaction Books.

JAMES, N. (1992a) 'Care, work and carework: a synthesis?', in ROBINSON, J., GRAY, A. and ELKAN, R. (Eds) *Policy Issues in Nursing*, Milton Keynes: Open University Press.

JAMES, N. (1992b) 'Care = organisation + physical labour = emotional labour', *Sociology of Health and Illness*, **14**, pp. 488–509.

JAMES, N., ARTHUR, T. and PITTMAN, A. (1993) *Nursing Quality Counts: A Case Study of Neonatal Services 1990–1992*, University of Nottingham: Nursing Policy Studies 9.

JENSON, J. (1989) 'The talents of women, the skills of men: flexible specialization and women', in WOODS, S. (Ed.) *The Transformation of Work*, London: Unwin Hyman.

KLEIN, R. (1995) *The New Politics of the NHS* (3rd edn), London: Longman.

MACGUIRE, J.M. (1980) *The Expanded Role of the Nurse*, London: King's Fund.

MAINES, D. and CHARLTON, J.C. (1985) 'The negotiated order approach to the analysis of social organisation', in FABERMAN, H.A. and PERINBANAYAGAM, R.S. (Eds) *Foundations of Interpretative Sociology: Original Essays in Symbolic Interaction. Studies in Symbolic Interaction*, Supplement 1, pp. 271–308, London: JAI Press.

MELIA, K. (1979) 'A sociological approach to the analysis of nursing work', *Journal of Advanced Nursing*, **4**, pp. 57–67.

MELIA, K. (1987) *Learning and Working: The Occupational Socialisation of Nurses*, London: Tavistock.

NHSME (1991) *Junior Doctors: The New Deal*, London: NHSME.

PATON, C. (1993) 'Devolution and centralism in the National Health Service', *Social Policy and Administration*, **27**, pp. 83–108.

PEARSON, A. (Ed.) (1988) *Primary Nursing: Nursing in Burford and Oxford Nursing Development Units*, Beckenham: Croom Helm.

PORTER, S. (1991) 'A participant observation study of power relations between nurses and doctors in a general hospital', *Journal of Advanced Nursing*, **16**, pp. 728–35.

PORTER, S. (1992a) 'The poverty of professionalization: a critical analysis of strategies for the occupational advancement of nursing', *Journal of Advanced Nursing* **17**, pp. 720–26.

PORTER, S. (1992b) 'Women in a women's job: the gendered experience of nurses', *Sociology of Health and Illness*, **14**, pp. 510–27.

ROBINSON, J., STILWELL, J., HAWLEY, C. and HEMPSTEAD, N. (1989) *The Role of the Support Worker in the Ward Health Care Team*, Warwick: University of Warwick, Nursing Policy Studies Centre, Nursing Policy Studies 6.

SALVAGE, J. (1985) *The Politics of Nursing*, London: Heinemann Nursing.

SALVAGE, J. (1985) 'The New Nursing: Empowering patients or empowering nurses?', in ROBINSON, J. GRAY, A. and ELKAN, R. (Eds) *Policy Issues in Nursing*, Milton Keynes: Open University Press.

SAVAGE, J. (1995) *Nursing Intimacy: An Ethnographic Approach to Nurse–Patient Interaction*, London: Scutari.

SHAW, I. (1993) 'The politics of interprofessional training – lessons from learning disability', *Journal of Interprofessional Care*, **7**, pp. 255–62.

SMITH, P. (1992) *The Emotional Labour of Nursing: How Nurses Care*, London: Macmillan Education.

STACEY, M. (1981) 'The division of labour revisited or overcoming the two Adams!', in ABRAHAMS, P., DEEM, R., FINCH, J. and ROCK, P. (Eds) *Practice and Progress: British Sociology 1950–1980*, London: Allen and Unwin.

STRAUSS, A.L. (1978) *Negotiations: Varieties, Contexts, Processes and Social Order*, London: Jossey-Bass.

STRAUSS, A. *et al.* (1963) 'The hospital and its negotiated order', in FREIDSON, E. (Ed.) *The Hospital in Modern Society*, New York: Free Press.

STRAUSS, A.L., SCHATZMAN, L., BUCHER, R., EHRLICH, D. and SABSHIN, M. (1964) *Psychiatric Ideologies and Institutions*, New York: Free Press.

STRAUSS, A., FAGERHAUGH, S. and SUCZET, B. (1985) *Social Organisation of Medical Work*, Chicago: University of Chicago Press.

UKCC (1987) *Project 2000: The Final Proposals*, London: UKCC.

UKCC (1992) *The Scope of Professional Practice*, London: UKCC.

WALBY, S. (1989) 'Flexibility and the changing sexual division of labour', in WOOD, S. (Ed.) *The Transformation of Work*, London: Unwin Hyman.

WALBY, S. and GREENWELL, J., with MACKAY, L. and SOOTHILL, K. (1994) *Medicine and Nursing: Professions in a Changing Health Service*, London: Sage.

WHITE, R. (1986) 'From matron to manager: the political construction of reality', in WHITE, R. (Ed.) *Political Issues in Nursing: Past, Present and Future*, New York: Wiley.

WOOD, S. (1989) 'The transformation of work?', in WOOD, S. (Ed.) *The Transformation of Work*, London: Unwin Hyman.

WRIGHT, S. (1995) 'The role of the nurse: extended or expanded?', *Nursing Standard*, **9** (33), pp. 25–9.

Chapter 12

Doing the Right Thing? Managerialism and Social Welfare

John Clarke

This chapter summarizes recent work about the relationship between managerialism and the restructuring of social welfare and draws out a number of issues. These concern: the problem of how to evaluate the impact of managerialism; the character of managerialism as a 'discursive strategy'; the 'perverse effects' of managerialism for social welfare; and finally, the political problem of identifying what 'right thing' it is that managerialism may have been doing.

It is clear that managerialism has formed part of a sustained attempt to reform the old institutional arrangements of the welfare state in Britain. Most significantly, managerialism promised to transform old organizational patterns and practices (Pollitt, 1993a; Taylor-Gooby and Lawson, 1993; Clarke, Cochrane and McLaughlin, 1994; Waine and Cutler, 1994; Clarke and Newman, 1997). In particular, it promised to discipline those embodiments of 'producer power', the welfare professionals. I do not want to get bogged down in a discussion of whether such occupational and organizational formations are or are not 'real' professions, or even whether they are semi-, pseudo- or quasi-professions. As the next section will show, however, there are reasons to take seriously the public representation of such formations as professions. For the moment, however, I think it is more useful to consider the characteristic forms of organizational co-ordination in the practice of state welfare work.

Colleagues and I have found it useful to treat professionalism and bureaucracy as the characteristic modes of organizational co-ordination that dominated the institutional arrangements of the old welfare state (Clarke and Newman, 1997; see also Cousins, 1987). By 'modes of co-ordination', I intend to refer to the complex set of rules, roles and regulatory principles around which the social practices of organizations are structured. These modes generate typical patterns of internal and external social relationships and, in particular, privilege certain types of knowledge. We have used this idea of modes of co-ordination partly because it undercuts the naturalizing effect of the word 'managing', in which the commonsense meaning of 'running things' is elided with the more specific prescriptions of a managerialist mode of co-ordination (this is taken up later). By starting from these ideas of bureaucratic and professional modes of co-ordination, it is possible to develop a view of welfare agencies as organizational regimes in which different modes of co-ordination co-existed – in the characteristic form of 'bureau-professional regimes'. The reason for this rather circuitous approach to treating social welfare organizations as combining professionalism and bureaucracy is that much discussion of welfare restructuring has proceeded as if the old welfare state was either dominated by professionals or was entirely bureaucratic. The effect of emphasizing either one of these is to miss the internal complexity of the organizational forms, labour processes and significant intra-organizational struggles that characterized the bureau-professional regimes of state welfare (Clarke, 1994; Cochrane, 1993).

There are two further uses of this conceptual framework that are significant for what follows. The ideas of modes of co-ordination and organizational regimes provide a way of thinking about differences of organizational form within the welfare state – for example, the different sorts of organizational structures, cultures and processes that characterized the range between the NHS, on the one hand, and (what used to be) the Department of Health and Social Security on the other. In this range the co-existence of professional and bureaucratic modes resulted in very different forms and distributions of power and privileged different sorts of organizationally-valued knowledge. The second value of the framework is that it allows some degree of analytical grip on the (uneven) combinations between these regimes and a third mode of co-ordination – that of political representation. The effects – and discomforts – of this articulation have tended to be most visible at the level of the local state – around education, social services and housing, for example (Cochrane, 1993). The 'bureau-professional' character of the post-war welfare state in Britain also had significant ideological dimensions that are the focus of the next section.

Welfare Bureau-professionalism and the Public Good

Given that we have all learnt to be sceptical about the grandiose and self-advancing mystiques through which both rational administration and professionalism sought to impose themselves on the social world, it is perhaps worth taking a step back to think about how and why they came to be installed as the dominant organizational principles of the post-war welfare state. I want to suggest that each of them contributed a distinctive ideological strand to the construction of the welfare state. At the core of this process was the Fabian or social democratic conception of the state, in which the state stood for society or the collective interests of the people, and was the agency for social reform or improvement. What both 'administration' and 'professionalism' contributed to this ideological formation was the capacity to be neutral. Bureaucratic administration had, at its heart, the promise of dispassionate organizational and social regulation (du Gay, 1994). The bureaucrat – in this scenario – was a heroic figure, able to separate personal interest or attachment from the performance of organizational duty. The systematic organization of public services through bureaucratic means promised that all citizens would be dealt with on their merits and according to their statutory rights, rather than because of who they were, who they knew or how much they were worth. This conception of 'egalitarian due process' provided a vital ideological underpinning for post-war conceptions of social citizenship.

Professionalism presented a matching ideological imagery, encapsulated in conceptions of impersonal service. It, too, promised to transcend narrow social or personal concerns in the pursuit of the public good by making specialist knowledge available to those in need. Professionalism was seen as being in the service of individual or collective progress. In their different ways, the ideologies of bureaucracy and professionalism enshrined a commitment to the public good in the organizational infrastructure of the welfare state. Together with the emergence of bipartisan political consensus on the need for a welfare state, they formed an ideological trinity which celebrates the social neutrality of the welfare state in the service of the nation. There are, of course, some troubling concerns about these ideological conceptions of the citizenry and the nation which subsequently came to haunt this celebration of neutrality, but in the construction of the post-war welfare state, bureau-professionalism was a powerful force both organizationally and ideologically.

The Dimensions of Crisis

The crisis of the welfare state has been conventionally located in the intersection of economics and politics: the underlying weakness of the British economy in the context of global recession, allied to the rise of New Right politics. The New Right, typically involving a mix of neo-liberal views of deregulated markets as the basis of human freedom and neo-conservative concerns about moral decay and social disorder, broke with the post-war 'social democratic consensus'. In both the UK and the USA,

New Right politics and ideology challenged the old structures, cultures and assumptions of the state, particularly in relation to social welfare (see also Hughes and Lewis, 1998). Conventional accounts stress the ways in which the economic and political 'settlements' associated with the social democratic welfare state came apart, but they are less attentive to the problems in what might be called the 'social' and 'organizational' settlements of the welfare state (Clarke and Newman, 1997). The social settlement is the one eloquently described by Fiona Williams as the intersection of 'family, work and nation', with its distinctive assumptions about the gendered and racialized formations of British society and their consequences for social policy (Williams, 1989; 1993). The interplay of social changes – in the make-up of households, workers and the people – and new forms of social, cultural and political movements disturbed the social settlement profoundly, but also called into question the nature of the welfare state's neutrality. The much-prized neutrality did not extend to the sexual division of labour, or to the racialized structuring of social relations, since these had been consigned to the realm of the extra-social. Nor were 'citizens' intended to play an active part in defining their own needs in the face of state definitions constructed and administered by experts.

The crisis of all three settlements – economic, political and social – imploded into the 'organizational settlement'. The organizational regimes of the old welfare state (and their dominant modes of co-ordination) became a central site for the playing out of the multiple problems and conflicts associated with all three of the 'external' settlements. Enforcing a thoroughly racialized and patriarchal set of norms, embedded in legislation, regulations and professional practice, exposed the claims to neutrality of bureau-professional regimes. It also led to internal tensions as welfare organizations attempted to adapt to or compromise with such challenges – expressed in the search for and struggles over feminist, multi-cultural, anti-racist, anti-homophobic or non-discriminatory forms of welfare practice (Newman and Williams, 1996). As Hoggett (1994, pp. 42–3) has argued, bureau-professional regimes also proved to be relatively weak institutional arrangements for the exercise of the fiscal discipline thought to be needed after 1976. Attempts to impose such discipline frequently provoked lines of internal fracture, especially between administrators and professionals.

The rise of the New Right and their dismantling of the political consensus on state welfare certainly intensified and dramatized these problems of the 'organizational settlement'. Indeed, one of the striking features of the 1980s and 1990s was the way that the New Right turned these organizational issues into potent public stories, 'morality tales', that were woven as a central thread in the narratives which the New Right constructed about the monstrous power of the state and how it subjugated and oppressed the people. These stories were peopled by representatives of the characteristic modes of co-ordination of the post-war welfare state. 'Bureaucrats' sat in their offices plotting their budget and empire growth, hiding behind rules and regulations. Impersonality became the 'depersonalized' mistreatment of individuals. Professionals acted arrogantly and overbearingly, always insisting that they knew best, even when this meant flying in the face of 'common sense'. They constantly interfered unnecessarily or inappropriately in people's lives. Politicians, driven by outdated dogma, failed to represent or protect the people from this machinery of domination. They also failed to run it efficiently. It should be noted that 'politicians' did not, of course, include those of the New Right. One consistent accomplishment of the New Right was simultaneously to reinvent 'ideological politics' and to position themselves as 'beyond politics' – as the representatives of popular common sense and as on the side of the people against government (even when they *were* the government). These stories – and the related narratives about costs, choice and dependency – have been mobilized as the preconditions for restructuring welfare services around 'markets' and 'managers' as the guarantors of efficiency, choice, dynamism and responsiveness (Clarke and Newman, 1997).

Naturalizing Managerialism

In part, the new role for management derived from the New Right's ideological insistence on the innate superiority of the market over the state as a means of allocating resources. In this view, 'managers' inhabited the world of market action, and were thus the natural bearers of its entrepreneurialism, its dynamism and the full gamut of 'good business practices' from which organizations in the public sector needed to learn. To some extent, this imagery of management was concerned with rather old-fashioned virtues of organizational co-ordination – the 'hard-headed' control of costs in the pursuit of greater efficiency, not least through intensified labour productivity. But it also drew on the more dynamic celebration of the manager-as-hero being articulated in the new managerialism – particularly in those new conceptions of the manager as leader and corporate culture shaper, inspiring the unending pursuit of quality and excellence (Clarke and Newman, 1993a; Pollitt, 1993a; Flynn, 1994). Both, however, centred on one essential precondition for 'transforming' the dull professional bureaucracies into modern organizations – the establishment or enhancement of 'the right to manage'.

The legitimation of managerialism as a new mode of co-ordination for social welfare organizations involved a double discursive tactic. On the one hand, public sector organizations were subjected to a *logic of universalism.* This defined all organizations as essentially the same. It suggested that all organizations face similar tasks; all need to be co-ordinated to pursue their goals efficiently; managers have the capacity to create efficiency; therefore, all organizations need to be managed. On the other hand, public sector organizations were also subjected to a *logic of isomorphism*. This implied that successful organizational performance is to be found in the private sector, and since public sector organizations deviate from the 'norm' of the private sector, so public sector organizations must become more 'businesslike'. Managers provide 'good business practices', so public sector organizations need to be managed. In the process, the demand that public services need 'more and better management' was legitimised.

These legitimizations of the 'natural' desirability of management as the obvious way of running organizations (reflected in the increasing use of the phrase 'well-managed' to describe successful organizations) were supported by a further discursive tactic. This involved the articulation of the differences between management and the other pre-existing forms of co-ordination in the welfare state, juxtaposing the virtues of managers with the failings of bureaucrats, professionals and politicians. So, where bureaucrats were rule bound, inward-looking and inert, managers were innovative, externally-oriented and dynamic. Where professionals were paternalistic, self-regulating, building a mystique to protect their power, managers were customer-centred, created transparent organizations and were tested in the 'real world' of the marketplace. Finally, where politicians were dogmatic, interfering and changeable, managers were realists, capable of taking a strategic view and – if given the 'freedom to manage' – able to 'do the right thing'.

It is difficult to find any reform of social welfare in the 1990s which did not draw on and contribute to this installation of a managerial mode of co-ordination – from the creation of agencies (Benefits, Child Support, etc.) to the reorganization of health and social care. I have tried to summarize the main dimensions of the ideological and organizational salience of managerialism and managerialization.

Managerialism is:

- *an ideology* centred on expanding the right to manage in the pursuit of greater efficiency in the achievement of organizational and social objectives;
- *a calculative framework* which orders knowledge about organizational goals and the means of their achievement, typically around an internal calculus of efficiency (inputs–outputs) and an external calculus of competitive positioning within a field of market relations;
- *a series of overlapping discourses* which articulate different – even divergent – conceptions of how to manage and what is to be managed (Total Quality Management; Excellence; Human Resource Management; Business Process Re-engineering and so on).

Managerialization is:

- a process of *establishing managerial discretion/authority* over corporate resources (material, human, symbolic) and decision-making about them;
- a process of *establishing calculative frameworks* that define the terms and conditions of decision-making, and are embedded in patterns of internal and external processes;
- a process of *creating forms of managing and types of managers*. It might be suggested that there are three forms of 'managing' visible in the restructuring of social welfare: managers; hybrids; and a 'dispersed managerial consciousness'.

I want to concentrate here on the last point, about creating forms of managing. The most obvious indicator of the impact of managerialism in social welfare is the rapid growth in the number of people who are employed as 'managers' – for example, in the NHS. These are either 'imports' or 'converts': the former brought in from elsewhere (probably the 'real world'); the latter manufactured 'in-house' through management training or development programmes and making a career shift to a clearly identified managerial role. Although such numbers may be the most obvious indicators of managerialization, the other two forms may be of at least equal importance. The 'hybrid' form is now widespread in what were formerly bureau-professional services. We have used the phrase (Clarke and Newman, 1997) to identify the incorporation of professional workers, characteristically through processes of devolution and delegation, into the new structures of corporate co-ordination (see also Fitzgerald, Ashburner and Ferlie, 1995). Clinical directors, ward managers and fundholding practices in the NHS; head teachers under LMS; care management in social services; devolved operational management in policing, and so on, all rest on the construction of articulations between professional and managerial modes of co-ordination. Such 'hybrids' evoke a complex set of motivations, since they draw on 'service values' or commitments to underpin engagement with corporate management.

At the same time, they require that these commitments are subjected to the disciplines contained in accepting the 'realities' and 'responsibilities' of corporate management. They are often an uncomfortable place to be, because they are subject to conflicting demands and expectations in a field of tensions between the 'service' and 'corporate' concerns. In an earlier article, Janet Newman and I argued that such hybrid formations were the focal point for 'devolved stress', as significant organizational tensions and conflicts came to be embodied in single individuals:

> Devolved management has sought to dissolve the characteristic problem of managing professionals . . . not by subjecting them to

> more management but by turning them into managers. In the process, the tension between organisational and professional commitments becomes internalised rather than external. Such new managers become the focal point for conflicting identities and loyalties, struggle to reconcile in their identities and practice the previously separated commitments. This process takes place in the context of devolved resources, which carry with them the devolution of resource limits, such that 'hard choices' are pushed down the organisation towards the front line, bringing with them the stress that accompanies trying to balance service commitments and resource limits. (1993b, p. 55)

The final effect of managerialization is the creation of a 'dispersed managerial consciousness': the embedding of the calculative frameworks of managerialism throughout organizations. This refers to the processes by which all employees come to find their decisions, actions and possibilities framed by the imperatives of managerial co-ordination: competitive positioning, budgetary control, performance management and other initiatives. The use of the word 'consciousness' is not meant to imply that people think of themselves as 'managers' (although the rhetorical devices of 'we are all responsible now' clearly seek such an effect). But it marks the way in which people have become increasingly conscious that the managerial agenda and the corporate calculus condition their working relationships, conditions and practices and need to be negotiated.

Lost for Words or Empty Rhetoric?

The impact of managerialism on social welfare raises some issues about the discursive constitution of subjects that may be worth further attention. Critics of managerialism in social welfare have tended to categorize it as merely 'empty rhetoric' intended to disguise or distract attention from the 'real' changes taking place (cuts in welfare resourcing, privatization, etc.). By contrast, its proponents tend to talk about it in terms of bringing about 'cultural change' in organizations: installing new paradigms, visions, corporate missions and commitments. In this they tend to have the inadvertent support of at least some practitioners of discourse analysis who have treated the new managerialism as constructing new subjects in the work place (e.g. Rose, 1990). I want to suggest that none of these views will quite do. The 'empty rhetoric' view of managerialism fails to take account of the real effects which the process has produced. Welfare organizations operate differently as a consequence of its impact – both in the way they address and interact with users and other organizations and in their internal processes and practices. It is certainly true that these changes are not exactly those claimed for the model by its protagonists and, equally, their connection with improved benefits and services in social policy is tenuous – but there has been something more than rhetoric at stake here.

The alternative view has tended to treat such rhetoric as part of a process of discursive subjection – the construction of new subjects within organizations. This view is embraced by both the adherents of managerial approaches to 'cultural change' who wish to create new motivational attachments between employees and organizations and, from a rather different starting-point, by post-Foucauldian discourse analysts. Both are united in the view that subjects can be produced by cultural or discursive transformations. There are a number of problems with these theories and practices of subjection. The first is that older discourses and the subject positions and identities associated with them have not gone away. They linger on, not just out of nostalgia, but because the *specific* practices of welfare provision continue to require particular combinations of skills, competences and orientations which outrun the discourse of business, management and enterprise. What has been constructed is a field of tensions within which people manoeuvre – calculatingly, passionately, politically. Some of the central tensions are visible in simple but potent competing representations: 'being business-like' versus 'public service'; 'managers' versus 'professionals'; 'competition' versus 'collaboration'; 'customers' versus 'patients' or 'students', and so on. No discourse – even one as apparently engaging and compelling as the new managerialism – is uncontested.

None of this is intended to deny that managerialism has its enthusiasts and converts. It promises release from stifling or troublesome conditions that characterized the 'old ways' – bureaucratic inertia, professional conservatism or political interference. Ideas of 'quality', 'excellence' or even 'liberation management' (Peters, 1993) have created profound resonances in public service cultures – either in their old forms or in what Newman (1996) has called the 'impoverished cultures' resulting from two decades of becoming 'lean and mean'. The appeal of the new managerialism in social welfare was that it offered both the prospect of being able to 'get on with what really matters' (sometimes called the 'core business') instead of being held back by inappropriate forms of organization, and the opportunity to be 'real managers' and act decisively. It is also underpinned by the reconfiguration of career structures in such organizations in which the old lines of professional advancement have tended to become truncated and had managerial routes superimposed upon them. Nevertheless, not everyone has 'come on board' and there remain widespread anxieties about, and hostility to, the spread of the 'business culture'. These anxieties are so widespread that they have even become a feature of popular entertainment, as in the TV series *Health and Efficiency* and *Cardiac Arrest*, both of which have used the tension between professional and managerial orientations as a central narrative focus. One recurrent theme has been the inappropriateness of managerial values, and the 'ungrounded' feel of the managerial discourse as 'empty rhetoric'. One way of thinking about the emptiness of this 'empty rhetoric' is that it results from the inability of the managerial discourse to colonize its own terms of reference. It cannot *fix* the meanings of the words that it deploys as a discursive strategy. This is not just an abstract observation that all words are polysemic. Rather, it is that specific words in particular contexts are subjected to attempts to articulate them to divergent projects. In the context of managerialization, such 'key words' might include 'the customer', 'loyalty', 'motivation', 'needs' and 'quality'. In thinking about managerialism as a discursive strategy, it might be worth looking at some of the more localized 'tactics' that are at play in the attempt to dominate the fields of organizational meaning. I want to put forward three such tactics which, I suggest, have been significant: displacement; subordination; and co-option.

Displacement might be identified in the rise of the idea of the customer (Clarke, 1997). The customer displaces the imagery (and the implied relationships) of older ideological representations of the citizen and the client (or service-specific variants such as patient or student). The image of the customer challenges the authority of professionals or politicians to 'speak for' the needs and interests of service users. In the process, it (discursively) empowers the customer (as an active agent capable of making choices) and managers (who are intrinsically 'customer-centred'). The apparatuses of customer surveys and feedback produce the new organizationally-valued, informational currency in place of the implicit or informal knowledges claimed by professionals and others about users.

Subordination has predominantly taken the form of framing the exercise of 'professional judgement' by the requirement that it take account of the 'realities and responsibilities' of budgetary management. Increasingly, professional assessment encounters budgetary implications at an earlier stage, so that the assessment of need no longer takes place prior to – and separate from – the resourcing of the response, but alongside it. This is most clearly visible in the fields of health and social care. The combination of devolved budgets and care assessment and planning in community care was an attempt to discipline the 'irresponsible' exercise of professional judgement about needs, by making it coterminous with the allocation of resources. Where 'need' was once the product of the intersection of bureaucratic categorization and professional judgement, it is now increasingly articulated with, and disciplined by, a managerial calculus of resources and priorities.

Co-option refers to managerialist attempts to colonize the terrain of professional discourse, constructing articulations between professional concerns and languages and those of management. The most obvious example is to be found in the epidemic of quality (Kirkpatrick and Martinez-Lucio, 1996). Quality appeared to be the 'home ground' of professionals, committed as they were to the maintenance of standards, the production and dissemination of 'good practice' and the delivery of 'service'. Nevertheless, as a number of authors have demonstrated, quality is also a central mechanism for disciplining professional autonomy (Pollitt, 1993b; Jackson, 1994). The systematization of quality through the production of indicators, comparable information and evaluation has sought, in Peter Jackson's delightful phrase, to 'curb the promiscuity' of quality.

The effect of these discursive tactics is to leave old professional or service discourses marginalized – in the condition of being 'lost for words'. The old languages have lost some of their purchase on organizational realities and their capacity to mobilize power and resources. That sense of loss is intensified by the fluidity of managerial discourse in its attempts to stake out the high moral ground of organizational command. Who can deny that organizational commitments to efficiency or quality are desirable objectives? This is probably best manifested in the Peters and Waterman-derived demand that we 'learn to love change' – a clarion call that has been taken up across the public services. Being 'against change' is a rather difficult discursive position to occupy, especially when the urgency of organizational change is legitimized by reference to the pace and scale of change in the turbulent 'external environment', as evidenced in the opening paragraphs of any strategic plan. To be a 'conservative' (or resister) in such circumstances carries the risk of being identified as outmoded, defending elitist or sectional interests, against progress, or threatening the future of the organization. The fluidity of the discourse of change is an essential precondition of its deployment as a discursive tactic, since any particular change is subject to a process of elision with the (epochal) Need For Change (Clarke and Newman, 1997, Ch. 3). Where managerialism may be concerned to curb the 'promiscuity' of quality, it is also intent on promoting the promiscuity of 'learning to love change' (or at least a condition of serial monogamy, since a new corporate initiative should soon replace the last one in employees' affections).

The final issue here concerns the conditions under which the discourse of managerialism works – its ability to transform the world of social welfare effectively. I have suggested that there are ways in which it has been potent, but I think it is arguable whether this has been reflected in a capacity to produce new subjects. This is itself a rather tricky theoretical and methodological issue, in that it is difficult to establish how one would know if such subjects were being constituted in practice. But I do want to insist that there are some dangers attached to simply reading them off from the discourse itself. It is, of course, possible to find the bearers of the new managerialism – in both its trained products and its enthusiastic converts within welfare organizations. It is equally possible to find those who use the discourse conditionally or calculatingly: performing compliance, as it were (Hopfl, 1992). Finally, it is possible to see those who 'do not believe a word of it' but whose behaviour is nevertheless constrained and constructed by the institutional embeddedness of the discourse. Indeed, I am tempted to argue that what has been most striking about the impact of managerialism is its ability to produce behavioural compliance at the same time as inducing scepticism, cynicism and disbelief. For many people working in social welfare the problem about the discourse is not that it constructs them as subjects, but that they find it offensively transparent (or transparently offensive). There is a difference between being subjected to a discourse and becoming a subject through it.

A rather different way of thinking about the success of the managerialist discourse is to consider how it has accomplished the TINA effect ('There Is No Alternative'). This means paying attention to the transformations in the fields of relationships, processes and practices in which welfare work is embedded and not merely to representations of them. The reworking of organizational regimes, the conditions of inter-organizational relationships, the architecture of power within and between them, the preferred modes of calculation and control and the allocation of resources, create a new terrain in which people behave in an increasingly managerialized fashion. They compete for contracts, engage in decentralized decision-making, prepare business plans and interact with customers because those are the logics of the organizational and inter-organizational field of relationships (see also Hoggett, 1996). These are, so to speak, the new rules of the game, and to play the game means acknowledging those conditions (however conditionally).

'Perverse Effects': Managerialism and Social Welfare

This section traces some of the consequences of managerialism for the provision of welfare services. What follows is highly selective, and is focused on four specific shifts that are intimately linked to the arrival of managerial regimes. The four shifts are encapsulated in the ideas of 'core business', 'ownership', 'audit' and 'corporate culture'.

The idea of an organization's *core business* is a corollary of processes of service fragmentation (between providers) and forms of quasi-market competitiveness. It represents the managerial attempt to define the focus of attention of the organization – either externally-oriented in terms of competitive positioning, or as the internal management of 'waste and inefficiency'. Such specifications order the priorities of different potential calls on organizational resources and are formulated within a range of possibilities that are constructed by external or statutory requirements and internal organizational politics. Perhaps more important, the specification of core business legitimizes withdrawal from previously undertaken activities that become redefined as 'inessential'. Recent examples might include extra-curricular provision by schools, accident and emergency facilities of hospitals, response to burglar alarms by police forces, and so on. In the process, there is a question about what happens to those activities and services that fail to form part of any agency's 'core business' when they do not fit either the competitive position or the survival strategy of the organizations involved.

The effects of defining core business overlap with the issue of *ownership*. The creation of ownership – of missions, targets, and responsibilities – has been one of the most sought-after effects of the managerial revolution. Its aim is to construct commitment and motivation among staff in the pursuit of corporate objectives (Clarke and Newman, 1993a). Nevertheless, there is a conception of ownership which highlights a darker side of such initiatives: this is the view of ownership as 'proprietorialism' or 'possessive individualism'. Owners tend to stake out property rights – the rights to the exclusive use of what they own. It is, therefore, not surprising to find the new field of welfare provision being characterized by ownership conflicts: over who owns customers (their needs and the resources that might accompany them); who owns service responsibilities and the resource implications that they bring; and who owns those practices that take place in the interstices between organizations or departments. So, the 'boundary disputes' between health and social care raise questions about who owns types of needs as well as who has the definitional power over how needs are to be categorized (Charlesworth, Clarke and Cochrane, 1996). There are intra-organizational tensions about internal markets or recharging policies, particularly exposing the 'overhead' costs of central services. There is also the 'commodification' of inter-agency or inter-professional goodwill, with attempts to recharge the cost of contributing to joint initiatives (for example, in child protection work). In the present conditions, promoting 'ownership' of a budget may create a new sense of fiscal discipline and responsibility, but it is also likely to create competitive manoeuvring to maximize income and reduce expenditure. The general tendencies towards proprietorialism also underpin more specific tactics, such as 'cream skimming', identified in the growing literature on quasi-markets (Le Grand and Bartlett, 1993).

What Michael Power (1993) has referred to as the *audit explosion* indicates the growth in both internal and external evaluations of performance and compliance. In part, such processes may reflect the increasing impossibility of 'trust' between citizens and service providers, between government and its agencies, or between purchasers and providers (Walsh, 1995). But they are also strategic responses from the centre aimed both at extending the disciplines available to regulate the periphery, and overcoming the dislocating relationships of an increasingly fragmented or, perhaps more accurately, dispersed state (Clarke, 1996a). Nevertheless, they also have perverse effects on welfare services. They transfer scarce organizational resources from what Power calls 'Level 1' to 'Level 2' activities: from service production or delivery to information and monitoring systems (with an emphasis on guaranteeing procedural correctness). In the public sector context, they have become increasingly enmeshed in the intensification of competitiveness (rankings, league tables) despite the acknowledged problems both of comparability and identification of appropriate indicators. Such evaluative scrutiny has become an essential component of the TINA effect discussed above. It may be that no-one believes them – either the supposed beneficiaries of the information or the service providers subjected to them – but they are taken seriously in practice, since to fail to do so has competitive or resourcing consequences. As a result, organizations, units and individuals are likely to find themselves pursuing objectives and targets in which they may have little confidence (waiting list reductions or telephone answering rates) and which may even draw attention and resources away from activities perceived as more significant to the service in question.

Finally, it is possible that the growth of audit, in its many forms, also contributes to isomorphic tendencies in the current system, impelling organizations towards the idea that there is 'one best way' of running things. In part, this tendency is the effect of demands for organizations to possess systems that will generate comparable information to facilitate the process of evaluation. But it is also the result of some degree of blurring between the evaluative functions of audit and the concerns of 'organizational design'. Some of this is visible in the trajectory of the Audit Commission which has increasingly developed a prescriptive agenda about organizational and management structures for public service organizations, exemplified in its definition of the 'cultural revolution' needed to make a success of community care (Audit Commission, 1992; also see Gray and Jenkins, 1993; Langan and Clarke, 1994).

The enthusiasm for creating new *corporate cultures* poses rather different problems (Newman, 1996). At a mundane level, this enthusiasm seems to have inversely proportionate effects on staff motivation and morale, producing credibility gaps and collective cynicism. More significantly, the attempt to elaborate corporate cultures reflects the processes of fragmentation and dispersal and the impact of competitive field of relationships, so that individual fortunes (what used to be called careers) are seen as increasingly tied to the success – or at least survival – of the particular organization rather than a professional field. One counter-tendency to this is to be found in the combination of competition and the growing possibilities of local wage bargaining which has the potential for creating 'transfer markets' for high performers. A second counter-tendency is to be found in the search for increased managerial authority over labour – in particular over its disposability – since affective attachment or loyalty to corporate cultures may be undermined by the lack of evidence of corporate loyalty to employees (British Gas has probably been the most 'successful' example).

Despite such problems, it is clear that public sector managements have discovered the attractions of corporate cultures and their enthusiasm (or missionary zeal) has once more put professionalism in social welfare at the centre of tensions. Whatever other flaws it might have had, welfare professionalism always contained threads of 'collegiality' (or 'horizontalism', as organizational texts now refer to it) and 'cosmopolitanism', which, to some extent, ran counter to hierarchical, centralizing and localizing organizational regimes. At their most minimal, such tendencies towards collegiality and cosmopolitanism evoked a sense of belonging to something other than a particular organization, department or unit. In more developed forms, these trans-organizational connections have been a fertile ground for some of the significant politics of social welfare over the last two decades (the varieties of radical social work, anti-discriminatory or access policies, and so on). Welfare professionalism has not just been defensive or imperialist. Collegiality and cosmopolitanism represent a problem for corporate cultures, because they sustain a sense (or an illusion) that there is an 'elsewhere' beyond the organization to which people may form loyalties or affective identifications. Such attachments are problematic for attempts to engage in symbolic management, since they are the source of disruptive or dislocatory symbols that are not generated 'in-house'. One of the most forceful articulations of these corporate claims was made by Roy Lilley (Chairman of the Homewood Trust in Surrey), when he argued that doctors' first duty was to the organization in which they worked (*The Guardian*, 14 November 1994). Corporate cultures are always likely to strive to discipline or diminish potentially conflicting loyalties, simply because they *are* corporate cultures. They embody a retreat from the older expansive conceptions of 'public service' or even of generic fields of public provision (such as education or health). The identification of 'niches' makes it harder to sustain conceptions of life beyond the organization which are not merely the 'external environment'. This environment is an unpleasant place. As mapped by strategic plans, it is split into threats and opportunities and peopled by cut-throat competitors. Corporate cultures, in short, are antithetical to conceptions of a public realm. Welfare professionalism, in however attenuated a form, articulated such ideas of public service (Clarke, 1996b). Taken together, these 'perverse effects' of managerialization reflect both a political agenda and the unintended consequences of new organizational regimes. Trying to disentangle the relationships between managerialization and the political project of the New Right is the focus of the final section.

Doing the Right Thing? The Politics of Managerialism

The title of this chapter derives from the frequently quoted assertion that the difference between administrators and managers is that where 'administrators do things right, managers do the right thing'. But it also raises the question of whether, in the context of welfare restructuring, managerialism has been doing the Right's thing. Managerialism has been both the beneficiary of and the conduit for Conservative policies for social welfare and the wider reconstruction of the relationship between state and society. The New Right's obsession with dismantling the institutionalized forms of social democracy led to a view of managerialism as a lever to break open the power bloc that the old welfare state represented. As I have suggested earlier, 'management' performed a double role as the organizational proxy of the market (embodying 'good business practices') and as a means of disrupting and disciplining the old forms of organizational co-ordination – bureaucratic, professional and political.

The conditions for managerialism playing this role can be traced back to the mid-1970s in the points of overlap between the emergent agendas of both the New Right and the new managerialism. As we have argued elsewhere (Clarke and Newman, 1993a; 1997), there were a number of affinities between these projects. They shared: a hostility to bureaucratic organization; a commitment to entrepreneurial dynamism and competition; a drive towards deregulation; and, above all, a demand for the 'freedoms' necessary to give managers 'the right to manage'. Such affinities created the grounds for an alliance between the political and the organizational forces for change. But I am not convinced that it is satisfactory to treat managerialism simply as the organizational 'proxy' of the New Right. This does not mean that managements have not pursued elements of the Conservative reforms with great enthusiasm, since they clearly have. But thinking of the relationship between managerialism and the New Right as an alliance (rather than a hierarchical structure of strategists and implementers or leaders and subalterns) opens up issues both about the limits of the alliance and the prospects of managerialism after the New Right.

There are a number of potential sites of antagonism or tension within this alliance that have been particularly visible in recent years. The first concerns the allocation of responsibility. Several authors have seen the managerialization of social welfare as a way of moving (or attempting to move) hard choices out of the political arena into the realm of managerial responsibility (see, for example, Salter, 1993). This dispersal of decision-making (through agencies and quangos, and into multiple or fragmented sites) has applied most to the problems of budgetary management and service priorities. But it has not always been successful, since questions of services and priorities have tended to resurface at the political level despite government attempts to gloss them as 'operational' or 'managerial' matters. Indeed, some of the issues have returned to the political realm precisely because those in managerial roles have refused 'responsibility' (in community care and the Gloucestershire test case; in the 1995 conflicts over school budget setting, and so on).

There are also problems about how managements choose to exercise their new-found freedoms to manage, since the pursuit of local objectives may not deliver the nationally-desired aims. Consequently, political intervention has been required in what had been identified as the realms of the market or NHS management as the 'wrong results' appear (for example, in the 1993 'over-achievement' on contracts, leading to ward closures). In a rather more dramatic way, the 'Romeo and Juliet' saga in Hackney highlighted the potential for local management to produce unintended consequences. 'Local' management contains the permanent possibility of new alliances or of managements being themselves co-opted to local values, objectives or missions. As the organizational hinge between government policy and 'local' users – staff and other 'stakeholders' – managements find themselves trying to reconcile potentially conflicting interests. Although, as Taylor-Gooby and Lawson put it, the twin strategy of centralization and decentralization aims to ensure that 'power over the essentials is retained centrally while the management of inessentials is decentralized' (1993, p. 133), it is harder to guarantee that the choice of what to decentralize can anticipate what will be 'essential' in practice.

Finally, there are continuing problems about the 'freedom' of managers to manage. For the New Right, this has primarily been interpreted as needing the combination of deregulation and the removal or reduction of trades union 'interference'. But there has been a tension between the political concerns of policy-making and the wish of managements to be able to behave like 'real managers'. So, the decision to retain a role for Regional Health Authorities provoked dismay among Trust managers who saw it as an unwanted inhibition of their autonomy (see also Harrison *et al.*, 1992, pp. 122–8). Similarly, many 'business units' in local authorities and other public sector institutions complain of being artificially confined by wider corporate agendas, policies and costs which stop them from getting out there and 'doing the right thing'. At a number of different levels, the dispersal of the state and decision-making has established instabilities at the intersection between centrifugal and centripetal forces – or between pressures towards further fragmentation and stronger integration.

I raise these issues because they serve as reminders that managerialism was not simply or solely a proxy for New Right policies. It is also a social and organizational force with its own trajectory that was not wholly circumscribed by Conservative programmes. Recognizing that difference also requires us to consider the longer-term salience of managerialism for the future of social welfare. Treating managerialism as a Conservative proxy would leave us with the comforting assumption that the creation of a 'new Labour' government might see the end of both the policies and their means of implementation. This seems to me not to be very helpful – or very likely. Alternatively, we could view managerialism as 'apolitical' and subscribe to the claim that it is merely the technical means of implementing whatever objectives the 'national board of directors' decides upon. There are clearly attractions to this view, not least the implication that social policy becomes a matter of deciding on new 'targets' and embedding them in the nexus of corporate missions, strategic plans and indicators for performance audit.

And yet, I confess I cannot quite bring myself to believe in this vision of managerialism's technocratic innocence. In the end, I return to the view that all modes of organizational co-ordination are implicated in the construction of particular regimes of power. While the managerialist mission may be to 'empower everyone', I lack a sense of trust (in my multiple identities as a social scientist, a service user, a manager and one who is managed). As a result, I am left with a series of as yet unanswered questions. Is it possible to discipline managerialism as a form of social and organizational power – and how might this be accomplished? Put another way, the problem with the claim to 'do the right thing' is that it is self-referential. By what means can the rest of us judge whether it is 'right', or exercise control over the managerial autonomy legitimated by the claim? Is it possible to overcome the perverse effects of dispersal and fragmentation without reverting to centralization? Is it possible to restore some collective conception of the public, the public good and public service which does not reproduce the post-war mythology of the one-dimensional nation, which at the same time escapes treating diversity as the individual differences of autonomous customers? Is it possible to develop a conception of management as stewardship, responsible for the preservation and enhancement of the public realm, rather than management as entrepreneurialism, chasing the next big transformation?

Note

As usual, I have drawn heavily on collaborative work with a number of people, especially Janet Newman, Allan Cochrane and Eugene McLaughlin, whose efforts to keep me thinking are gratefully acknowledged. They are not, however, responsible for the idiosyncratic uses I have made of those collaborations.

References

AUDIT COMMISSION (1992) *The Community Revolution: Personal Social Services and Community Care*, London: HMSO.

BURROWS, R. and LOADER, B. (Eds) (1994) *Towards a Post-Fordist Welfare State?*, London: Routledge.

CHARLESWORTH, J., CLARKE, J. and COCHRANE, A. (1996) 'Tangled webs? Managing local mixed economies of care', *Public Administration*, **74**, pp. 67–88.

CLARKE, J. (1994) 'Towards a post-Fordist welfare state?', *Local Government Studies*, (Winter).

CLARKE, J. (1996a) 'The problem of the state after the welfare state', in MAY, M., BRUNSDON, E. and CRAIG, G. (Eds) *Social Policy Review 8*, London: Social Policy Association.

CLARKE, J. (1996b) 'Public nightmares and communitarian dreams: the crisis of the social in social welfare', in EDGELL, S., HETHERINGTON, P. and WARDE, A. (Eds) *Consumption Matters*, Oxford: Blackwell/The Sociological Review.

CLARKE, J. (1997) 'Capturing the customer? Consumerism and social welfare', *Self, Agency and Society*, 1, pp. 55–73.

CLARKE, J. and NEWMAN, J. (1993a) 'The right to manage: a second managerial revolution?', *Cultural Studies*, **7** (3), pp. 427–41.

CLARKE, J. and NEWMAN, J. (1993b) 'Managing to survive: dilemmas of changing organizational forms in the public sector', in DEAKIN, N. and PAGE, R. (Eds) *The Costs of Welfare*, Aldershot: Avebury.

CLARKE, J. and NEWMAN, J. (1997) *The Managerial State: Power, Politics and Ideology in the Remaking of Social Welfare*, London: Sage.

CLARKE, J., COCHRANE, A. and MCLAUGHLIN, E. (1994) 'Mission accomplished or unfinished business? The impact of managerialisation', in CLARKE, J., COCHRANE, A. and MCLAUGHLIN, E. (Eds) *Managing Social Policy*, London: Sage.

CLARKE, J., COCHRANE, A. and MCLAUGHLIN, E. (Eds) (1994) *Managing Social Policy*, London: Sage.

COCHRANE, A. (1993) *Whatever Happened to Local Government?*, Buckingham: Open University Press.

COUSINS, C. (1987) *Controlling Social Welfare*, Brighton: Wheatsheaf Books.

DU GAY, P. (1994) 'Making up managers: bureaucracy, enterprise and the liberal art of separation', *British Journal of Sociology*, **45**, pp. 655–74.

FITZGERALD, L., ASHBURNER, L. and FERLIE, E. (1995) 'Professions, markets and managers: empirical evidence from the NHS', paper for ESRC seminar on 'Professionals in late modernity', University of Warwick.

FLYNN, N. (1994) 'Control, commitment and contracts', in CLARKE, J., COCHRANE, A. and MCLAUGHLIN, E. (Eds) *Managing Social Policy*, London: Sage.

GRAY, A. and JENKINS, B. (1993) 'Markets, managers and the public service: the changing of a culture', in TAYLOR-GOOBY, P. and LAWSON, R. (Eds), *Markets and Managers*, Buckingham: Open University.

HARRISON, S., HUNTER, D., MARNOCH, G. and POLLITT, C. (1992) *Just Managing: Power and Culture in the National Health Service*, Basingstoke: Macmillan.

HOGGETT, P. (1994) 'The politics of the modernisation of the UK welfare state', in BURROWS, R. and LOADER, B. (Eds) *Towards a Post-Fordist Welfare State?*, London: Routledge.

HOGGETT, P. (1996) 'New modes of control in the public service', *Public Administration*, **74**, pp. 9–32.

HOPFL, H. (1992) 'The making of the corporate acolyte: Some thoughts on charismatic leadership and the reality of organizational commitment', *Journal of Management Studies*, **29**, pp. 23–34.

HUGHES, G. and LEWIS, G. (Eds) (1998) *Unsettling Welfare*, London: Routledge.

JACKSON, P. (1994) 'Curbing promiscuity: constructing total quality in an Acute Hospitals Trust', paper presented to ERU conference on 'The Contract State', Cardiff.

KIRKPATRICK, I. and MARTINEZ-LUCIO, M. (Eds) (1996) *The Politics of Quality in the Public Sector*, London: Routledge.

LANGAN, M. and CLARKE, J. (1994) 'Managing in the mixed economy of care', in CLARKE, J., COCHRANE, A. and MCLAUGHLIN, E. (Eds) *Managing Social Policy*, London: Sage.

LE GRAND, J. and BARTLETT, W. (Eds) (1993) *Quasi-Markets and Social Policy*, Basingstoke: Macmillan.

NEWMAN, J. (1996) *Shaping Organisational Cultures*, London: Pitman.

NEWMAN, J. and CLARKE, J. (1994) 'Going about our business? The managerialization of social welfare', in CLARKE, J., COCHRANE, A. and MCLAUGHLIN, E. (Eds) *Managing Social Policy*, London: Sage.

NEWMAN, J. and WILLIAMS, F. (1996) 'Diversity and change: gender, welfare and organizational relations', in ITZIN, C. and NEWMAN, J. (Eds) *Gender, Culture and Organisational Change*, London: Routledge.

PETERS, T. (1993) *Liberation Management*, New York: Knopf.

POLLITT, C. (1993a) *Managerialism and the Public Services* (2nd edn), Oxford: Basil Blackwell.

POLLITT, C. (1993b) 'The struggle for quality: the case of the National Health Service', *Policy and Politics*, **21**, pp. 161–70.

POWER, M. (1993) *The Audit Explosion*, London: Demos.

ROSE, N. (1990) *Governing the Soul*, London: Routledge.

SALTER, B. (1993) 'The politics of purchasing in the National Health Service', *Policy and Politics*, **21**, pp. 171–81.

TAYLOR-GOOBY, P. and LAWSON, R. (1993a) 'Where we go from here? The new order in welfare', in TAYLOR-GOOBY, P. and LAWSON, R. (Eds) *Markets and Managers*, Buckingham: Open University Press.

WAINE, B. and CUTLER, T. (1994) *Managing the Welfare State*, London: Berg.

WALSH, K. (1995) *Public Services and Market Mechanisms: Competition, Contracting and the New Public Management*, Basingstoke: Macmillan.
WILLIAMS, F. (1989) *Social Policy: A Critical Introduction*, Cambridge: Polity Press.
WILLIAMS, F. (1993) 'Gender, "race" and class in British welfare policy', in COCHRANE, A. and CLARKE, J. (Eds) *Comparing Welfare States*, London: Sage.

Chapter 13

Reflections

Liz Meerabeau and Pamela Abbott

Introduction

In this book we have been considering occupations that have at best an ambivalent status in the hierarchy of occupations. Developing out of Victorian philanthropy, occupations such as nursing, primary-school teaching and social work were seen as providing an appropriate opportunity for middle-class women to enter the public sphere of paid employment. The hope of many middle-class women at the close of the nineteenth century was that they would provide occupations for women on a par with the professional occupations of their husbands, brothers and sons. However, from the outset these occupations were more controlled and perceived as being of lower status than the then established professions. The occupants of these occupational roles lacked the autonomy and the educational credentials of the established (male) professions and enjoyed neither their salaries nor their conditions of service. Indeed, the work undertaken by these occupational groups was seen as using the 'natural' qualities of women, and training as necessary only to permit the full development of these qualities. However, these roles did provide, and continue to provide, high-status core occupations in the female occupational hierarchy, although women are often concentrated on the lower rungs with men disproportionately occupying senior and managerial positions.

During the course of the twentieth century these occupations have been engaged in struggles to enhance their status, using both trade union and professionalizing strategies. Professionalizing strategies have been challenged by other occupational groups (especially, in the case of nursing, by medical doctors) and by some within the occupation itself. Nevertheless, there *has* been a move from an apprenticeship and training mode to education, generally resulting in higher education credentials, although these have often been at diploma rather than degree level, and an emphasis on the acquisition of practical skills as opposed to theoretical knowledge has been retained. However, the tight bureaucratic mode of control has remained, with practitioners managed and controlled within bureaucratic structures. Accountability has generally been to managers.

The development of New Managerialism, while tightening managerial control over occupations such as medicine, has only resulted in two parallel forms of management for occupations such as nursing and social work. Dominelli (1997) suggests that just over a third of social work time is spent meeting administrative demands imposed by new managerialism. Among these demands she mentions time spent processing client records and inputting information on to IT systems which in turn facilitate more intensive and invasive management surveillance of individual cases. These same managerialist strategies reduce the potential for professional relationships as opposed to bureaucratic procedures. Dominelli suggests that

> . . . the case management approach to social work has reduced the space for professionals to explore the needs of the 'person-in-the-situation'. This trend is most evident in community care where social workers have become engrossed in chasing other professionals and service providers to deliver 'packages of care' which focus on a discrete aspect of a 'client's' life rather than addressing their circumstances in a holistic way. (p. 118)

In drawing the threads of this book together, we will examine both the similarities and the differences between the occupational groups. Some of the similarities have been discussed: their origins at a similar point in time in what has been termed the disciplinary society; the construction and maintenance of a knowledge base; the effects of patriarchy, either externally (medicine) or internally due to the high percentage of men in upper management. All, regardles of whether they are in the UK or Australia, have been affected by the same macro-environment, in particular the 'new managerialism'. Like Clarke in this volume, we feel that the Zeitgeist is unlikely to change in the foreseeable future, despite a change of government in the UK.

Developing the Knowledge Base

Torstendahl (1990) argues that in any definition of 'professions', knowledge systems will play an important role. There are debates as to whether this knowledge actually serves to solve problems or has a largely symbolic purpose, acting as social capital by excluding others from providing a service (Larson, 1990). Abbott (1988, p. 9) claims that a key factor is the degree of abstraction, which enables the occupation to 'redefine its problems and tasks, defend them from interlopers, and seize new problems'. For Macdonald (1995), there needs to be a balance between knowledge and technique, between 'mere formalism' and craft. The new managerialism includes a refusal to take occupations at their own face value, and a requirement for them to spell out what they do; this has impacted differently on different occupations, and Jamous and Peloille's (1970) concept of the indeterminacy:technicality ratio has been used in this book as a useful analytic tool. Both social work and probation had a well-developed knowledge base, with a large amount of indeterminacy. Much of the work was, however, based on values, and therefore vulnerable to shifts in the political climate, and both could be construed as counter to 'common sense'. May and Annison argue that probation work was based on technical knowledge, but that the concept of what it is to be a probation officer has changed, with the shift to a more punitive model.

Health visiting has also been particularly vulnerable, in that much of the work is around prevention and health promotion: for many years, health visitors rather complacently stated that it was not therefore possible to assess its effectiveness, and claimed that they were 'practitioners in their own right', not dependent on the GP for acquiring their caseload. When research was commissioned on the effectiveness of health visiting, in the NHS Health Technology Assessment programme, health visitors were not the main drivers in prioritizing the topic, or in commissioning the research. The introduction of the new GP contract in the early 1990s enabled GPs to purchase health visiting and district nursing services, putting the onus on both groups to spell out what they did, and also creating anxieties that contracts might be switched (Hiscock and Pearson, 1996). At the same time GPs were recruiting large numbers of practice nurses (Atkin *et al.*, 1993) who were under their direct management.

> Community nursing changed from being a loose grouping of diverse professionals to a commodity, shaped and driven by the market. (Gough, 1997)

As Kirkham notes in this volume, midwifery in the UK has sought an (uneasy?) alliance with medicine in developing its knowledge base, as has mental health nursing. General (now termed adult) nursing has behaved rather differently. Having developed in the shadow of medicine, it now has the dilemma of how to construct a knowledge base and role which are independent of medicine, particularly since the latter has been spectacularly successful in colonizing biology, one of the underpinning disciplines of both medicine and nursing. One route is to develop the 'expanded role', taking on medical tasks such as the insertion of intravenous infusions, but construing this as being part of the holistic delivery of care, not merely undertaking a task. Another is to develop a knowledge base around ongoing patient problems in which doctors show no great interest, such as wound care; however, medical interest may reawaken and they may take the subject back, as has happened in palliative care. A third is to construct a knowledge base from the social sciences and humanities: there is, for example, a thriving Heidegger industry in nursing. The risk of this is that it is not knowledge which is readily perceived as useful. It is high in indeterminacy, but low on technicality, and, as Hugman points out, both are needed. A fourth approach is to reclaim and attempt to theorize previously undervalued tacit knowledge of the body (Lawler, 1991). This is a sophisticated ploy if, as Macdonald (1995) states, nursing is generally more practice- than theory-oriented. Some of this knowledge will be close to lay knowledge: nursing must then patrol its borders, and try to argue that seemingly unskilled or semi-skilled care work in fact requires underlying expertise. (A commonly used argument is that bathing may not seem a skilled activity, but it is an opportunity for the skilled worker to observe and diagnose.) Such knowledge lacks the abstraction which enables an occupation to 'redefine its problems and tasks, defend them from interlopers' (Abbott, 1988). Since the knowledge base on outcomes of nursing care is so embryonic, it is difficult to link outcomes of care to the level of skill of the carer. This is exploited by the enthusiasts for skill-mix, who have the knack of presenting themselves as entrepreneurial and far-sighted, in contrast to the unimaginative and self-serving professionals (DOH, 1996). Nursing is also ambivalent in its relationship to less skilled staff, particularly if they are part of the same team, since many nurses do not wish to draw a boundary between themselves and less trained staff. The RCN Congress has, for example, debated whether health care assistants should be allowed to join the Royal College of Nursing.

As Kirkham discusses, midwifery is a long-established occupation originally independent of medicine, but in order to achieve occupational closure (registration) it had to accept regulation by medicine. As in nursing, the majority of practitioners were working- or lower-middle-class, and middle-class women moved rapidly into management, a problem which persists today, in that neither occupation has been able to develop a career structure for those who wish to stay in direct patient care (Davies, 1995). Midwifery has not had to defend itself against the incursions of less skilled workers in quite the same way as nursing, but has had difficulty in defining (or redefining) its role and knowledge base as separate from medicine. In some ways, Kirkham claims, the knowledge base may have actually *decreased*, and she recommends developing knowledge based on normality. One of midwifery's most problematic boundaries is with nursing. In the recent past, the majority of midwives were trained nurses, but this has changed radically in the last ten years; at the same time midwifery has moved into higher education and is therefore required to share some of its teaching and much of its education management with nursing.

It is difficult for midwifery and nursing in the UK to emerge from the shadow of medicine. Robinson (1991, pp. 141–2) used the metaphor of the nurses' house, rather dilapidated, and 'positively squashed between a very big house on one side' (the women's house) and 'a posh house on the other' belonging to the doctors. A few stay in the nurses' house and try to get over their boredom by going up to the attic (into management); a few peep into the doctors' house and offer to undertake the jobs which they do not do, or do badly:

> But as soon as the doctors hear about this they start shouting back through the hole in the wall. 'You can't do that', they bellow, 'it's illegal, it's our job, keep off.'

A recent example of the slowness of change in the doctor–nurse interface is nurse prescribing, which was mooted in 1986, introduced in eight pilot projects in 1994 for specially-trained health visitors and district nurses, and is only very gradually being extended (although one of the chief deterrents is the fear that nurses may inflate the drugs bill, rather than anxiety about their competence).

Nursing and midwifery often seem to be trying to find a small voice in a discourse which has been created by other, far louder, voices. This may be partly because nursing has not known how to play the game (Scott, 1994), and also the difficulty of speaking the language, or trying to use a different language. A parallel could be drawn here with 'Man-Made Language' (Spender, 1980), in which until recently the term 'man' could refer to women as well, but it was often not clear whether it did. The term 'clinician' serves a similar function, since it is usually used by doctors but could mean nurses as well. 'Medicine' is sometimes used in a similar way. A case in point is evidence-based medicine (Sackett *et al.*, 1996), discussed by Robinson. This can be construed as the epitome of high modernity, in which for all interventions the existing research is collated and evaluated, and only interventions with a sound knowledge base are undertaken. However, much of the research and other knowledge in nursing and midwifery does not lend itself to being summarized in this way, and is not in the form of randomized, controlled trials.

Changes in Higher Education

All of the occupations discussed in this book have been affected by developments in higher education, in particular the advent of the new managerialism and the increasing emphasis on competences and transferable skills

(NCIHE, 1997). Their history in academe is different, but as the recent removal of probation training from higher education illustrates, it may not be secure. (Although the new Government are proposing higher education accreditation but not social work training for new entrants to probation.) Social work training was established at the London School of Economics and Political Science in 1912, but it has since 1997 ceased to provide it, because of the pressures of running a practically-oriented course in a research-led institution (Midgley, 1997). One of the triggers for the course closure was reported to be the decision of the Home Office to stop funding social work students intending to work in the probation service, and concerns were reported that the Department of Health might also be considering on-the-job training for social workers. It has recently been reported (Brindle, 1997) that the Secretary of State in the Department of Health has announced plans to regulate social work and to tackle 'excessive political correctness'.

As discussed in Chapter 1, many nursing and midwifery courses are recent entrants to higher education, but are unlike any other part of HE in that the diploma courses are purchased by local consortia for a local market and they put a considerable emphasis on 'fitness for purpose'. Webb (1992) argues that there are a number of convergences in the structure of nursing and social work education, and that the current discourse on inter-professional working, more recently embodied in the White Paper *A Service with Ambitions* (Department of Health, 1996) is part of occupational deregulation. As Allen points out in this volume, such flexibility is encouraged by post-Fordism, but flexible workers are not seen as skilled.

Consumerism

As several of the contributors to this volume have commented, the caring professions are ambivalent about whether they wish to be fully-fledged professions, or whether as Davies (1996) argues, the 'cloak of professionalism' is an anachronism more appropriate to a nineteenth-century gentleman. Until recently, much of the discourse was of 'empowerment'; this has been superseded by consumerism. We have not been able to explore the meaning of the growth of consumerism (Gabriel and Lang, 1995) in this volume. Like managerialism, it grew in the 1980s as a perceived remedy for the shortcomings of public services. Abercrombie (1994) argues that authority has now shifted from the producer to the consumer, leading in health care to anxiety about the possibility of complaints and litigation (Dingwall, 1994; Annandale, 1996).

Gabriel and Lang (1995, p. 2) state that in the late twentieth century, the term 'consumer' has such a 'readiness to act as an obedient and polite guest in almost any discourse' that as a concept it is in danger of imminent collapse. Consumerism is also a slippery concept. Gabriel and Lang refer to five broad groups of meanings: as a vehicle for power and happiness; as the ideology of conspicuous consumption; as an economic ideology for global development; as a political ideology; and as a social movement to protect the rights of consumers.

Hugman (1994) argues that in the UK health and welfare contain three main elements of consumerism: taking responsibility and making provision to meet one's own needs where possible; residential state provision; and access to corporate services mediated by professionals, working within clearly defined limits. Consumerism assumes that the interests of professionals and service users can be harmonized, and that the range of services is sufficient and appropriate. It is difficult to see how the term 'consumer' could be meaningfully applied to the recipient of the probation service, since the professional has the power to define social reality, and the recipient of the service may be far from willing.

In health care, the following points can be made:

- There is often uncertainty about outcomes, and consumers find it difficult to judge the quality of technical care.
- In the market, consumers seek the best buy for themselves and do not damage others' interests by doing so, whereas public sector marketing involves managing demand since resources are finite.
- At the point of contact, consumers of health care are often vulnerable. The concept of the consumer can become overly abstract and cognitive, whereas in health care there are many emotional aspects.

The recipients of midwifery care may the nearest to full-blown consumers, and as Kirkham notes, they are not passive consumers, but involved in the 'ultimate productive act'.

The discourse on consumerism and that on the panoptic society may be parallel discourses, or they may intersect – for example, in the recognition that consumers of health care are also producers of health care, and are involved in their own surveillance. Gabriel and Lang (1995) refer only briefly to surveillance, in the context of the consumer as identity seeker (identity checks and surveillance cameras help to establish 'forensic identity') and as a check against shoplifting (the consumer as rebel). In commercial terms, the capacity for surveillance of the customer increases with the use of credit rather than cash, and our buying habits may be monitored via Electronic Point of Sale machines. In health care, the Electronic Patient Record has been hotly debated (and resisted) in the medical press, but has received less attention in nursing. Despite the rhetoric of the previous UK government about the Patient's Charter (Department of Health, 1992) the concept of the consumer of health care is a slippery one.

Conclusion

Burrage and Torstendahl (1990) argue that there are four main actors involved in determining the nature of a profession: practising members, the state, users, and universities. Macdonald (1995) adds a fifth – professional bodies. In Johnson's (1972) terminology, the caring professions are mediative, in that a third party, the state, defines needs and how they are met: as Torstendahl (1990) and Johnson (1995) point out, the state has been an important actor with many professions, particularly in Europe. Certainly the state continues to take a keen interest, and to maintain a tight control, in the caring professions: in recruitment; in defining what counts as relevant knowledge; and in commenting upon practice. Davies (1996) argues for a new concept of professionalism, in which intuitive, experiential knowledge is valued, users are empowered, and care is seen as a team-based phenomenon. As indicated earlier, the rhetoric is there (Department of Health, 1996), but the space for professional artistry becomes increasingly cramped.

References

Abbott, A. (1988) *The System of Professions: An Essay on the Division of Expert Labor*, Chicago: University of Chicago Press.

Abercrombie, N. (1994) 'Authority and consumer society', in Keat, R., Whiteley, N. and Abercrombie, N. (Eds) *The Authority of the Consumer*, London: Routledge.

Annandale, E. (1996) 'Working on the front-line: Risk culture and nursing in the new NHS', *The Sociological Review*, **44**, pp. 416–51.

Atkin, K., Lunt, N., Parker, G. and Hirst, M. (1993) *Nurses Count: A National Census of Practice Nurses*, York: Social Policy Research Unit.

Brindle, D. (1997) 'Dobson seeks care shake-up', *The Guardian* (1 November).

Burrage, M. and Torstendahl, R. (1990) *Professions in Theory and History*, London: Sage.

Davies, C. (1995) *Gender and the Professional Predicament in Nursing*, Buckingham: Open University Press.

Davies, C. (1996) 'A new vision of professionalism', *Nursing Times*, **92** (46), pp. 54–6.

Department of Health (1992) *The Patient's Charter*, London: HMSO.

Department of Health (1996) *A Service with Ambitions*, London: Department of Health.

Dingwall, R. (1994) 'Litigation and the threat to medicine', in Gabe, J., Kelleher, D. and Williams, G. (Eds) *Challenging Medicine*, London: Routledge.

Dominelli, L. (1997) *Sociology for Social Work*, London: Macmillan.

GABRIEL, Y. and LANG, T. (1995) *The Unmanageable Consumer: Contemporary Consumption and its Fragmentation,* London: Sage.

GOUGH, P. (1997) 'From profession to commodity', *Nursing Times,* **93** (30), pp. 34–7.

HEALTH SERVICE MANAGEMENT UNIT (1996) *The Future Health-Care Workforce,* Manchester: University of Manchester.

HISCOCK, J. and PEARSON, M. (1996) 'Professional costs and invisible value in the community nursing market', *Journal of Interprofessional Care,* **10**, pp. 23–31.

HUGMAN, R. (1994) 'Consuming health and welfare', in KEAT, R., WHITELEY, N. and ABERCROMBIE, N. (Eds) *The Authority of the Consumer,* London: Routledge.

JAMOUS, H. and PELOILLE, B. (1970) 'Changes in the French university-hospital system', in JACKSON, J.A. (Ed.) *Professions and Professionalization,* Cambridge: Cambridge University Press.

JOHNSON, T. (1972) *Professions and Power,* London: Macmillan.

JOHNSON, T. (1995) 'Governmentality and the institutionalization of expertise', in JOHNSON, T., LARKIN, G. and SAKS, M. (Eds) *Health Professions and the State in Europe,* London: Routledge.

LARSON, M. (1990) 'On the matter of experts and professionals, or how impossible it is to leave nothing unsaid', in TORSTENDAHL, R. and BURRAGE, M. (Eds) *The Formation of Professions: Knowledge, State and Strategy,* pp. 24–50, London: Sage.

LAWLER, J. (1991) *Behind the Screens: Nursing, Somology and the Problem of the Body,* Melbourne: Churchill Livingstone.

MACDONALD, K. (1995) *The Sociology of the Professions,* London: Sage.

MIDGLEY, S. (1997) 'Out of social work', *The Guardian* (5 August), p. 23.

NATIONAL COMMITTEE OF INQUIRY INTO HIGHER EDUCATION (1997) *Higher Education in the Learning Society,* London: HMSO.

POLLITT, C. (1993) *Managerialism and the Public Services* (2nd edn), Oxford: Basil Blackwell.

ROBINSON, J. (1991) 'Power and policy-making in nursing', in SALVAGE, J. (Ed.) *Nurse Practitioners: Working for Change in Primary Health Care Nursing,* London: King's Fund.

SACKETT, D., ROSENBERG, W., MUIR GRAY, J., HAYNES, R. and RICHARDSON, W. (1996) 'Evidence based medicine: What it is and what it isn't', *British Medical Journal,* **312**, pp. 71–2.

SCOTT, E. (1994) *The Influence of the Staff of the Ministry of Health on Policies for Nursing 1919–1968,* PhD Thesis, University of London.

SPENDER, D. (1980) *Man-Made Language,* London: Routledge and Kegan Paul.

TORSTENDAHL, R. (1990) 'Introduction: Promotion and strategies of knowledge-based groups', in TORSTENDAHL, R. and BURRAGE, M. (Eds) *The Formation of Professions: Knowledge, State and Strategy,* London: Sage.

WEBB, D. (1992) 'Competencies, contracts and cadres: Common themes in the social control of nurse and social work education', *Journal of Interprofessional Care,* **6**, pp. 223–30.

Index